Deaf Education in the 21st Century

Topics and Trends

Nanci A. Scheetz
Valdosta State University

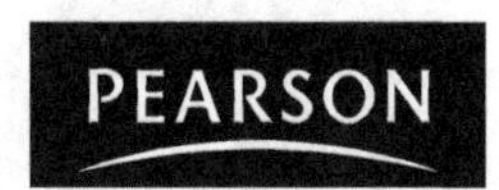

Boston Columbus Indianapolis New York San Francisco Upper Saddle River
Amsterdam Cape Town Dubai London Madrid Milan Munich Paris Montreal Toronto
Delhi Mexico City Sao Paulo Sydney Hong Kong Seoul Singapore Taipei Tokyo

Vice President and Editorial Director: Jeffery W. Johnston
Executive Editor and Publisher: Stephen D. Dragin
Editorial Assistant: Jamie Bushell
Vice President, Director of Marketing: Margaret Waples
Marketing Manager: Weslie Sellinger
Senior Managing Editor: Pamela D. Bennett
Production Editor: Kerry Rubadue
Production Manager: Susan Hannahs
Senior Art Director: Jayne Conte
Photo Coordinator: Carol Sykes
Cover Designer: Bruce Kenselaar
Cover Art: Fotolia
Full-Service Project Management: Sudip Sinha/Aptara®, Inc.
Composition: Aptara®, Inc.
Text and Cover Printer/Bindery: North Chelmsford Digital, LSC Communications
Text Font: 10/12 Times

Library of Congress Cataloging-in-Publication Data
Scheetz, Nanci A.
Deaf education in the 21st century : topics and trends / Nanci A. Scheetz.—1st ed.
p. cm.
Includes bibliographical references and index.
ISBN-13: 978-0-13-815444-8
ISBN-10: 0-13-815444-9
1. Deaf—Education. 2. Hearing impaired children—Education. I. Title.
HV2430.S34 2012
371.91′2—dc22 2010053448

11 17

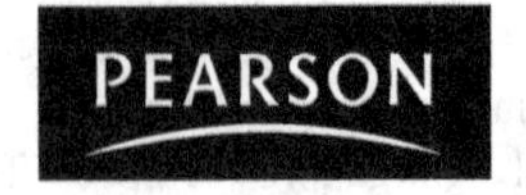

www.pearsonhighered.com

ISBN 10: 0-13-815444-9
ISBN 13: 978-0-13-815444-8

Dedicated to Faye and Connor,
the next generation of scholars

PREFACE

Deaf education in the 21st century has and will continue to undergo a rapid transformation primarily due to the advent of technological advances, innovative educational opportunities, and shrinking cultural boundaries. As it evolves into a complex and multifaceted discipline, both future and current professionals are being charged to provide this student population with the foundation to succeed academically, socially, and vocationally. While providing instruction and support services to students who are deaf and hard of hearing, highly qualified educators, interpreters, and other related support personnel are being challenged to raise the bar and alleviate the achievement gap often exhibited by this student population. This book has been written with those goals in mind.

Today's professionals are working with students in a multiplicity of settings, from residential schools to included classrooms. They encounter students who are as diverse as the settings in which they work. Representing individuals from a variety of ethnic, cultural, and linguistic backgrounds, they bring their personal skill sets with them as they enter the educational environment.

This text has been written to provide professionals, preservice teachers, interpreters, counselors, and other related personnel with a broad and balanced perspective on current topics and trends germane to the field today. In the coverage of a wide array of topics that include educational perspectives, psychosocial precepts, communication modes, cochlear implants, advances in hearing-aid technology, and other timely and relevant topics, the reader is exposed to a panoramic view of a complex field rather than an in-depth analysis of each of the major dimensions.

This text is a sourcebook on the many dimensions found within the field of deaf education. Designed as a teaching–learning vehicle, basic concepts recur in varying situations, and illustrations and some concepts are repeated in diverging contexts to promote comprehension and enhance retention.

When professionals from the field of deaf education convene and share their concerns and their vision for the future, the stories they tell and the backgrounds from which they come form a colorful mosaic. Among the participants are Deaf individuals who represent a rich cultural, linguistic heritage as well as hearing and Deaf professionals who are passionate about how to best serve this population. Their backgrounds are as varied as the individuals that they encounter. Writing a foundation text that addresses the needs of this diverse group of consumers and professionals presents a challenge for any author. It is hoped that the content that follows will spark the interest of the reader to further explore some of the topics discussed in the pages that follow.

No text is ever written in isolation; it takes the support of many to bring any major undertaking to fruition. With that in mind, I wish to express my deep appreciation to the following Valdosta State University graduate students: Lydia S. Evans, Kelly H. Williford, Stephanie N. Akers, Kristina A. Cornell, and Kelsey Rapp Halpern. All of them assisted with research and editing and their help remains greatly appreciated.

I also want to extend my heartfelt thanks to Marie Scheetz for all of her excellent illustrations. She applied her talents patiently, cheerfully accepted the task of creating and modifying the drawings, and was always willing to do "just one more."

I extend special thanks to Glenna Ashton for her insights on the Deaf community, Cecil Bradley for reviewing the chapter on employment, and M. Tish Consolini for reviewing the chapters on hearing loss and hearing-aid technology and for contributing the audiograms.

I also extend special thanks to Dr. Barbara Stanley for granting release time and offering support to this project. Her encouragement, words of wisdom, gentle prodding to finish the manuscript, and sense of humor provided further impetus to complete the book in a timely fashion.

I extend continued thanks and an expression of deep appreciation to Steve Dragin, Jamie Bushell, Kerry Rubadue, and the staff at Pearson. Their attention to detail has made this a stronger manuscript.

I also appreciate the input and feedback I received from the following reviewers: James Blair, Ph.D., Utah State University; Brenda Cartwright, Lansing Community College; Helen Morrison, Texas Christian University; Jean Plant, Georgia Perimeter College; and Barbara Strassman, The College of New Jersey.

Finally, I wish to acknowledge my daughters, Melissa, Marie, Megghan, and Monique, for all of their support, encouragement, and suggestions throughout the duration of this project, and to little Ms. Faye for her "You can do it" video, which provided a bright spot throughout the long process of writing and revising the manuscript. Most important, I express my heartfelt thanks to my husband, Rich, for his continuous support, encouragement, and the many hours he devoted to reading the chapters, as well as for all of the suggestions he offered for enhancing the content.

CONTENTS

Chapter 14 EDUCATIONAL INTERPRETING TO SERVE INDIVIDUALS WHO ARE DEAF OR HARD OF HEARING: ROLES AND RESPONSIBILITIES 253

Chapter 15 EPILOGUE 272

1

Deaf Education in the 21st Century

Topics, Trends, and Technology: A Brief Overview

OVERVIEW

With a few twists and turns of a kaleidoscope, the pattern rapidly changes while the colors remain the same. Sometimes the new design is more appealing than the prior motif; sometimes we prefer the configurations that have been produced previously, whereas other times we hesitate to make any changes at all for fear of what appears to be the perfect artistic representation. The field of deaf education can also be viewed through the lens of a kaleidoscope reflecting tremendous changes that have occurred throughout the course of history.

One of these changes is the use of people-first language. Although the author is cognizant of this trend and recognizes that some of the current literature in the field is written to adhere to people-first language, other contemporary articles and texts continue to refer to "deaf individuals," "deaf children," or "deaf students." When possible, people-first language is being used; however, when this change creates undue wordiness, making the meaning of the text difficult to comprehend, the word *deaf* appears first. Furthermore, the uppercase term *Deaf*, as in Deaf community, is used to refer to individuals who share a distinct mode of communication, American Sign Language (ASL), while striving to preserve and foster the development of their culture. Those who identify with the Deaf community are usually people who were born deaf or lost their hearing during childhood (Schein, 1989). The capital *D* is used when referring to those individuals who have assumed a Deaf identity and declare membership within the Deaf community. Rather than viewing their deafness as a disability, they view themselves as whole individuals who cherish their valued heritage. The lowercase term *deaf* describes an audiological condition of those who experience difficulty hearing. In addition, the term *D/deaf* is used to designate both groups of individuals: those who are culturally Deaf as well as those who view their hearing loss as a medical condition.

Even though the field has experienced an abundance of twists and turns, the primary goal of deaf education, much like the colors of the kaleidoscope, remains the same. The beliefs about who deaf people are, the philosophy regarding how to best serve this population, and the way to best prepare future professionals to work with these individuals have evolved into ever-changing new patterns. These patterns are reflective of current advances that have transpired within the areas of medicine, technology, and education. Although some of the twists and turns along the way have produced some positive results, others, in hindsight, have proved to be extremely detrimental.

Since the International Convention in Milan in 1880, when American Sign Language was banned from the schools for the deaf and qualified Deaf professionals were not allowed to use their native language in the classroom, the course of deaf education has experienced a tremendous change. This change would revolutionize the way students who are deaf would be educated for the next several decades. Setting the stage for the dominance of oral education, very few Deaf administrators or teachers were employed by schools for the deaf. At the International Congress of Educators of the Deaf in 2010, a historic event took place and a formal statement was issued by the organization to reject what had been agreed on more than a hundred years earlier. Supported unanimously by those in attendance, hearing professionals would apologize for, and Deaf and hearing professionals alike would reject, the edict that had been formulated and handed down years before.

Throughout history academicians have witnessed a dramatic transformation with respect to how students who are deaf and hard of hearing are educated. This is predominantly due to shrinking global boundaries, advances in technology, travel, and easy access to international research. Collaborative projects have produced additional insights into the complex nature of the field, providing new perspectives on age-old topics. These findings have also had a significant impact on deaf education, challenging professionals to raise the bar with respect to educational standards and expectations for students who are deaf and hard of hearing. The educational arena has moved well beyond the oral manual controversy and has entered a new decade where bilingual and multilingual modes of communication, plurality, and diversity are all being addressed.

Change can be seen in all aspects of the field. As parents, teachers, and, professionals familiar with the discipline, as well as those unfamiliar with it, form new partnerships and alliances, the field of deaf education is entering a new era in which matters once thought to be impossible are becoming a reality. From the universal newborn hearing screening (UNHS) programs to bilateral cochlear implants, the opportunities for current and future generations are rapidly changing. Although at one time hearing loss was not diagnosed until a child was approximately 2 years of age or older, professionals can identify hearing loss in today's infants by 6 months of age or younger. This early identification, coupled with quality intervention services, is setting the stage for endless possibilities for future generations of individuals deaf.

With the advent of infant screenings, professionals are challenged to remain current in the field. Their roles are vital in providing parents with information regarding the wide variety of options that are available to them. Under the guidance of unbiased professionals, parents become better equipped to make informed choices. This is of paramount importance as these decisions will affect the life course that parents elect for their child. Furthermore, oftentimes these decisions must be made at a stressful time when parents are dealing with all of the emotions frequently experienced when the initial diagnosis of deafness is made. The lens through which parents perceive their initial contacts with professionals, what they are told, and how they are told will ultimately influence their feelings, perceptions, and expectations regarding their deaf child.

While some parents may feel comfortable making critical choices for their infants, others may flounder in the sea of information and need time and unbiased assistance as they strive to understand and process all the information presented to them. Professionals sensitive to the diverse nature and needs of the parent population are able to skillfully present information which recognizes that all parents are different and each one represents a set of values, priorities, and a lifestyle that is unique to that individual family unit. By listening to what parents want for their child and matching these requests with available services, the path is established for the child to grow cognitively, linguistically, socially, and academically. Those professionals who are cognizant of the fact that one size does not fit all, and that family units represent microcosms characterized by ethnic, educational, vocational, religious, and socioeconomic backgrounds, are better equipped to match services to the identified needs of the child as well as the entire family constellation.

WHAT WE KNOW ABOUT THE FIELD TODAY

The 21st century is an exciting time for professionals entering the field of deaf education. Teachers, interpreters, audiologists, counselors, speech pathologists, and rehabilitation counselors have at their disposal an array of resources engineered to meet the needs of today's students who are deaf and hard of hearing. From advances in sign language research to new developments in hearing-aid technology, professionals as well as consumers have access to information that was previously unavailable to them. Those entering and working in the field today are asked to gather data on what students need and want, and to use that data to deliver services of a caliber that fosters and promotes excellence in education.

As increasing numbers of professionals consult with Deaf professionals and learners who are deaf, insights are being gleaned with respect to how this population learns and what types of interventions and strategies these consumers feel are beneficial for them. Building on this fundamental knowledge, educators are able to provide direct instruction, collaborate with general education classroom teachers, and recommend support services that will ultimately maximize opportunities for students who are deaf to flourish in the academic arena. While striving to change any negative attitudes that general education teachers might hold toward the capabilities of deaf and learners who are deaf and hard of hearing and assisting them in making their classroom instruction and activities accessible for this diverse population, the stage is being set for these individuals to successfully compete alongside their hearing peers.

The changing landscape of where the school-age deaf population is being educated is as dramatic as the changes affecting the professionals entering the field. Residential schools that once spawned a sense of Deaf community and belonging for the majority of the nation's deaf and hard-of-hearing population have been replaced by included classrooms in neighborhood schools. With 85% of students who are deaf and hard of hearing receiving their education in public settings, rather than in residential settings, the opportunities for socialization with their peers who are deaf may be virtually nonexistent. Although larger cities, due to the mere fact of demographics, may provide more opportunities for students who are deaf to find camaraderie and socialization with several peers who experience similar degrees of hearing loss, this is not always the case in smaller school districts or rural areas. In these instances students, especially those who rely on ASL to communicate, may seek solace and companionship in their sign language interpreters who can engage easily and fluently in conversations with them.

While some of these students will succeed academically and socially, others will struggle in included settings only to return to the residential setting years later after losing valuable time and ground while sitting alongside their hearing peers. It is critical that we recognize that each student, regardless of his or her individual hearing status, represents a unique entity characterized by an individual set of attributes that will influence and contribute to his or her ability to compete and succeed in the classroom. By acknowledging that Deaf students represent a cultural and linguistic group of individuals, it becomes imperative that teachers find ways to incorporate Deaf studies into the general education curriculum.

One venue for incorporating Deaf studies into the curriculum is through technology. Technology is changing the world daily, opening up new vistas for accessing information and connecting with others globally inside as well as outside of the classroom. From netbooks to handheld devices, PCs and laptops, those with state-of-the-art equipment and software have at their disposal endless avenues affording them unlimited access to information not previously accessible. As teachers rely on interactive whiteboards, captioned media, the World Wide Web, and so forth, they are able to engage young learners with a wide array of course materials, adding a new visual dimension to learning while connecting students with their rich cultural heritage (Stinson, 2010).

The classrooms of today are continuously being shaped by technology, academic rigor, and expectations for universal achievement. Schools are being challenged to provide all students with the scholastic foundation they need to become academic achievers. With an impetus for providing quality educational services for students who are deaf and hard of hearing, members and staff of the Commission on the Education of the Deaf (COED) set forth to design an agenda that would identify and prioritize goals that, if followed, could be instrumental in alleviating the achievement gap experienced by this population. With the publication of *The National Agenda: Moving Forward on Achieving Educational Equality for Deaf and Hard of Hearing Students* (Martin, 2005), eight goals were set forth to provide local schools with the foundation to enhance educational programming for this group of unique and diverse learners.

The eight goals focus on (a) early identification and intervention; (b) communication, language, and literacy; (c) collaborative partnerships; (d) systems responsibility: accountability, high stakes testing, assessment, and standards-based environments; (e) placement and programs; (f) technology; (g) professional standards and personnel preparation; and (h) research (Martin, 2005). Developed by a coalition of professionals, consumers, and parent groups, this agenda strives to address and improve educational programming so that the doors to a fair and equal education remain open to all students who are deaf and hard of hearing. Although many of these issues have been paramount in the field for decades, they are being viewed with a new perspective with the hope of enhancing student achievement, rather than maintaining status quo by focusing more on the abilities instead of the disabilities of this population of learners.

The future of Deaf education will continue to be shaped by consumers and parents as well as by present and future educators. As we turn to learners who are deaf for input regarding how they learn, what strategies work best for them, and what mode or modes of communication they are most comfortable using, we will continue to unlock the key to the curriculum. While looking through the kaleidoscope at the many changes the field has experienced, it is critical to remain cognizant of the impact that Deaf professionals have had on the field. From the early Deaf teachers of the deaf to the Deaf President Now movement, deaf education has witnessed a transformation and has arrived at a time when Deaf professionals are not only recognized for their accomplishments but also for the rich dimension they bring to the field. Through Deaf poetry, storytelling, and theatrical performances, an added cultural dimension is shared through the beauty of American Sign Language.

In the midst of change, it is essential that practitioners reflect on the past while moving forward. By casting a critical eye on past mistakes and reaping the benefits from that body of knowledge, future pitfalls can be avoided, thus providing new insights into the current state of the field today. Furthermore, while conducting research and garnering evidence with respect to best practices, fresh perspectives can be gained that will benefit current and future generations of individuals who are deaf and hard of hearing. Although professionals entering the field today will, in all likelihood, continue to encounter a multiplicity of programs that embrace various modes of communication, educational strategies, and philosophical differences, the parents they meet and work with will radiate the same fundamental concerns that lie at the heart of all caregivers who have children who have experienced varying degrees of hearing loss.

Recurrent themes expressed by these parents include concerns regarding communication, socialization, and academic preparation. Parents will want to know if the professionals dealing with their children will be able to communicate with them using the communication mode of their choice. Will their children have friends and be able to develop a sense of belonging and acceptance? Will they be taunted or ridiculed because of the ramifications of their hearing loss? Will they be able to access the curriculum and succeed academically? Will their talents be tapped to allow them to capitalize on their strengths rather than being reminded of their weaknesses? Will they leave the educational arena as independent young men and women with a sense of self-confidence, ready to continue their postsecondary education or enter the competitive world of employment?

Professionals as well as parents are equally committed to finding the answers to these complex questions. While researchers continue to explore topics such as language and literacy, educational program development, cochlear implants and auditory management, as well as preparation of qualified teachers and sign language interpreters, practitioners are concurrently striving to provide the highest quality of service to this population. It is a well-established fact that the field has experienced a dramatic paradigm shift since the 1970s. Moving from a medical to a cultural–linguistic model, students who are deaf and hard of hearing are being viewed as a diverse population of learners who have the potential to succeed academically when provided with instruction that matches their individual learning needs and styles. Recognizing that one "size" does not fit all, the field is being challenged to meet the discrete needs of this vibrant population.

Several of these critical topics are addressed in the chapters that follow. Although it is important to gain an understanding of the auditory process and the complexities involved in comprehending information transmitted through the auditory channel, it is equally important to become knowledgeable of the dynamic group of individuals who refer to themselves as members of the Deaf community. The goal of this text is to provide readers with a balanced and broad overview of the field, being mindful that no one text can provide an in-depth comprehensive discussion of each of these topics. Rather, numerous texts have been devoted to any one of the subjects, and readers are encouraged to explore additional resources.

As the kaleidoscope of deaf education continues to produce remarkable and rapid changes in the field, it is anticipated that several questions will be answered while an infinite number more will be asked. With research and evidence-based practice on the horizon, current professionals as well as future graduates will be provided with new answers to many of these age-old questions. While some of the concerns and issues will remain at the forefront in the field for several decades to come, others will be resolved based on new findings. Staying abreast of the research, utilizing state-of-the-art technology, and implementing differentiated instruction will provide students who are deaf and hard of hearing with opportunities not only to access but, more importantly, to master the curriculum. The future holds promise for them. By recognizing their abilities and deemphasizing their disabilities, this multivariate group of students will be able to concentrate on capitalizing strengths and maximizing capabilities.

2

Myths and Misconceptions About People Who Are Deaf

Dispelling the Myths

It is well documented in the literature that deafness is a low-incidence disability. Although many individuals are familiar with someone who has lost hearing due to the aging process, it is not uncommon for those who can hear to arrive at adulthood never having encountered a culturally Deaf person. Therefore, skewed perceptions of the Deaf community and Deaf individuals are formed by what hearing people have read, what they have observed, and what other hearing individuals have told them. Through a series of misunderstandings and misinterpretations, erroneous information is perpetuated, and stereotypes as well as faulty perceptions are commonly formed, shared, spread, and believed by those outside of the Deaf community.

In general, few hearing people are familiar with the ramifications of hearing loss, especially those who are born with severe to profound losses. As a result, when they encounter individuals who are deaf, they may have many preconceived ideas that are completely inaccurate. It is common for the hearing population to assume that persons who are deaf cannot read or drive and that they rely on Braille for communication. Upon encountering an individual who is deaf for the first time, the hearing person, sensing a breakdown in the communication process, may first resort to shouting, hoping that the person will be able to hear. Upon realizing that this mode of communication will not work, the hearing person will attempt to discover if the person who is deaf can read. Sensing frustration with the communication process, those involved may leave the encounter with the hearing person blaming the person who is deaf for the communication breakdown, failing to recognize or accept the fact that he or she was mutually responsible for the success or failure of the transmission of information.

Furthermore, when those outside the field encounter individuals with cochlear implants or wearing hearing aids, they may assume that these devices will cure deafness and therefore assume that anyone taking advantage of technology can hear, not recognizing the magnitude of the loss, the demands on the individual's residual hearing, and the environment in which listening occurs will all impact the effectiveness the hearing device affords them. In the ensuing pages, several of the more common myths and misconceptions associated with people who are deaf are addressed; the goal is to dispel the myths and replace them with accurate information that can be disseminated both inside and outside the field of deaf education.

MYTH: PEOPLE WHO ARE DEAF CANNOT HEAR ANYTHING

It is not uncommon for members of the lay community, upon encountering an individual who is deaf for the first time, to assume that the person cannot hear anything. As a result, phrases such as "stone deaf" and "deaf as a post" become incorporated into the hearing person's vernacular. The word choices, which are of a derogatory nature, represent one of the fallacies associated with deafness.

The cause, type, and severity of one's hearing loss and the age at onset all contribute to the extent to which the disability becomes a handicapping condition. Losses range from mild to profound and affect various frequencies. Although one individual may experience a loss in the high-frequency range, others may hear those sounds satisfactorily but be unable to differentiate sounds produced at lower frequencies.

In addition, two individuals may produce audiograms that appear identical; however, the effect the loss has on each of the individuals is strikingly different. Although some may be able to compensate for their hearing deficits, utilize their residual hearing, and function as hard of hearing, others may find their loss to be significant and feel isolated from interactions within their social environment. The term *hard of hearing* refers to a score on an audiological evaluation and is not reflective of the individual's functioning ability. Therefore, even though two individuals may have identical audiograms, it is possible that they will function in completely different ways when they encounter various environmental situations.

The term *hearing loss* is broad, encompassing the hard of hearing at one end of the continuum and the profoundly deaf on the other end. It represents a heterogeneous group comprised of unique individuals. Individuals' hearing losses differ, the sounds they are able to hear are diverse, and they vary in their abilities to capitalize on their residual hearing.

MYTHS SURROUNDING THE CAUSES OF HEARING LOSS

Although the majority of those who are diagnosed as having a hearing loss are provided with a medical explanation for their loss, some cases have unknown etiologies. As a result, parents, as well as concerned family members and friends, attempt to find reasons to justify why the person cannot hear speech or sounds within the environment.

Misconceptions surrounding the causes of hearing loss include blows to the head, "brain fever," and high fevers that have "burned up the nerves" (Mindel & Vernon, 1987). These reasons may appear logical to parents when no other medical explanations are available. Nearly all parents can remember when their children have been sick and run a high fever or have taken a tumble. When searching for a reason for their child's deafness, they may feel that these events have contributed to their child's hearing loss.

However, fever alone does not cause hearing loss. In the event that the child contracts a disease, such as spinal meningitis, and runs a high fever, a loss may occur; but the fever by itself will not generate "burned up nerves" or create an auditory dysfunction. A blow to the head is not likely to create a loss either, unless it is severe enough to fracture the bones of the skull that protect the auditory mechanism. It is a rare occurrence when fractures occur simultaneously and damage both ears. At best, when people cite these reasons for causes of hearing loss, it is because the true medical diagnosis is unknown.

MYTH: ALL CHILDREN WHO ARE DEAF HAVE PARENTS WHO ARE DEAF

Deafness is a low-incidence disability affecting only a small percentage of the total population. Information provided by the National Institute on Deafness and Other Communication Disorders (NIDCD) indicates that approximately 17% or 36 million Americans encounter varying degrees of difficulty hearing (NIDCD, 2010). Furthermore, about 2 to 3 out of every 1,000 children in the United States are born deaf or hard of hearing (NIDCD, 2010). Of those who have difficulty hearing, as many as 2 million have been diagnosed as having a severe to profound loss (NIDCD, 1990).

Frequently the assumption is made that deaf parents produce children who are deaf and, therefore, all children who are deaf have parents whose hearing loss mirrors that of their offspring. However, this is generally not the case. Although between 150 and 175 types of hereditary or genetic deafness and hearing loss have been identified (Bess & Humes, 1995), congenital deafness is prevalent in only a small percentage of families (Moore & Levitan, 2003). Research indicates that 9 out of every 10 children born to deaf parents hear normally (approximately 88%). Although hearing loss can be attributed to genetic causes, it does not occur frequently, affecting only a small percentage of the population.

In reality only 3 to 4% of children who are deaf are born into families with two parents whose hearing loss reflects the same degree of loss that is evident in their children. Furthermore, fewer than 10% are known to have at least one parent who is deaf, and approximately 30% have a relative who is deaf or hard of hearing (Moores, 1996). Research pertaining to the genetic causes of deafness indicates that most hereditary deafness is attributed to a recessive genetic trait rather than a dominant genetic trait. Therefore, according to Northern and Downs (1991), "the marriage of two deaf persons gives only a slightly increased risk of deafness in their children because there is small chance that two such persons would be affected by the same exact genetic deafness" (p. 90).

MYTH: ALL PEOPLE WHO ARE DEAF CAN READ LIPS

The term *lipreading* has been used to denote the process that individuals who are deaf engage in while attempting to comprehend what the speaker is saying. However, upon closer examination, the term was changed to *speechreading*, thus signifying the comprehensive scope of the process. Speechreading, unlike lipreading, includes not only lip movements but also facial expressions, eye movements, and body gestures (Bevan, 1988). All these factors assist individuals who are deaf and hard of hearing as they attempt to comprehend what the speaker or group of participants is saying. Speechreading, therefore, becomes a supplement to the communication process, assisting individuals in their receptive skills. It is not a substitute for one's hearing but, rather, a technique that can be incorporated to enhance communication and promote understanding of the spoken message.

Members of the professional community have debated whether speechreading itself is an innate ability individuals possess or, rather, a skill that can be developed. Although there is no consensus on this point, certain issues within the domain of speechreading are generally agreed upon. Almost all professionals support the premise that speechreading has certain limitations. These limitations can be summarized as follows:

1. Between 40 and 50% of speech sounds encountered in the English language are not visible on the lips. Sounds such as *i, e, g, h, a,* and *k* remain hidden when they are vocalized, thus preventing the speech reader from receiving words in their entirety.
2. Only 16 mouth movements are distinguishable in the English language. These 16 movements represent the 38 English phonemes. Therefore, the mouth movements for differing

speech sounds may look the same; the distinguishing features for these sounds are made by the tongue, or the larynx, both of which are invisible (Schein & Stewart, 1995). As a result, some of the sounds are homophonous (look alike on the lips) such as *p, b,* and *m*, and add confusion as one tries to determine if the word is *mat, bat,* or *pat.*

3. To benefit from speechreading, individuals must have a fairly extensive language background. Without this they are unable to fill in the gaps with information that cannot be obtained through speechreading or hearing (Bevan, 1988, p. 106).
4. Additional factors that can ultimately impact and influence one's ability to effectively comprehend speakers while relying on speechreading include the following:
   a. ***Placement of the speaker.*** In optimal situations the speaker will directly face the deaf individual and will refrain from turning his or her head from side to side while speaking. Attempting to speechread the profile of a face is extremely challenging, if not altogether impossible.
   b. ***Lighting.*** Conversations or presentations should take place in rooms that are well lit to facilitate ease in speechreading; speakers should refrain from standing with their backs to light sources. This will result in extreme eye strain as the individual who is deaf looks directly into the light while trying to focus on mouth movements and facial expressions.
   c. ***Obstructions while speaking.*** It is critical that when talking to an individual who is deaf that speakers avoid placing their hands over their mouths and refrain from placing objects in their mouths (pens, pencils, cigarettes). These items interfere with the visibility and production of speech sounds and thus hinder the ability of the individual to comprehend the message.
   d. ***Volume, inflection, and prosody.*** Discourse should be delivered with appropriate volume for the situation. Shouting and presenting information with exaggerated facial expressions distort the face and minimize the effectiveness of the message. Furthermore, when speakers pay attention to pace, phrasing, and word choice they can be instrumental in assisting the person attempting to speechread. It is important to remain cognizant of the fact that ambiguous sentences are oftentimes rendered effective when they are rephrased for the listener.

Hearing individuals outside of the field of deaf education frequently assume that all people who are deaf can speechread and fully comprehend what they are saying when they are communicating with them. This is a misconception, and individuals who cannot hear speech and clearly distinguish one word from another are faced daily with frustrations as they attempt to understand what the speaker is saying. Although some individuals who are deaf and hard of hearing are excellent speachreaders, most are not, and they find themselves struggling in their efforts to comprehend what is being said.

When trying to surmount a breakdown in communication with a person who is deaf or hard of hearing, hearing people frequently resort to other methods in their attempt to convey their message. Oftentimes, the first question to arise in the mind of the hearing person pertains to whether or not the deaf or hard-of-hearing person has the ability to read.

MYTH: PEOPLE WHO ARE DEAF CANNOT READ

Although the majority of individuals who are deaf and hard of hearing can read, their levels of comprehension vary dramatically. Some who are hard of hearing (possessing a mild to severe loss) achieve reading levels that are comparable to their hearing counterparts; however, others who experience a severe to profound loss rarely become veritably skilled readers.

National surveys, individual studies of reading achievement, and studies of specific aspects of the reading process all indicate that most children who are deaf (those who have a severe to profound loss) have difficulty reading the English language (Quigley & Paul, 1984). This can be attributed, in part, to their depressed general knowledge bank resulting from the isolation they experience on a daily basis. Hearing children have the benefit of gathering a substantial knowledge base as they interact with parents and significant others. These experiences are internalized through the spoken language process and become part of the hearing child's practical knowledge. As a result, hearing children enter the reading process with a language base from which to draw. Children who are born deaf, or lose their hearing prior to the development of language patterns, and who encounter communication problems with those significant others, frequently enter the domain of reading with a very impoverished knowledge base (Quigley & Paul, p. 137).

Studies conducted by the Office of Demographic Studies (ODS) at Gallaudet University provide the most comprehensive information on reading achievement levels. Throughout the years, various studies have been undertaken and cited in the literature. They consistently reveal that those students with a severe to profound loss do not perform well at any age level on tests of general ability to read standard English text. The results of these studies are notable.

These seminal studies represent the findings of the larger body of research and reflect the reading problems experienced by the population comprised of students who are deaf and hard of hearing. Beginning with research conducted in the 1960s and 1970s, they highlight some of the findings and characteristics of readers who are deaf and hard of hearing. Current research studies pertaining to literacy are included in Chapter 9. The studies listed here depict a history of research pertinent to the field:

- In the 1960s, national norms for reading levels of deaf children were supplied by Wrightstone, Aronow, and Moskowitz (1963). They administered the elementary level battery of the Metropolitan Achievement Test to 5,307 deaf students between the ages of 10½ and 16½ years.
- Furth (1966) conducted an analysis on the data from that study and determined that only 8% of the national sampling of deaf and hard-of-hearing students read above the fourth-grade level.

In addition, reading grade levels for the sample increased as follows:

> "A mean improvement to only 2.7 years between the ages of 10 and 11 increasing to only 5.5 between 15 and 16 years of age, representing an increase of less than one grade level in five years." (Quigley & Paul, 1984, p. 115)

In the 1970s, studies revealed that over a 10-year period, students who were deaf and hard of hearing between the ages of 8 to 18 increased their vocabulary, on the average, only as much as the average hearing child does between the beginning of kindergarten and the latter part of second grade.

Studies during this period also revealed that the reading ability of students who are deaf in special education increased very little between the ages of 13 and 20; furthermore, only 10% of the young deaf adult population could easily read a newspaper written at the eighth-grade level (Benderly, 1980, p. 88).

- An additional study conducted by Trybus and Karchmer reported reading scores for a stratified random sample of 6,871 deaf students. They found that the median reading level at age 20 was a grade equivalent of only 4.5, a score that is reflective of the reading level they had obtained at age 14. Only 10% of the very best students enrolled in the reading group (consisting of 18-year-olds) could read at or above the eighth-grade level (Trybus & Karchmer, 1977).

- During the 1980s, Allen analyzed data from the two norming projects (1974 and 1983) involving the Stanford Achievement Test scores normed on hearing-impaired students. His analysis revealed that although deaf students as a group acquired reading comprehension skills more rapidly in 1983 than in 1974, they showed little or no gain in relation to their hearing cohorts (Allen, 1986).

The results of these studies reveal the difficulties experienced by individuals who are deaf and hard of hearing when presented with written material. Although they possess the intellectual abilities needed for comprehension to occur, they frequently lack the experiential, cognitive, and linguistic base required for fluency to develop.

MYTH: PEOPLE WHO ARE DEAF CANNOT TALK

Hearing people typically assume that everyone can hear and speak. Upon encountering individuals who have hearing losses and observing them sign or write, hearing individuals automatically assume that all people who are deaf are unable to speak. Speech is equated with language; the hearing person may surmise that without speech language does not develop and thought processes do not occur. Therefore, the individual who is deaf is perceived as lacking the resources to think, develop language, and use oral expression. Nothing could be further from the truth.

Unless an abnormality occurs in the speech mechanism, such as the larynx, vocal cords, or structures within the mouth involving the articulators, individuals have the capability to produce sound. However, the process involved in imitating speech sounds and producing intelligible words is highly complex. To produce accurate vocal utterances, air must pass through the mouth, and the individual must alter the flow of the air by changing the shape of the mouth or obstructing the airflow by utilizing the teeth or the tongue (Mindel & Vernon, 1987, p. 114).

Infants who have normal hearing listen to speech for an extended time before they are able to speak intelligibly. At the earliest stages, babies begin babbling, store the sounds they make in their memory, and retrieve them at will. By initiating these sounds and listening to them, they begin to monitor their own production of sound. As they develop, their babbling becomes incorporated into the elements of speech sounds that will later be used to form words. Their ability to hear themselves speak and to monitor sound production is critical to the development of the speech process. Through this form of feedback, children can determine how accurately they are producing any given sound. Throughout this process they rely on the acoustic images they hear, strive to imitate those speech sounds they perceive, and vocalize them as accurately as possible (Mindel & Vernon, 1987, p. 114).

Consequently, children who are prelingually deaf often face an insurmountable struggle as they strive to develop comprehensible speech sounds. This occurs for two reasons: First, they cannot receive speech sounds auditorily and, second, they have no way to monitor their production of sounds, thus interfering with the critical feedback process. Although amplification for these children may be somewhat beneficial, it does not clarify speech sounds, and the individuals who are deaf are left wondering if they are saying things in the right manner.

Hearing individuals who have enrolled in a foreign language class understand the importance of speaking the language accurately. They spend hours mastering word order, accent, and vocabulary choice to guarantee that their message will be understood and that no one will ridicule them. Those wishing to utilize their language in a foreign country want to ensure that they will be able to express themselves without the fear of embarrassment.

Individuals who are deaf experience the same challenge as they attempt to speak. Nonetheless, their task becomes more difficult as they rely almost exclusively on their visual channel for cues. Individuals who can hear have the advantage of hearing the foreign language spoken and can match their responses accordingly. However, children and adults who are unable to hear speech through the auditory channel must master English, which for many of them is a foreign language. Although some reap the benefits of assistive listening devices, hearing aids, and cochlear implants, others are unable to access spoken communication through this technology. As a result, they are challenged to develop clear, articulate speech within the confines of a restricted sound environment.

Among those who cannot hear how they sound or monitor how loudly or softly they are speaking, many prefer not to use their voices. Others will attempt to speak and either realize that they are not being understood or feel ridiculed and, therefore, refrain from talking.

MYTH: AMERICAN SIGN LANGUAGE IS JUST ENGLISH ON THE HANDS

Members of the majority culture—the hearing community—who have either observed Deaf individuals signing or have watched a sign language interpreter facilitate communication may have a preconceived idea that American Sign Language (ASL) is just English on the hands. Because they are unfamiliar with the language, they may attempt to assimilate what they see into their schemata of language and unknowingly assume that the motions they observe are designed to depict word-for-word representations of the English language. Later, if and when they enroll in formal coursework, they discover that ASL is an independent language complete with its own vocabulary and syntax.

One of the most striking differences between ASL and English is that English is an aural/oral language that was developed within a community of hearing and speaking individuals, while ASL, on the other hand, is a visual/gestural language comprised of its own vocabulary and syntax. This language has been developed within a community that relies on its sight and body movements for communication. Like other languages, it provides a systematic means for communicating thoughts, ideas, and feelings through the use of conventional symbols (Schein, 1984). American Sign Language uses the visual representations of concepts utilizing three-dimensional space to transmit information (Borden, 1996).

While spoken languages follow a linear order, sound by sound, word by word, ASL is produced visually with signs simultaneously communicating additional information (i.e. number, adverbials, questions versus statements, and other grammatical information). This simultaneous additional information is conveyed through signs, spatial relationships, sign movements, facial expressions, and non-manual signals (Scheetz, 2009). One cannot derive the entire meaning from a signed message from the hands alone. Rather, the listener must be attentive to nonmanual expressions such as raised eyebrows, puffed cheeks, and eye glances. These facial expressions contain significant linguistic signals; although these signals are frequently incorporated together with signs, they also can be produced independently of any hand movement.

It is important to note that these nonmanual signals differ from the facial expressions and body postures that accompany speech. Although there are some similarities, the nonmanual markers in ASL serve a grammatical function that distinguishes them from the role similar behaviors play in spoken languages (Schein & Stewart, 1995, p. 44).

Within the English language, parts of speech, verb changes, and word order are incorporated to facilitate communication. Likewise, within ASL certain characteristics are unique to the language system. ASL incorporates tense indicators, classifiers, verbs utilizing directionality, placement of pronouns, and reduplication of signs to convey meaning (Wilbur, 1979).

As a result ASL becomes an interactive language. It is dependent on both the location of the signer and the recipient of the information. It relies on their eye contact, their use of signing space, the linguistic signals projected by their bodies, and their facial expressions. These features, coupled with the syntactical structure of the language, help distinguish it from English.

MYTH: AMERICAN SIGN LANGUAGE IS CONSISTENT THROUGHOUT THE UNITED STATES

Although ASL is used extensively throughout the United States and has achieved a considerable level of homogeneity, regional differences can and do exist. This is reflective of the various dialects that are prevalent in any language. As one travels throughout the United States, it is not uncommon to hear such terms as *y'all, yous,* and *yewns* for the word *you, redup* for *clean up*, *gum bands* for *rubber bands*, or *tumped over* for *fell over*. Likewise, in ASL, while traveling between different regions of the United States you can observe a variety of sign productions representing the same sign concept. Several different regional signs are known for such words as *birthday, Halloween, Christmas,* and *outside* (Moore & Levitan, 2003). (See Figure 2.1 for the regional sign differences for the word *cereal.*) As Deaf individuals and hearing professionals who work in the field interact with Deaf people from regions other than their own, they will frequently ask for clarification or an explanation for signs that are unfamiliar to them.

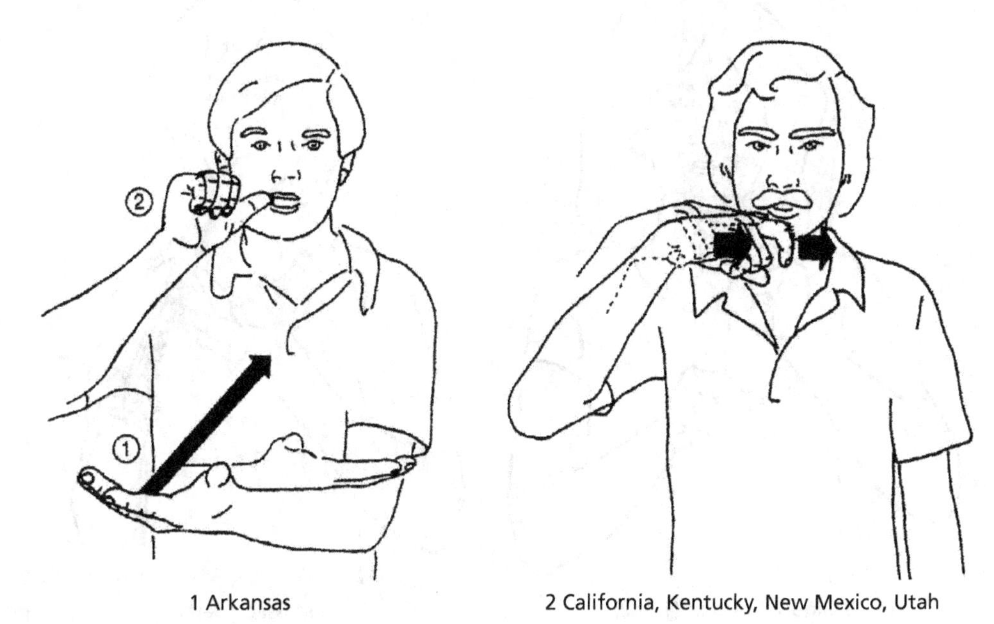

1 Arkansas

2 California, Kentucky, New Mexico, Utah

FIGURE 2.1 Regional signs for *cereal.*

Source: Gallaudet University Press.

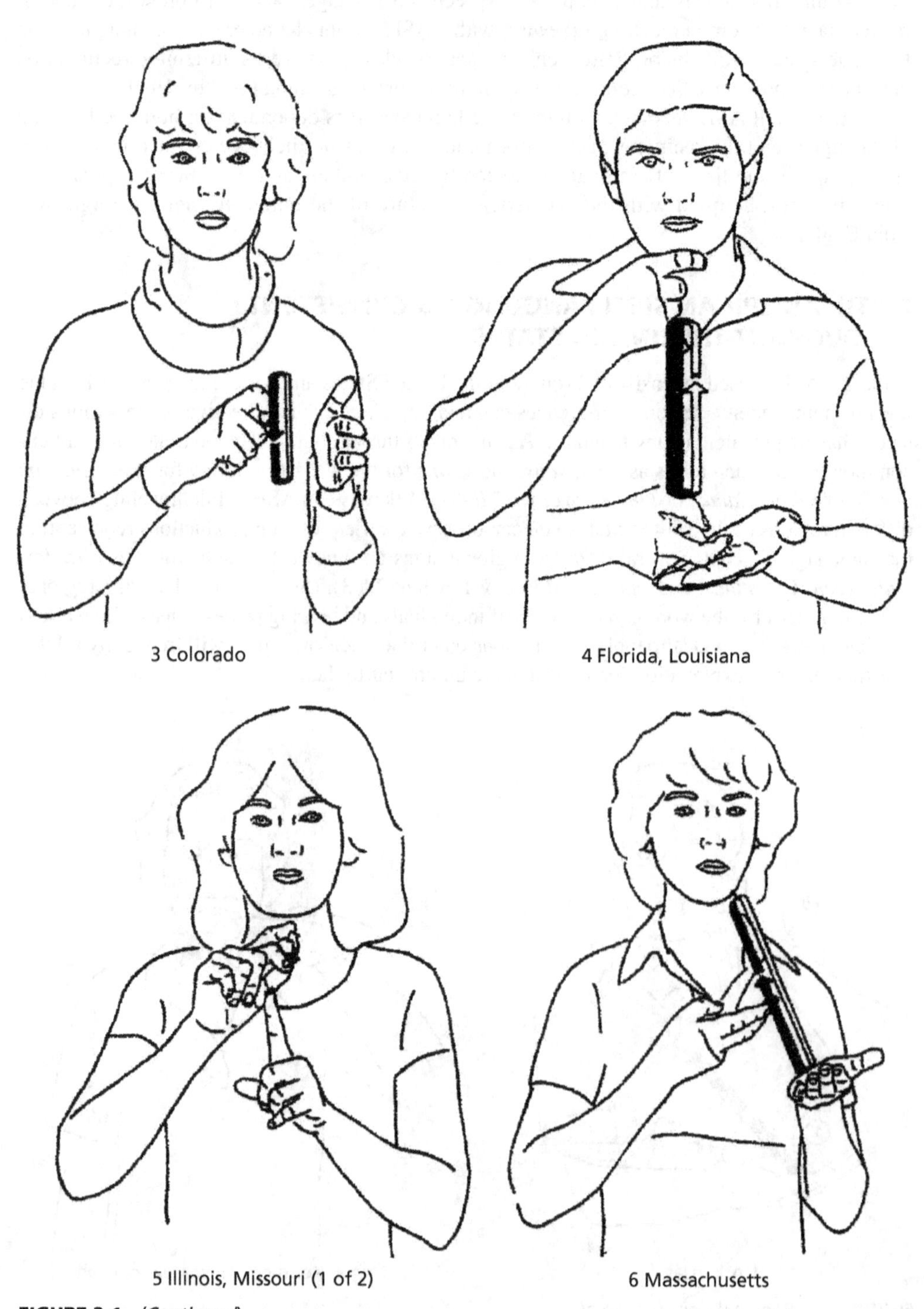

FIGURE 2.1 *(Continued)*

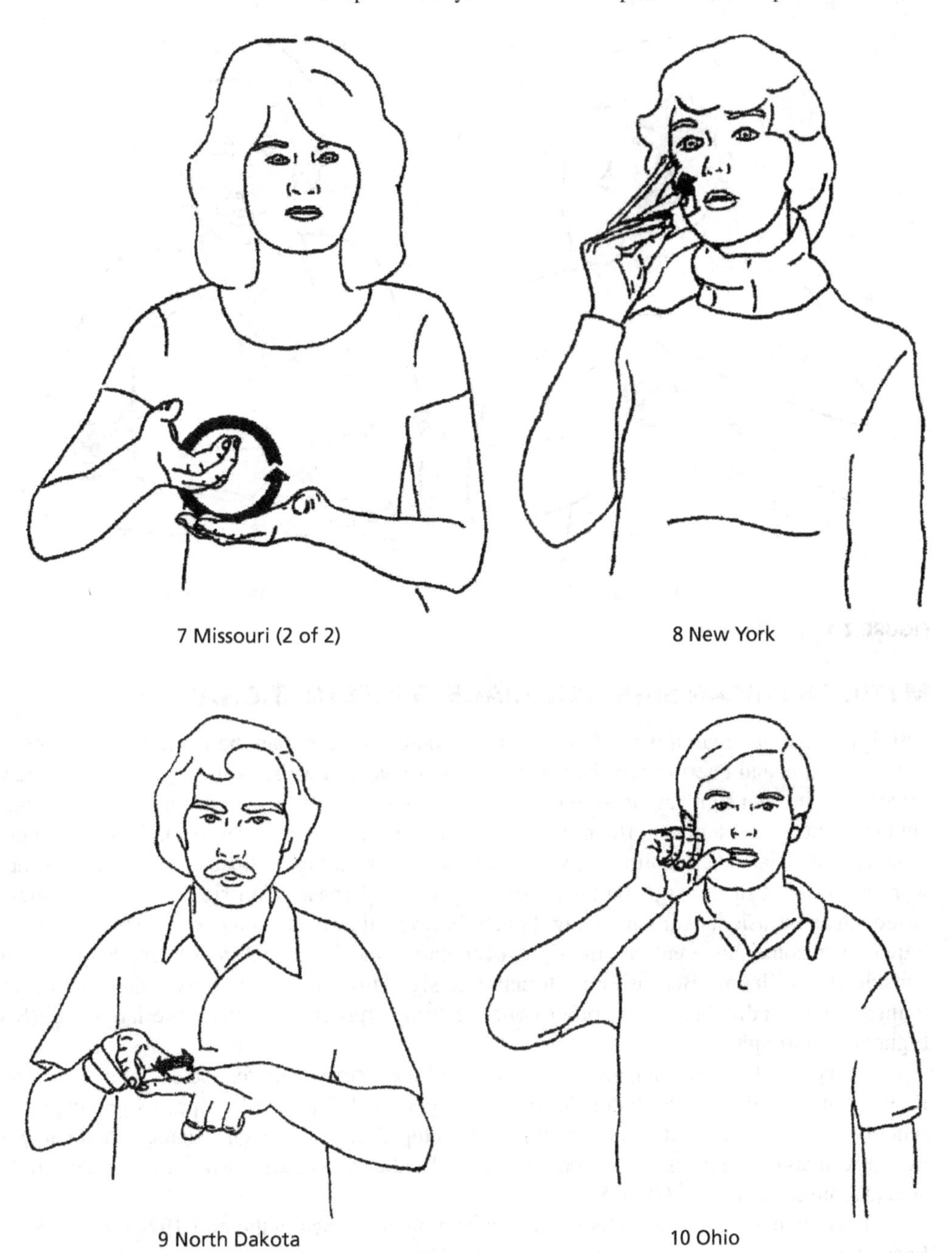

7 Missouri (2 of 2)

8 New York

9 North Dakota

10 Ohio

FIGURE 2.1 *(Continued)*

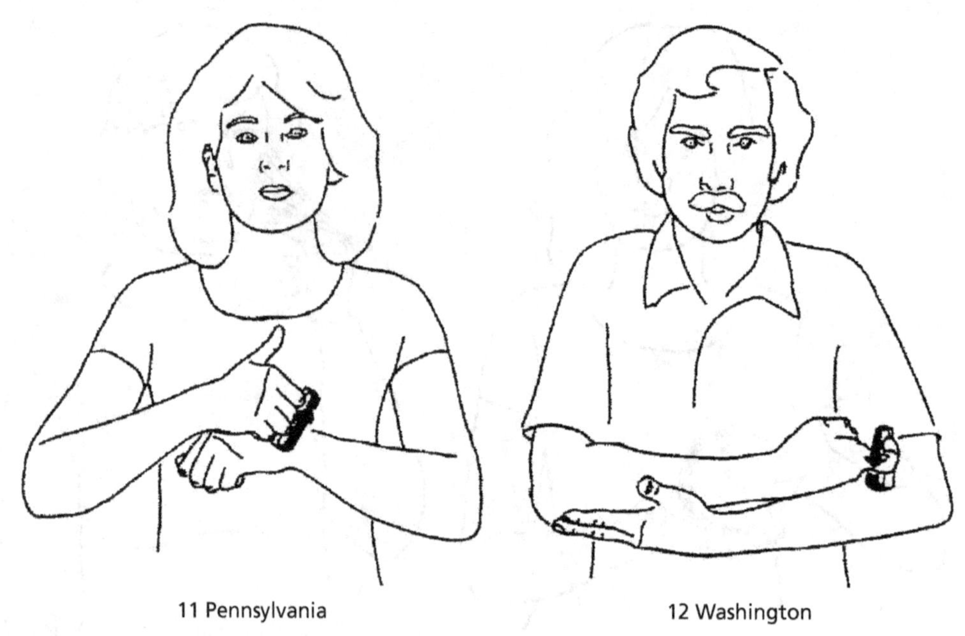

FIGURE 2.1 *(Continued)*

MYTH: AMERICAN SIGN LANGUAGE IS INTERNATIONAL

ASL is not international; it is used only in a few countries other than the United States, such as Canada, Guam, and Puerto Rico. Just as each country has its own spoken language, each country also has its own sign language. Each of these languages differs in sign formation and presentation. Therefore, someone fluent in ASL would not be able to travel to England, Germany, France, or Russia and communicate with native signers residing in those countries unless they were also fluent in the sign language used by each of these countries' Deaf individuals. Although an occasional similarity might occur between the signs from two different countries, it quickly becomes apparent that the sign vocabularies and fingerspelling of each language are considerably different. Because no international sign language exists, those wishing to communicate with individuals from other countries must master more than one language. (See Figures 2.2 through 2.4.)

Every country's sign language is reflective of the history, culture, and social mores of the Deaf community that resides there. Asian sign languages differ from European sign languages; schools across the Czech Republic each have developed their own sign language; and some of the African sign languages have been influenced by the missionaries who have worked in the area (Moore & Levitan, 2003, p. 50).

Even though ASL is not international, a committee formed in the mid-1970s by the World Federation of the Deaf's Commission on Unification of Signs was charged with developing an "artificial," international vocabulary. Initially referred to as *Gestuno,* it was designed to function as a kind of visual Esperanto for use at international gatherings. In 1992, the World Federation of the Deaf board recommended that the term *Gestuno* be changed to *International Sign* or *International Sign Language,* the terms that are currently used today (Y. Andersson, personal communication, 2010). Sometimes used for international conferences such as Deaf Way I and II, Deaflympics (Deaf Olympics), and numerous other national and international events,

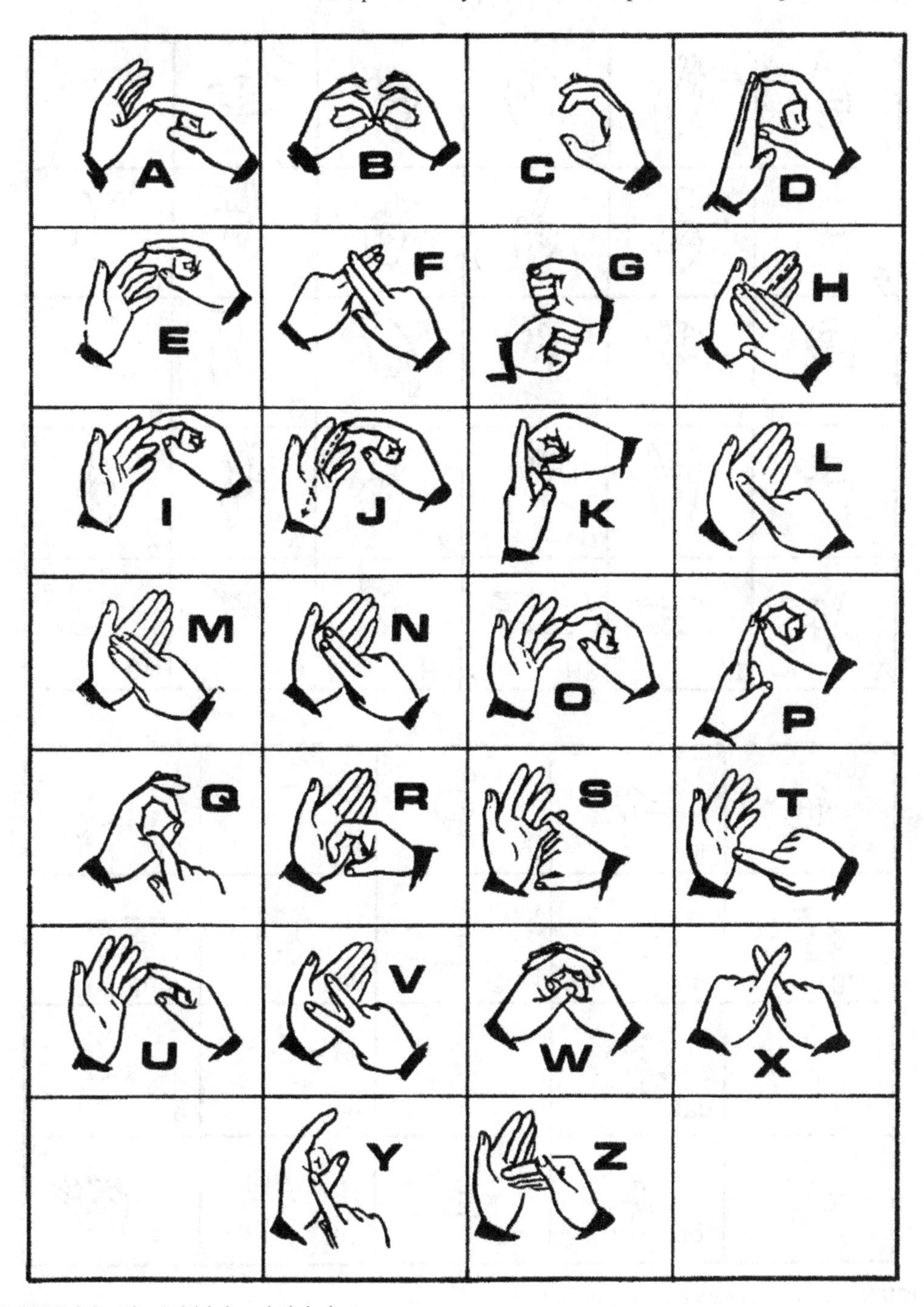

FIGURE 2.2 The British hand alphabet.

Source: Simon J. Carmel.

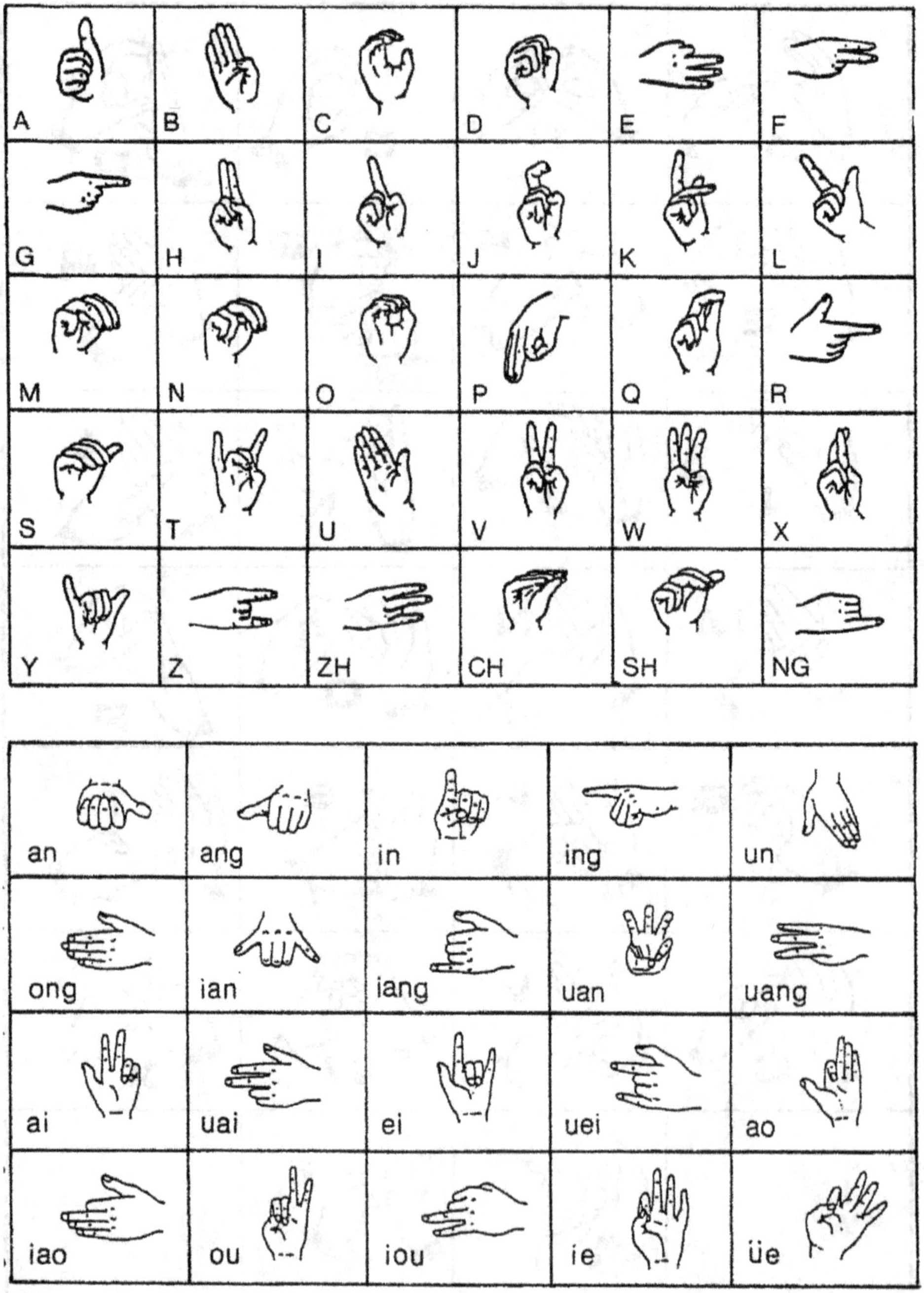

A	B	C	D	E	F
G	H	I	J	K	L
M	N	O	P	Q	R
S	T	U	V	W	X
Y	Z	ZH	CH	SH	NG

an	ang	in	ing	un
ong	ian	iang	uan	uang
ai	uai	ei	uei	ao
iao	ou	iou	ie	üe

FIGURE 2.3 The Chinese hand alphabet.

Source: Simon J. Carmel.

"Man"

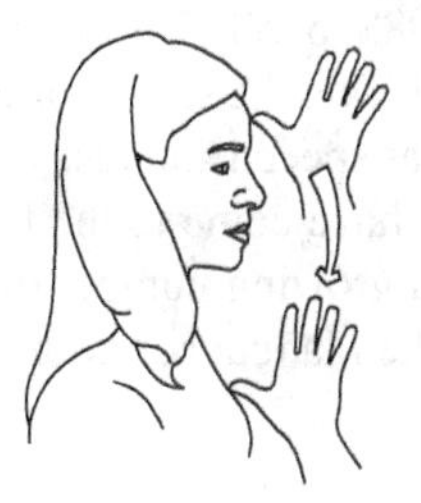

American Sign Language

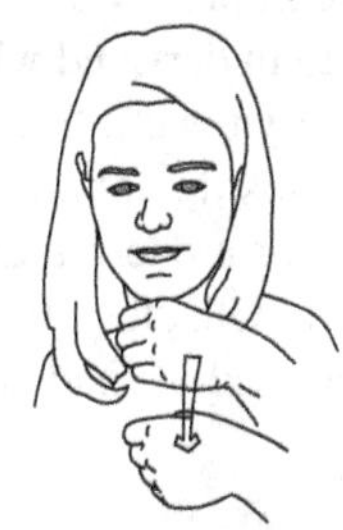

Australian Sign Language

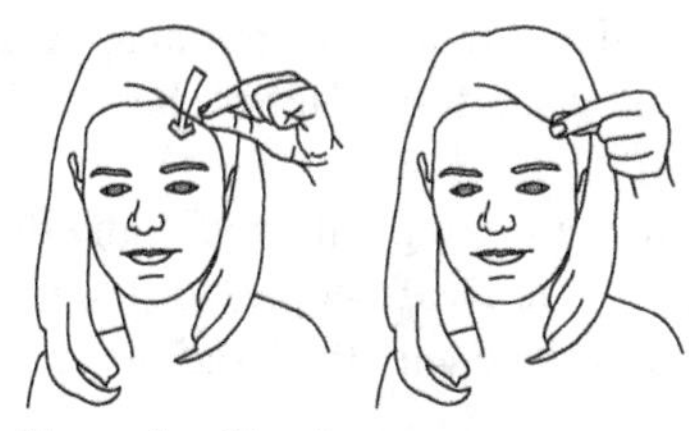

Hungarian Sign Language

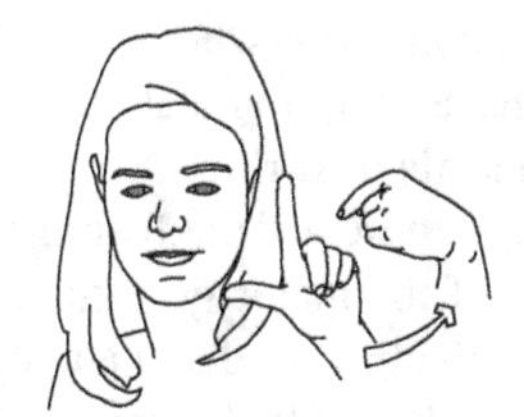

French Sign Language

FIGURE 2.4 Examples of signs from different countries.

Source: Courtesy of Marie A. Scheetz.

International Sign provides an avenue for Deaf individuals from different countries to communicate and access conferences and presentations (Moore & Levitan, p. 51).

MYTH: HEARING AIDS ENABLE PEOPLE WHO ARE DEAF TO HEAR SPEECH

One of the common misconceptions surrounding deafness lies in the area of amplification. Hearing aids are frequently purchased with the preconceived notion that they will restore normal hearing to the person who experiences difficulty in hearing. Older adults, particularly, may become frustrated when they purchase an aid. They may find that the quality of sound they receive falls far short of their expectations. Although their level of hearing may be enhanced, they may find that what they are able to understand varies considerably.

Hearing aids serve the purpose of amplifying sounds. Speech sounds become loud enough that they are within the range of the individual's hearing. However, an aid cannot replace damaged nerve fibers and cannot clarify speech. The type of loss experienced will determine how beneficial the aid will be. If the loss is mild, the increased volume provided by the aid may permit excellent clarity. However, if the individual has severe damage to the nerve fibers located in the inner ear, amplification received through traditional hearing aids will not provide the same effect; when using an aid, these individuals will experience the ability to hear speech and environmental sounds, but often they will not be able to clearly differentiate the speech sounds.

Those who have a sensorineural loss are unable to hear frequencies in the higher speech range, where the greatest amount of speech sounds are located. Even with a hearing aid, amplified speech may still be distorted. When too many nerve fibers located in the inner ear are damaged, speech will never be completely clear. As a result, individuals may be able to hear the sound, but they will not be able to understand what is being said (Bevan, 1988, p. 58). Those with profound hearing losses frequently benefit from an aid, as they are able to locate the source of environmental sounds. However, aids do not provide the individual with clear speech sounds.

With the advent of modern technology, cochlear implants have come to the forefront (see complete description in Chapter 7). These devices are used by a growing number of the school-age deaf population and adults and are designed to enhance spoken language acquisition.

MYTH: ALL PEOPLE WHO ARE DEAF WISH THEY COULD HEAR

To the outsider, the world of the Deaf often appears bleak, empty, and dismal. Hearing people tend to look upon those who are deaf with pity, surmising that they are unhappy and helpless. They make the assumption that all people who are deaf want desperately to hear and are not content living in a silent world.

Although these are the feelings expressed by some prelingually deaf individuals, they are not reflective of the majority of the adult Deaf population. Deaf people, for the most part, may struggle through childhood and adolescence as they interface with the larger hearing community but emerge as self-fulfilled, happy adults.

The Deaf community is comprised of dynamic, cheerful, and well-balanced people who live their lives and attend to business without much more visible distress than people who can hear. They attend Deaf socials, engage in athletic events, take advantage of technology to stay connected with one another, and enjoy face-to-face communication. All of these avenues provide them with opportunities to exchange stories and anecdotes (Becker, 1980).

Deaf people are frequently asked if they would take advantage of a procedure that would cure their deafness and restore their hearing. Their answers always vary. Younger members of this unique population periodically respond with an affirmative. However, those adults who have resided in the Deaf community for their entire life consider themselves members of a special culture and have no desire to hear. They enjoy their friends, participate in social activities, and dislike being pitied. Many feel there are advantages to being deaf and feel fortunate that they are not bothered with the cacophony of daily life bombarding hearing people. Others have become accustomed to their state of hearing and have no desire to experience the world from a hearing perspective.

Throughout history, Deaf individuals have shared their perspectives on what it means to be Deaf. Dating back to 1910 when George Veditz, an eloquent American Deaf leader described Deaf individuals as "first, last, and for all time, people of the eye" (McKee, 2001), the community has created and relied on a visual language to communicate their like experiences, values, and perspectives regarding what it means to be Deaf. When asked about being Deaf, those responding frequently describe their passion for the language and the camaraderie they feel when they have the opportunity to interact with other Deaf individuals. Comments, such as the following, reflect these feelings:

> "I really do love sign language. . . . I feel quite passionate about it. To me it's a beautiful language. I've never been embarrassed or ashamed of it. If a hearing person tries to put me down for signing in public, I just ignore them and carry on."
>
> "A Deaf person first took me along to the Deaf Club in 1945 when I was 13. Someone else took me to a Deaf Sunday school, and I liked that, because there were plenty of Deaf people to talk to." (Still, 2001)

"On the issue of Deaf identity, I think those who have difficulties with their Deaf identity are probably those who have some hearing, who aren't profoundly Deaf, and who are maybe in between two worlds. . . . I know I'm Deaf, and that's from my point of view." (Hamilton, 2001)

"When I'm in the Deaf world I feel different from when I'm with hearing people: the atmosphere among Deaf people seems happy, communication is great; things are always alive. There's always something to do there, and people to meet up with. In the Deaf community you learn from other people's life experiences . . . there's a natural bond with other Deaf people . . . in the Deaf world you enjoy things better, you feel more relaxed. The signing, the facial expression, and body language are amazing; I love it . . . hearing people seem dull the way they talk with a deadpan face, except for when they laugh occasionally. Deaf people are so alive! You feel part of everything so easily." (Smith, 2001)

MYTH: PEOPLE WHO ARE DEAF ARE NOT AS INTELLIGENT AS HEARING PEOPLE

One's intelligence is often confused with one's ability to communicate. Upon encountering individuals who have weak expressive skills, the tendency is to assume that the person has inferior intellectual functioning abilities. Hearing people place a high premium on communication skills, and the way individuals present themselves is often used as a baseline to determine how intelligent they are. Word choice, sentence structure, grammar, and presentation are all used as measures by the hearing population to ascertain who is intelligent and who is not. Unfortunately, many individuals are stereotyped based on these criteria.

When people who are deaf express themselves vocally and the sounds they produce do not make sense to the hearing observer, the assumption is made that something is wrong with them. In addition, if those who cannot hear repeatedly request the same information, the layperson frequently assumes that it is because they are "dumb," "stupid," or "uneducated," and not realize the difficulties encountered with speechreading.

Research findings indicate that individuals who are deaf perform at the same levels of intellectual functioning as their peers who can hear. Studies conducted by Braden concluded that the average IQ score on the performance part of the WISC-R was 96.89, only slightly lower than the hearing children's norm of 100 (Braden, 1985, p. 499).

Because speech and language are often confused with thinking, deaf individuals are perceived as being intellectually inferior. However, one's ability to speak and the content of what one has to say are two entirely separate processes.

MYTH: PEOPLE WHO ARE DEAF CANNOT DRIVE, FLY PLANES, OR OPERATE MOTORBOATS

People who can hear incorporate the use of their eyes and ears when they are driving, thus alerting them to their surroundings. Sirens, the sound of screeching tires, and horns honking all provide warning signals for the hearing driver.

Because hearing individuals rely heavily on both vision and hearing to drive defensively, many assume that if one is hearing is impaired, one's ability to drive is also impaired. Members of the general public are oftentimes surprised to discover that people who are deaf do indeed drive and maintain very safe driving records.

A study conducted in 1968 by Sherman G. Finesilver (President's Advisory Committee on Traffic Safety) concluded that across the United States individuals who are deaf are involved in only one fourth as many accidents as their hearing counterparts. In addition, when driver's licensing officials were surveyed in 49 states, 41 of the 49 responding ranked the driver who is deaf at least as good, and in many cases better, than the hearing driver (Finesilver, 1968).

Because 97% of the warning signals that reach drivers are gained through the visual channel (Greenmum, 1952), drivers who are deaf have the opportunity to survey their surroundings and respond accordingly. Their eyes become their primary information resource, and they frequently wait at intersections when the light turns green to observe if any vehicles are not heeding the directive to stop. Although several states require that the driver who is deaf or hard of hearing purchase a side mirror for both sides of the vehicle, generally no other restrictions are mandated.

Closely related to the myth that people who are deaf cannot drive is the misconception that they cannot, or are not allowed to, fly aircraft. Currently, the number of pilots who are deaf is few; however, the number is growing steadily. In the early 1900s these individuals began participating in the world of aviation. As early as 1910 Calbraith Perry Rodgers, deafened since the age of six, made his mark in the field of flight by winning the endurance prize at Chicago's International Aviation Meet. In 1911 he was recognized for completing the first transcontinental solo flight across the United States.

Today approximately 50 individuals hold membership in the Deaf Pilots Association (DPA). Founded in 1994, the association's members represent approximately one fourth to one half of the pilots who are deaf in America. Flying small, private aircraft, they rely on vision and skill rather than on radio communication to fly their aircraft (Moore & Levitan, 2003).

MYTH: INDIVIDUALS WHO ARE DEAF HAVE MORE SERIOUS EMOTIONAL PROBLEMS THAN HEARING PEOPLE

Although some people who are deaf suffer serious emotional disturbances, their rate of bona fide maladjustment is not excessive, considering the rigors of their youth and the frustrations that can occur throughout their daily lives. Within the realm of psychiatric disorders, very few empirical studies have explored incidence rates concerning the various types of psychopathology evident in the population consisting of deaf individuals. However, research conducted by Pollard (1994) indicates that for the most part these individuals reflect the same diagnostic rates for adjustment disorders, mood disorders, organic disorders, anxiety disorders, and personality disorders as those reflected in hearing individuals.

Members of the hearing community periodically observe behaviors exhibited by people who are deaf as being abnormal or socially unacceptable. They, in turn, surmise that some psychological deficiency is inherently characteristic in the person who is deaf. However, with accurate background information pertaining to this population, it becomes apparent that those behaviors, which may appear to be abnormal, are merely the result of deficiencies of social knowledge.

According to Yambert and Van Craeynest (1975), much of what people who can hear learn is based on what they overhear. This is particularly true in the area of social knowledge. A tremendous amount of what the child learns to be socially acceptable or unacceptable is gleaned through overhearing parental discussions. Being privy to information regarding someone else's behavior provides the opportunity to learn about cultural norms and expectations about behavior.

The majority of children who are deaf cannot "eavesdrop" on parental or sibling conversations. Based on the fact that very few of their parents sign, the benefits of incidental learning experiences may be limited, if not altogether stymied. Hearing children automatically assimilate information and mimic behaviors by observing events that occur within their environment. However, this same information that emanates from an auditory environment must be taught to the child who is deaf. Those behaviors that, for all intents and purposes, appear to be everyday common knowledge can escape individuals who are deaf if they are not directly addressed.

This environmental deprivation can result in the hearing public stereotyping the child who is deaf as immature, exhibiting unacceptable behaviors, or having severe emotional problems. However, when the child is provided with ready access to this information and is challenged to grow, the potential for developing socially acceptable behaviors is present. Livneh and Antonak (1997) contend that poor communication skills, the presence of additional disabilities and poor educational experiences in segregated school settings can contribute to the increased risk of inappropriate psychosocial behaviors. They posit that although psychosocial maladaptation is not a necessary concomitant of prelingual, profound to severe deafness, environmental factors can be instrumental in promoting or discouraging the development of acceptable behaviors. Children who are deaf, like their counterparts who can hear, are provided with opportunities to flourish emotionally and socially when they are raised in environments by parents who are supportive, caring, and understanding.

MYTH: PEOPLE WHO ARE DEAF CANNOT WORK

Because deafness is a low-incidence disability, many employees may never encounter a Deaf worker. As a result, their mind-set about adults may revolve around the old stereotypes of the adult who is peddling manual alphabet cards to earn a living. The general public may be unaware of the wide away of employment possibilities available to this population.

Historically, individuals who are deaf were employed as factory workers, as printers, as dry cleaners, and in other forms of manual labor. However, with the advent of the Vocational Rehabilitation Act (1973), myriad vocational opportunities were made available to disabled individuals. Training programs were developed, support services provided, and individuals who were deaf began entering the competitive job market. Occupational surveys from the 1980s indicate that individuals who were deaf began securing employment in the managerial/professional sector; obtained jobs in the technical, sales, and administrative support areas; and continued to be employed as operators and precision production managers while also working as fabricators (Welsh & Walter, 1988).

With increasing numbers of individuals who are deaf entering postsecondary settings, the number of college graduates employed in the professional sector has increased. Teachers, counselors, superintendents, program managers, and psychologists continue to enter the workforce. Although unemployment and underemployment still plague this population today, individuals who are deaf and hard of hearing can be comparably trained and equally capable of working in a comparative field. Such positions provide these individuals with a sense of accomplishment and also enable them to live independently within the community. They take great pride in being self-sufficient and self-supporting, and many abhor those individuals who resort to peddling as a way of life.

Within the Deaf community, peddling is perceived as deviate behavior. Those community members who have worked hard to gain their rightful place in employment see the peddlers as spoiling their image and jeopardizing their chances of being rightfully included in activities controlled by the hearing world (Higgins, 1980, p. 175; Moore & Levitan, 2003). Historically, individuals who are deaf were perceived as being capable of earning a living only by peddling, an image the Deaf community has worked hard to dispel.

A question that is frequently asked by hearing members of society is whether or not they should purchase ABC cards, cards with key chains, or other trinkets from peddlers who mingle among crowds or set up tables on busy street corners. The sentiment expressed by those who can hear is that they want to help those individuals who are less fortunate members of society. Moore and Levitan (2003) remind the lay community that some of these peddlers can actually hear and are using this as a gimmick to generate income. Although others are deaf or hard of hearing, they are employable, choosing this line of work as a profitable way to earn a living.

While some members of the Deaf community are tolerant of Deaf peddlers, many more resent them for "giving deaf people a bad name." They recommend that hearing individuals wanting to support the Deaf community do so by buying artwork, tickets to National Theatre of the Deaf performances, books, or other items made by Deaf college or residential school students. Generally speaking and for the most part, members of the Deaf community have worked hard to dispel the image that deaf people cannot work and are resigned to a lifetime of peddling to earn a living.

MYTH: PEOPLE WHO ARE DEAF ARE VERY QUIET

From a distance, or to the untrained eye, the first impression of a "Deaf social event" is that these individuals are very quiet. However, upon closer examination one realizes that this is not the case. Deaf social events provide the participants with the opportunity to share stories with each other, tell jokes, and engage in lively entertainment. Peals of laughter, strikes of excitement, and animated sounds are all characteristic of these events. It is not uncommon for one to pound on the table, shout out a name, or stomp the floor to get a bystander's attention.

When music accompanies these events, it is usually played at a level enabling the participants to feel the vibrations on the floor. The music, coupled with the typical sounds produced by Deaf individuals, provides the hearing participant with an auditory as well as visual experience.

MYTH: ALL PEOPLE WHO ARE DEAF KNOW SIGN LANGUAGE

Sign language has received considerable attention throughout the past several years. The general public has become more aware of interpreters and has observed them as they facilitate communication. Sign language classes are offered on a regular basis by some community centers and college programs as more people express an interest in learning the language.

As a result of this exposure, hearing individuals may assume that all people who are deaf can sign. Today, 95% of students with severe to profound hearing losses attend classes that incorporate some type of manual communication into their program (Mindel & Vernon, 1987, p. 149). However, not all of those who are deaf use sign language to express themselves. Hearing individuals may encounter a person who is deaf and does not know how to sign or prefers to communicate orally.

Although the majority of individuals who are deaf can and do sign, not all are skilled in ASL. Deaf children of hearing parents who receive their education in included classrooms from teachers specifically trained to work with this population, or through support personnel such as sign language interpreters, may be receiving their information through a manually coded English sign system (see Chapter 6 for additional information). These students may have limited exposure to ASL; upon meeting Deaf individuals who have attended residential school facilities, they may find that both they and the Deaf individuals must make some modifications to effectively communicate.

Summary

Hearing individuals who have not encountered members of the Deaf community often "freeze" and withdraw when they meet a person who is deaf for the first time. Communication may be strained; misunderstandings may develop, resulting in feelings of embarrassment. If the hearing person does not have the skills to permit a free exchange of ideas to occur, the person who is deaf remains on the outside, trying to comprehend what is being conveyed. As a result, the exchange may end with both parties having formulated misconceptions about each other.

Throughout history, such interactions have led to the development of myths and misunderstandings that are still evident today. Only recently have Deaf spokespersons come to the forefront, thus dispelling some of these preconceived ideas. However, the general public is frequently still in awe upon meeting a person who is deaf for the first time. Therefore, their uncertainty of what to expect and how to communicate interferes with their ability to relate effectively.

The number of individuals who are born with a significant hearing loss will, in all likelihood, continue to represent a very small percentage of the overall population. Consequently, the majority of hearing individuals who have not been trained or are not employed in deaf education or related fields may have little, if any, contact with the prelingually deaf population.

With the advent of modern technology, recent legislation, and support services, many more people have become aware of the abilities of this unique population. Although several myths and misconceptions remain, some have been dispelled as an awareness of the characteristics and attributes of this population spreads.

3

A Look at the Field of Deaf Education

Where We've Been—Where We Are Today

Today's world can be characterized by rapidly changing technology, medical advances, shrinking cultural boundaries, and innovative educational opportunities. Access to a wealth of information is at our fingertips, and with a quick click on the computer we can find answers to our questions, share information, and connect with friends, families, and colleagues as we take advantage of what the Internet has to offer. For those seeking answers to questions, the information superhighway provides an abundance of resources, references, and additional topics to explore almost instantaneously.

Just as the world is changing rapidly, transformation is also evident in the population comprised of deaf individuals. During the past three decades, medical advancements, technological breakthroughs, and legislative mandates have impacted the way people who are deaf are educated, how they communicate, and where they congregate. Who are America's deaf people today? What is the prevalence and what are the characteristics used to describe those who are deaf and hard of hearing? What etiologies contribute to the varying degrees of hearing loss, and how are they identified by the medical profession? How is being deaf identified by the Deaf community? What type of diversity is evident in this segment of the population?

Professionals entering the field today are challenged with providing services to a population that represents a wide spectrum of attitudes, beliefs, abilities, and unique needs. Even though some are garnering the benefits of early identification and technological innovations, others are living on the cusp of poverty where these resources are meager, if not altogether nonexistent. In addition, as this economic divide continues to grow between those who "have" and those who "have not," the landscape of the field is being faced with a myriad of stark realities. Professionals entering the field today are faced with new demands in addition to the ones formerly experienced by teachers, interpreters, early intervention service providers, and specialists from the social services sector. What are the characteristics of this population today? How does it differ from even 30 years ago?

PREVALENCE, ETIOLOGY, AND IDENTIFICATION

As discussed in Chapter 2, statistics provided by the National Institute on Deafness and Other Communication Disorders (NIDCD) (2010) indicate that approximately 36 million American adults report some degree of hearing loss. Furthermore, between 500,000 and 750,000

Americans experience a severe to profound hearing loss. These individuals encounter varying degrees of difficulty in receiving and processing aural communication. Adults comprise the largest sector of this population. It is estimated that 77% of adults over the age of 65 experience some degree of hearing loss (NIDCD, 2010). Because many of these individuals lose their hearing later in life, due to the aging process, their needs are as unique as the individuals who experience the loss. For the majority of these adults the loss is gradual, impacting their ability to recognize and understand various speech sounds. As a result, they may not even be cognizant of how debilitating their loss has become until it has progressed to a point where they can no longer engage in successful communication exchanges. Deafened adults frequently need to improvise their own unique communication strategies, and some avail themselves of the opportunity to participate in support groups.

Deafened adults merit special consideration as they are recognized as a distinct population within the field and they frequently have needs that are very different from those who are born with a profound hearing loss. Several excellent texts and periodicals have been devoted to an in-depth discussion of this group's characteristics and needs. Those wishing to learn more about this group of individuals should consult that body of literature. This text does not explore this population; rather, it focuses primarily on the prelingual deaf population, those who are born deaf or lose their hearing before speech and language are developed. To acquire language and develop cognitively, socially, and psychologically, infants and toddlers who are deaf, as well as their families, require a multiplicity of services from early intervention specialists. These professionals establish partnerships with the families while concomitantly providing support services that lead toward the development of the whole child.

Keep in mind that, within the United States, approximately 2 to 3 out of every 1,000 children in the United States are born deaf or hard of hearing (NIDCD, 2010). Today hearing loss is being identified at an earlier age due to the increased use of neonatal screenings. Forty-two states and the District of Columbia now have programs to screen neonates for hearing loss (www.professional.asha.org). Prior to such mandates, the average age at which United States children with significant hearing losses were identified was 2 years of age or older (Schirmer, 2001). Furthermore, estimates provided by the U.S. Public Health Service (1990) indicate that 83 out of every 1,000 of these children exhibit an educationally significant hearing loss, and 9 out of every 1,000 of them are identified as having a severe to profound hearing loss. For an in-depth discussion of hearing loss and audiological evaluations, see Chapter 4.

The incidence of profound early childhood hearing loss has declined over the past decades, due in part to widespread vaccinations against rubella (Moores, 2001). However, when children are born with profound losses exceeding 90 dB, they are considered to be functionally deaf. Members of this population do not generally develop speech and language skills spontaneously without the assistance of educational and therapeutic interventions (Carney & Moeller, 1998; Paul & Whitelaw, 2011).

The majority of children with significant hearing loss are considered prelingually deaf (Schirmer, 2001). This terminology is used to describe hearing loss that is present at birth or occurred before the child began to talk. In essence, when children are born with a hearing loss of this magnitude, their perception of sounds is limited to those sounds exceeding 60 decibels (dB), or about the intensity level of a baby's cry. Therefore, in general, they will not be able to rely on their hearing to develop spontaneous oral language that approximates that of typical children (Carney & Moeller, 1998). Other avenues will need to be explored to ensure that these children have full access to the wealth of information that is transmitted through spoken communication.

Spoken communication provides most people with a lifeline, thus connecting them with families, friends, and communities. Early in life it becomes an interactive pipeline that allows for the mutual exchange of feelings, wants, and desires. Later it becomes the conduit for transmitting beliefs, values, traditions, and dreams while contributing to the shaping of one's identity. Furthermore, the primary mode of communication used by one's early caregivers furnishes individuals with the initial foundation upon which the building blocks of formal education will subsequently be placed. In addition, it creates an avenue for incidental language/learning to occur. Incidental learning later becomes one of the vital components in the fundamental learning process, frequently providing members of society with information that is taken for granted but used to make sense of the world that surrounds them. When our primary communication channel is affected, it impacts our personal, social, and cognitive development. The focus of this text is to provide the reader with information that pertains primarily to the prelingually deaf population. The attributes and characteristics of these individuals represent the same array of diversity that is exhibited in any other cultural or ethnic group of people.

DIVERSITY IN THE UNITED STATES

The United States can be characterized as a mosaic of diversity. Diversity is evident in terms of race, ethnicity, national origin, culture, linguistic preferences, and economic status. According to the United States Census Bureau (Nieto & Bode, 2008), the United States population exceeded 300,000,000 in 2006 and is projected to grow to over 419 million people by 2050. Between now and then, it is estimated that the White population will experience an increase of 7% to comprise 50.1% of the total population. Further projections indicate that the African American population is expected to increase from 12.7% to 14.6% of the total population. The Latino population will grow to 24.4% of the total United States population, nearly doubling its 12.6% of the population. In addition, the Asian population is expected to increase substantially from 10.7 million to 33.4 million in the United States.

Diversity is also apparent in economic status. In a report published by the National Center for Children in Poverty in 2010, there are over 25 million children under the age of 6 in the United States. Of these children, approximately 11.7 million or 46% live in low-income families. Approximately 11.7 million, or 46%, live in low-income families, and 6.1 million, or 24%, live in poor families. Further statistics indicate that the following number of children, identified by race/ethnicity, live in low-income families: 73% American Indian, 65% Latino, 66% Black, 31% Asian, and 32% White (Chau, Thampi, & Wright, 2010). Demographics also demonstrate that children, under the age of 6, from low-income families, are represented in all of the geographic regions throughout the United States. An examination of the population indicates these children live in each of the four major geographic areas. Of the total number of children under the age of 6 living in the South, 49% reside in low-income families, while 46% of the total number of children living in the West are from low-income families. Furthermore, of the total number of children living in the Northeast, 39% represent this population, while in the Midwest, 47% of them are representative of this group (Chau et al., 2010).

DIVERSITY WITHIN THE DEAF COMMUNITY

For several years the Gallaudet Research Institute (GRI) has also been conducting a survey to collect data on diversity in the deaf student population. Data collected in 2008 indicate that less than 60% of the deaf student population is White, less than 16% are Black/African American; 17% are Hispanic/Latino; 0.2% are American Indian or Alaska Native only; and slightly more than 3% are Asian American. Furthermore, approximately 23.5% of students who are deaf speak and write languages other than English at home. Of this group using a language other than English at home, 21.9% use Spanish, and 9.4% use multiple languages. In addition, of those who responded, 36.8% reported that they were economically disadvantaged (GRI, 2008).

Where do these children attend school? How do these educational settings compare with those available to students prior to the 1970s? Are most of their teachers hearing or deaf? How does the ethnic makeup of the teachers and administrators compare to the population that they serve? What communication modes do they use in the classroom for instructional purposes?

EDUCATIONAL SETTINGS

Prior to 1975, educational opportunities were somewhat limited for children with special needs. During this time the majority of students who were deaf were sent to residential facilities, and these schools became a mecca for Deaf culture; in schools for the deaf, students received their education from Deaf teachers, had exposure to Deaf adults performing a variety of job functions, and were privy to the stories and traditions previously established by the Deaf community. In many of these settings ASL flourished, providing students with equal opportunities to engage in classroom discussions and activities.

In 1950, almost 85% of all deaf children attended schools for the deaf (Padden & Humphries, 2005). Many remained at the schools for extended periods, only returning to their families to celebrate holidays and family traditions. These institutions provided a cornerstone for their identities while setting the stage for the formation of friendships that would last a lifetime. (Additional information regarding educational settings is presented in Chapter 8.)

Although prior to the mid 1970s the majority of these students received their education in residential schools, some parents enrolled their children in public schools, and some elected to keep their children at home. Moreover, even though public schools admitted the students, administrators and teachers were not required to provide any special services for them. As a result, many experienced failure and withdrew from the educational system.

However, the educational arena was transformed in 1975 with the passage of Public Law 94-142 (The Education for All Handicapped Children Act of 1975). With the enactment of this law, public schools were mandated to provide a free and appropriate education for all students with disabilities. Consequently, a significant change occurred in the demographic pattern of the school-age deaf population. Touted as a blessing by some and a curse by others, it signaled a decrease in enrollments at the schools for the deaf across the country. No longer would the majority of students who were deaf have daily contact with Deaf teachers and other Deaf professionals traditionally employed in the educational setting fostered by the schools for the deaf.

According to Stinson and Antia (1999), from 1973 to 1984 private and residential schools experienced a 65% drop in enrollment. In contrast to the remaining 32% who attended residential schools in 1985, 1.9% of the population was reported as being fully mainstreamed and 6.2% of the students were partially mainstreamed. This trend continued through the 1990s and has remained constant today. By the mid-1990s, 91% of students who were deaf were being educated to some extent in their local schools. In addition, nationally, between 1970 and 2000 the number of students who were deaf attending schools or special centers for the deaf declined more than 60% as increased numbers of students began and continued attending neighborhood school programs (Moores, 2006). Currently, approximately three quarters of children who are deaf or who have severe hearing loss attend local public schools (Antia, Reed, & Kreimeyer, 2005). According to the Regional and National Summary provided by the Gallaudet Research Institute (2008), students who are deaf and hard of hearing are receiving their education in the following settings: 24% in deaf-centric or center schools, 39.1% in regular school settings with hearing students, 17.4% in self-contained classrooms in regular education settings, 9.6% in resource rooms, 2.1% at home, and 3.1% in "Other" settings (Gallaudet Research Institute, 2008).

Today, students who are deaf and hard of hearing attending residential and day schools for the deaf continue to receive the majority of their instruction, if not all of it, from teachers of the deaf in classes designed specifically for them. Within both of these settings, students have the opportunity to participate in extracurricular activities, sports, and other events with other students who are deaf and hard of hearing. However, unlike in residential schools, in day schools students do not have the option of living in dormitories and must return to their primary caregivers at the end of the school day. Within both of these settings and depending on the geographic location, students are sometimes afforded the opportunity to travel to their neighborhood schools for specific, designated classes. However, depending on the setting, their time in these schools can be limited.

Even though the majority of those who are deaf attend public schools, the communication mode, support services, and settings for delivering instruction there are as diverse as the students enrolled in the programs. Some of the students are included in the general education classroom for the entire day and receive support services in the form of interpreters, note takers, and tutors. They are also provided services by itinerant teachers specifically trained to work with them. Although some of these teachers provide consultative services to general education teachers, others form collaborative partnerships with them and are provided with the opportunity to co-teach the academic curriculum. Although some students attending included programs remain in the general education classroom for the entire day, others are pulled out and receive part of their instruction in resource rooms for one or more subjects throughout the day. This segment of the student population represents the same degree of diversity that is reflected in the larger hearing population. Who are the teachers serving these students? How many of them are deaf? Do these professionals depict the same ethnic diversity as their students? What are the characteristics of the teachers instructing these students?

Simms, Rusher, Andrews, and Coryell (2008) conducted a diversity survey in 2004 of 3,227 professionals in 313 deaf education programs to determine the characteristics of professionals working in the field. Their objective was to discover how many D/deaf teachers and D/deaf administrators worked with students who were deaf in included programs housed in K–12 public or residential schools or were enrolled in university teacher preparation programs. Of the 33% of those surveyed who responded, results indicated that 22.0% of the teachers and 14.5% of the administrators were deaf. This is reflective of less than a 10% increase in deaf professionals since 1993. In addition, 9.5% of teachers and 6.1% of administrators were professionals of color. Of these minority teachers, only 2.5% were deaf persons of color. Of those who responded, only 3, or 0.6%, of the deaf administrators were persons of color.

Results further reflect a teaching profession primarily consisting of White, hearing females, characteristic of the general teaching population today (Simms et al., 2008). These data further support previous studies that reflect the need for the field of deaf education to "diversify its professional force in order to utilize the intellectual, linguistic, and multicultural proficiencies of hearing teachers of color, deaf teachers, and deaf teachers of color" (Simms et al., p. 384). Within these classrooms several forms of communication are used for instructional purposes. What has historically been used in schools for the deaf? What are teachers relying on today to instruct their students? Have any significant changes occurred throughout the past 30 years?

MODES OF COMMUNICATION

Communication provides a lifeline by connecting us to people and our environment. Our exposure and interaction with the various forms of communication—print, spoken language, sign language, and others—promote personal growth and development. The essentials of communication lie in language, and for most members of the hearing population language development occurs naturally. Modeling their mother tongue, children acquire these building blocks without giving much, if any, thought to the process.

However, for the prelingual deaf population this is not the case. The 90% of children who are deaf born to parents who can hear find they have entered a world filled with barriers to the spoken language that is used in the home. Parents of these children struggle to determine the best avenue to use to communicate with their children who are deaf. Although a few hearing parents advocate for sign language and elect to use this form of communication, the majority commit to using speech as their primary means for interacting with their child.

The decision to sign or rely on spoken communication is almost always a difficult one for parents who can hear. Many are already feeling very overwhelmed when they receive the initial diagnosis that their child is deaf. In coming to terms with this reality, they are also confronted with making a communication choice that will significantly impact the child's development. Many feel they do not have adequate information to make this decision. Frequently, they find they have more questions than answers as they grapple with all of the information. Struggling to make the right choice, they hope that the decision they make will be in the best interest of their child and will positively impact their future growth and development. (Chapter 5 takes an in-depth look at family dynamics.)

Parents are not the only ones who have endeavored to ascertain which mode of communication they should or should not use. Since the inception of deaf education in this country, specialized schools have discussed, debated, and fought over the use of an oral/aural approach, or one that supports a manual form of communication such as ASL, one of the sign systems (SEE I, SEE II, CASE, Signed English, etc.), or, more recently, adopting a bilingual/bicultural (Bi-Bi) approach. In the United States, the heated controversy about this has resulted primarily in the establishment of two types of programs: those that embrace the philosophy of using a totally oral/aural method and those that believe in using ASL or a form of one of the sign systems.

Historically speaking, throughout the United States the oral/aural approach is the oldest of the communication approaches that has been used in the education of students who are deaf (Easterbrooks & Baker, 2002). Proponents of this approach to deaf education believe that children who are deaf are best served by instruction in lipreading and in maximizing use of their residual hearing (through amplification and auditory training) (Easterbrooks & Baker). Although this approach has a long-standing history within deaf education, some educators became dismayed in the 1960s and 1970s by the relatively poor academic achievement of graduates of older, orally focused programs and began developing approaches to support oral language input with manual sign systems.

Committed to making the curriculum accessible to students who were deaf, several teachers and administrators began experimenting with a variety of instructional techniques. These included teaching methods and sign systems. Although some of the schools introduced sign systems such as SEE I or SEE II into their classrooms, others combined these systems with speech for both instructional and conversational purposes. The goal was to provide students with a total form of communication, and the term *Total Communication* quickly became a catchword in the professional community (Scheetz, 1998).

During the same period that Total Communication came to the forefront, so did several forms of manual communication. Most of these systems share some common features: They generally adapt some ASL signs for vocabulary, invent new signs to convey grammatical concepts not expressed by discrete signs in ASL (such as articles, auxiliary verbs, and inflectional morphology), and produce sentences that duplicate the syntactic structure of English (Tye-Murray, 1998).

In the 1980s, Mindel and Vernon (1987) estimated that 95% of students with severe or profound hearing impairments utilized some form of manual communication in their educational settings; however, more recently, Schirmer (2001) reported that Total Communication "has gone somewhat out of style" and "did not increase literacy levels as hoped" (Easterbrooks & Baker, 2002).

During the 1980s, another form of manual communication, *Cued Speech*, was developed. Based on the hypothesis that several of the speech sounds in our spoken language look similar when produced on the lips, Cued Speech was devised to present a visual indicator of what sound is being produced. This manual system is distinct in its orientation and is more closely associated with oralist approaches to deaf education. It is used by relatively few children who are deaf and their teachers and parents.

Today, three primary communication methods are used in deaf education: oral/aural, total communication, and Bi-Bi. Each has undergone relative waves of popularity (Schirmer, 2001). The approach that focuses on amplification and auditory training (oral/aural) is now typically associated with the label *auditory verbal therapy* (Easterbrooks & Baker, 2002). Although relatively new, the Bi-Bi approach is proving to be efficacious, particularly in the education of children who receive cochlear implants (Rhoades, 2006). Bi-Bi programs emerged some time after Total Communication stopped being practiced and are modeled after English as a Second Language (ESL) (Easterbrooks & Baker, 2001; Moores, 1999). By adhering to many of the principles of ESL and foreign language immersion programs, Bi-Bi programs teach the language while emphasizing the positive aspects of Deaf culture. Recent data collected by the Gallaudet Research Institute (GRI) in 2008 indicate that auditory/oral-only approaches are currently used with 52% of deaf and hard-of-hearing children in the United States, sign and speech approaches with 34.9%, and sign-only approaches with just 11.4% (GRI, 2008). (A more detailed discussion of modes of communication is included in Chapter 6.)

Over the past 40 years the field of deaf education has witnessed a dramatic shift in the educational domain. This is depicted both in classroom settings and the communication mode selected to deliver instruction. Students who are deaf are being afforded numerous opportunities while being challenged to achieve the same standards as their hearing peers. Through these endeavors they are being prepared for a future that holds endless possibilities that were previously unavailable to them. Although educational institutions have served a vital role in shaping the lives of children who are deaf, they constitute only one of the many entities that have been instrumental in influencing their development. What other segments of society have made an impact on their lives, influencing them throughout their progression from childhood into adulthood? What role has technology played in the ways these individuals interface with the larger hearing population?

HEARING AIDS AND COCHLEAR IMPLANTS

One of the most dramatic changes within the field of hearing-aid technology lies in the development and implementation of the cochlear implant. This implantable device has revolutionized the way children who are deaf are receiving amplification. (See Chapter 7 for a discussion of cochlear implants and hearing-aid technology.) Approved by the U.S. Food and Drug Administration in December 1984, cochlear implants have been steadily gaining in popularity. Evidence of this can be seen in the increased number of individuals who have undergone this procedure.

In 2000, a survey was distributed to students who are deaf and hard of hearing receiving support from special education services throughout the United States. Results from the survey indicated that fewer than 2,000 were identified as having cochlear implants (Mitchell, 2004). However, by 2005, the U.S. Food and Drug Administration estimated that approximately 15,000 U.S. children had received such implants (NIDCD, 2006). Currently, the best estimate of cochlear implant prevalence appears to be 13.7% nationally, though this varies by region from 9.9% in the West to 14.7% in the South. Nationwide, 15.4% have had a second cochlear implant, with 20.5% being implanted in the Northeast and 16.6% in the South. Of those previously implanted, 92.4% report that they are currently using their devices (GRI, 2008). Termed "the most educationally and socially significant technological change for deaf children" (Wilkins & Hehir, 2008, p. 153), evidence in the literature suggests that children who are deaf and using cochlear implants present distinct educational challenges and opportunities compared with children who do not use them (Blamey et al., 2001; Hammes, Novak, Rotz, Willis, & Edmondson, 2002, as cited in Wilkins & Hehir, 2008).

Probably no other form of technology has caused more of a furor in the Deaf community than the cochlear implant. Opponents and proponents have engaged in frequent debates, often heated, regarding the merits of implanting young children. Originally, the National Association for the Deaf (NAD) voiced strong opposition to pediatric implants. In 1991 NAD issued a position statement stating, "[The NAD] deplores the decision of the Food and Drug Administration [to approve implantation in children aged 2–17] which was unsound scientifically, procedurally, and ethically." The NAD further declared that "The parents who make the decision for the child are often poorly informed about the deaf community, its rich heritage and promising futures" (Cochlear Implant Taskforce of the NAD, 1991, p. 1).

In 2000 NAD released a new position paper on cochlear implants. The position has been modified and currently reflects a more accepting philosophy of parents who elect to have their children implanted. According to the position paper released in October 2000, "Cochlear implantation is a technology that represents a tool to be used in some forms of communication, and not a cure for deafness." In addition, "The NAD recognizes all technological advancements with the potential to foster, enhance, and improve the quality of life for all deaf and hard of hearing persons." One other statement that merits attention addresses the rights of the parents to make informed decisions. "The NAD recognizes the rights of parents to make informed choices for their . . . children, respects their choice to use cochlear implants and all other assistive devices, and strongly supports the development of the whole child and of language and literacy" (NAD, 2002).

As the age of implantation continues to drop, the number of implants continues to rise. Worldwide an estimated 5,000 individuals received implants in 1990 (Christiansen & Leigh, 2002); by 1997 the number had increased to 16,000; by 2002 there were almost 60,000 recipients, and according to 2005 data almost 100,000 had received implants (NIDCD, 2002, 2006). Furthermore, both nationally and internationally more and more infants are being implanted, with an estimated 90 to 95% of all children born deaf receiving the device (Komesaroff, 2007).

The increasing global distribution of cochlear implants has been accompanied by a proliferation of research articles. Professionals are examining trends in educational placement as well as consumer attitudes and acceptance of the device. In addition, the communication abilities of children with implants as well as their levels of social interaction are being evaluated. Research studies are being conducted with older children that investigate Deaf identity issues as well as bilingual proficiency of both spoken and signed languages. (An in-depth look at this research is explored further in Chapter 6.)

What other forms of technology have played a significant role in the lives of children and adults who are deaf? Without a doubt, personal computers, handheld devices including two-way pagers, and texting telephones have had a powerful impact on communication. In addition, the advent of closed captioning, vibro-tactile devices, visual alerting devices, video interpreting services, and amplification devices have played an important role in leveling the communication field by opening avenues that were not previously available.

CLOSED CAPTIONING TECHNOLOGY

The inception and implementation of closed captioning marked a new era for individuals who are deaf and hard of hearing. Laying the groundwork in the 1970s, closed captioning in the United States would officially begin in 1980 (Gregg, 2006). The National Captioning Institute (NCI) spearheaded the effort to encode captions into commercial programs. Established by Congress in 1979, this nonprofit organization was instrumental in leading the nation toward providing individuals who are deaf and hard of hearing with access to social and political arenas broadcast through the media (Gregg). Largely through technology pioneered by NCI, the first closed-captioned television series was broadcast in 1980. This signaled the beginning of the captioning era. With an increased awareness of this technology and public demands, networks were encouraged to continue pursuing the development of real-time captioning. As a result, in 1982, the first live captioned program was broadcast (Gregg). By 1984 CBS had also agreed to transmit closed captions, and in 1989 closed captions, through the use of a decoder, were available for all prime-time programs and the majority of all major sporting events (DuBow, 1991; Gregg). These captions were initially viewed by installing a set-top box; however, the set-top box was expensive and difficult to install.

By 1990, decoders had been available for 10 years and were selling for between $150 and $180. Nonetheless, they were being used only in 300,000 homes across the United States. Even though the national census indicated that approximately 24 million Americans who were deaf or hard of hearing were living in the United States then, television manufacturers were still not inclined to integrate a microchip into sets to provide captioning possibilities for such a limited number of users, even though doing so might push the price lower than the set-top decoders (Gregg, 2006).

A breakthrough in the captioning industry occurred in 1990 when Congress approved the Television Decoder Circuitry Act. This legislation mandated that all television sets 13 inches or larger for sale in the United States be manufactured with caption-decoding microchips. This technology paved the way for individuals who were deaf and hard of hearing to gain access to information, thus allowing them to participate in the social, cultural, political, and economic experiences taken for granted by the larger hearing society (Gregg, 2006).

Provided with an avenue to stay abreast of local, national, and international developments, individuals who were deaf could now take advantage of the same news broadcasts as their hearing counterparts. Furthermore, they could also enjoy programming previously available solely to those who could hear. However, it quickly became apparent that the television would remain only one avenue for individuals who were deaf to access information. With the advent of personal computers, they too would soon have access to the information superhighway.

USE OF COMPUTER TECHNOLOGY

If one were to conduct a survey to identify the one piece of equipment that has revolutionized the way we communicate with others and conduct daily business, the personal computer would undoubtedly be mentioned most frequently. From the early onset of computer development in the late 1930s to the availability of the earliest commercial, nonkit personal computer in 1974 to personal computers being integrated into the workforce in 1977, personal computers became a basic tool in homes, schools, and businesses around 1984 (www.computerhistory.org/timeline/?category=cmptr).

In October 1984, the U.S. Census Bureau began including a section in the Current Population Survey (CPS) to assess ownership and use of computers. Results of the 2003 survey indicate that of the majority of American households, 70 million, or 62%, had one or more computers. This was a substantial increase from 22.8% in 1993, 15.0% in 1989, and 8.2% in 1984 (Kominski & Newburger, 1999). Although home computer use has been on the increase since the survey was first compiled, those using computers at home are most likely families with yearly incomes of $100,000 (97%), while only 47% of households with incomes below $25,000 report owning this technology.

Furthermore, race and educational attainment of the householder, as well as geographic region, all seem to have a strong influence on the presence of a computer in the household. Statistics indicate that children from non-Hispanic, White, or Asian families were more likely to have a computer at home (85%) as were children who grew up in households where the householder had a bachelor's degree (94%). In addition, children living in the South were less likely than those living elsewhere to have a computer at home (59% had a computer, and 52% had an Internet connection). Adults and children alike depend on computers to complete their work and access information. Of the more than 55 million children enrolled in school programs, 9 out of every 10 used a computer at school (Kominski & Neuberger, 1999).

This proliferation of computer availability has opened up a whole new avenue for individuals who are deaf and hard of hearing. From the connectivity with others using video conferencing technology to the videos posted by Deaf individuals on YouTube, global boundaries have grown smaller, and the Deaf are now able to engage in conversations with other community members, thus fostering a sense of a collective identity.

Research conducted by Rogers (1998) indicates that Deaf individuals began using the Internet in much the same fashion as their hearing counterparts. Exposed to the technology at work, in schools, and oftentimes at home, they have participated in Web surfing, e-mail, text messaging, and blogging. Zazove et al. (2004) surveyed Deaf individuals in Michigan and reported that 63% of those responding to the survey are active users of computer technology. Bowe (2002) noted that Deaf and hard-of-hearing people preferred the use of e-mail and instant messaging as forms of communication; the use of these two modalities has far exceeded the use of teletypewriters (TTYs) and other relay services.

From a historical standpoint, the advent of TTY technology provided people who are deaf and hard-of-hearing with viable access to telephone services. With the evolution of the acoustic coupler (modem), translated TTY signals could be transmitted over the phone. This provided the Deaf community with a way to connect to each other as well as the hearing world (Hogg, Lomicky, & Weiner, 2008). Research by Belcastro (2004) and Austin (2006) further highlights how electronic technologies can help students in rural areas who are deaf obtain services and provide connectivity with students in residential settings.

Hogg, Lomicky, and Weiner (2008) conducted a study focusing on Deaf students attending Gallaudet, as well as alumni, to determine the type of computer-mediated communication they utilized when wanting to express their views. Nearly all those surveyed indicated their favorite devices included T-Mobile's Sidekick, desktop computers, and laptops. T-Mobile's Sidekick is a messaging device that features a flip-out color screen with liquid crystal display (LCD) technology and a thumb keypad. The Sidekick was introduced to the general public in 2003. Allowing users to connect instantaneously with others, it began featuring a MySpace application in 2007.

Those who own a Sidekick can surf the Web, send e-mails, play games, and share photos (T-Mobile, 2010).

Furthermore, of those responding, half indicated they use some form of a video device, and almost all reported that they use e-mail (97%), and they engage in Web surfing (73%), text messaging (69%), and blogging (48%). This supports previous research by Bowe (2002) that revealed that e-mail and instant messaging were used to a far greater extent than TTY or other relay services. Replacing the TTYs of the 1960s and 1970s, video technology has come to the forefront in the form of video phones, video relay services (VRS), and video relay interpreters (VRI).

VIDEO RELAY SERVICES AND VIDEO RELAY INTERPRETERS

Several companies provide Video Relay Services (VRSs). Employing interpreters across the nation, they provide year-round services 24 hours a day. Although the companies vary, they all rely on video phones or video conferencing equipment that includes a camera, display screen, video conferencing software, a microphone and speaker, and a high-speed Internet connection. Deaf individuals wanting to communicate with hearing individuals, businesses, and so on, in remote locations, can do so using a VRS. For example, a D/deaf person wanting to order a pizza or make an appointment could do so by contacting one of the companies that provides VRS service. Interpreters working for these businesses, located in call centers throughout the country, are trained to provide services via video conferencing technology.

Video Relay Interpreters (VRIs) also rely on video conferencing technology to provide interpreting services. However, unlike a VRS, which provides interpreting for hearing and D/deaf individuals located in two different places, those receiving services from a VRI are in the same location with the interpreter provided remotely. For example, when a D/deaf person has been hospitalized in a rural location, the doctor could come into the room and talk with the patient through VRI. In this instance, both consumers are located within the same room, with the interpreter facilitating communication through video conferencing equipment. Although the equipment needed for VRS is provided free of charge to D/deaf consumers, allowing them to make point-to-point video phone calls in addition to using the relay service, the equipment used for VRI is purchased by businesses strictly for interpreting purposes.

Other forms of technology used for communication purposes are computer programs that utilize point-to-point video conferencing technology. Programs such as iVisit, Skype, Polycom, and Oovoo allow individuals at remote locations to use the Internet anywhere in the world to connect and communicate face-to-face through sign, speech, or shared documents. This has provided another communication option for consumers who are deaf and hard of hearing.

SPEECH-TO-TEXT TECHNOLOGY

Another form of technology that has come to the forefront in the last three decades is speech-to-text technology for use with this population. Software programs such as Communication Access Realtime Translation (CART), C-Print, and Type-Well are all designed to provide communication access and notes for people who need alternative or additional support accessing spoken communication. This form of technology is used in nonbroadcast settings for students enrolled in educational programs (fifth grade through graduate school) and for adults attending meetings, workshops, professional development activities, business or community events, conferences, and some churches.

Relying on a software program that converts spelling-based abbreviations, captionists, also referred to as transcribers, type in spoken information. The text is then converted to full text and can afterward be displayed on a computer or separate LCD screen for multiple users to view. The transcription can be saved, printed, and ultimately shared with the consumer. This software provides one more inroad into accessing spoken communication.

Professionals providing this service often consist of individuals who have elected to choose this as a career field, including sign language interpreters who have received cross-training as well as courtroom reporters who also do live captioning. Individuals working as captionists are trained in the software application and become skilled at typing abbreviations that appear as words and phrases for the consumer who is deaf or hard of hearing. These abbreviations reduce the number of keystrokes needed, allowing the captionist to provide as much spoken information as possible in text form. Although the message is not rendered verbatim, it is generally representative of the meaning being presented.

Technology, medical advances, and educational settings are only some of the factors that are impacting the lives of children and adults who are deaf. Legislation has also played an eminent role in the institutions that have had a significant impact on people's lives. Legislation mandates where children who are deaf are educated, what support services are available for them and for adults, and how those in need access communication today.

LEGISLATION

Legislation that was enacted in the early 1960s with the passage of Public Law 87-276 provided funds to prepare professionals to train teachers to work with students who are deaf or hard of hearing. This was followed by Public Law 89-10, the Elementary and Secondary Education Act, which allotted funds to states and local school districts for the purpose of developing programs for both economically disadvantaged and children with disabilities. Subsequent legislation described in Public Law 93-112, Section 504 of the Rehabilitation Act, further added that no individual could be excluded on the basis of disability alone from any program or activities that received federal funding.

Passed in 1973, Section 504 of the Rehabilitation Act of 1973 clearly states, in part, that "no otherwise qualified handicapped individual shall, solely by reason of his handicap, be excluded from the participation in, be denied the benefits of, or be subjected to discrimination in any program or activity receiving federal financial assistance." The Rehabilitation Act is not designed to provide any federal money to assist people with disabilities. Furthermore, it was not created to provide states with funds to serve individuals with disabilities; rather, it imposes a duty on every recipient of federal funds to treat all individuals fairly and equitably regardless of their disability.

Although this early legislation set the tone for what was to follow, the landmark legislation that was responsible for changing the face of education in this country can be attributed to Public Law 94-142, the Education of All Handicapped Children Act (EAHCA), which Congress passed in 1975. Since 1975, when it became law, several reauthorizations and amendments have been enacted. Public Law 94-142 mandated free and appropriate public education for all children with disabilities between the ages of 6 and 21. It protected the rights of children with disabilities and their parents in educational decision making and required that each child with a disability have an Individualized Education Program (IEP). It further stated that students with disabilities must receive educational services in the least restrictive environment.

Although certain populations served by IDEA embrace the ideology and the concept of a "least restrictive environment" by including students in general education classrooms, educators within the field of deaf education and some parents have held fast to the opinion that included settings may not always be the best environment for educating these students. Even though advocates for other disability groups viewed this legislation as a civil right, advocates for children who are deaf have often perceived these settings as a violation of their civil rights. Viewed as "a source of contention and controversy . . . most stakeholders [are of the opinion] that this type of placement could not meet the needs of all deaf children educationally, socially, emotionally, or culturally" (Schirmer, 2001). Subsequently, this legislation prompted many professionals within the field to believe that enactment of this legislation signaled the end of an era when deaf education was viewed as an independent entity. Today, deaf education has become incorporated into special education, which itself has been subsumed within general education. Students who are deaf and hard of hearing are provided with access to the regular curriculum in general education classrooms and are expected to successfully complete all the requirements leading to graduation.

Further legislation was passed by Congress in 1986, whereby provisions were included in Public Law 99-457, the Education of the Handicapped Act Amendments, for the expansion of services for infants and toddlers with disabilities from birth through age 2. The intent of this legislation was to provide early intervention services to children with developmental delays and those diagnosed with having a physical or mental impairment that could contribute to developmental delays. These early intervention services are prescribed and implemented according to an Individualized Family Services Plan (IFSP).

Other legislation that has impacted the field of deafness is Public Law 101-336, the Americans with Disabilities Act (ADA), which was signed into law in 1990. The ADA extends civil rights protection of persons with disabilities to private sector employment, all public services, public accommodations, transportation, and telecommunications.

One other piece of legislation that has made a major impact on the educational system, including children with disabilities, is the No Child Left Behind (NCLB) Act of 2001. The law's stated purpose is to close the achievement gap with accountability, flexibility, and choice so that no child is left behind. The specific goal of the law is to ensure that all students are 100% proficient in reading and language arts and mathematics by 2013. However, when this law was designed, no consideration was given to the needs of children who were deaf or severely hard of hearing.

Of all the requirements outlined in NCLB, probably the most stringent and controversial is the law's accountability system (Yell & Drasgow, 2009). NCLB mandates that each state establish rigorous academic content standards for every student served, assess all students' academic progress, and report results on an annual basis. Each state designs statewide assessments based on measurable objectives and defines how it will measure student progress toward meeting these standards. To measure Adequate Yearly Progress (AYP), states collect data on achievement scores obtained on statewide assessments, graduation rates, and other indicators of student achievement. Within the public schools, personnel in each of the states continue to grapple with managing AYP, administering assessments, and meeting the requirements for highly qualified teachers. As a result, the long-range effects of this legislation remain to be seen. Built on an apparent "one size fits all" concept, the future looms with additional doubts and concerns for those individuals who are deaf and hard of hearing. Will their needs be met? Will they fall through the cracks as the schools focus on the majority achieving AYP? The impact NCLB will have on future generations of children who are deaf and hard of hearing remains unknown.

When NCLB was implemented, it was supposed to take precedence over IDEA. Nevertheless, with the glaring omission of any language that specifically relates to children with disabilities, the needs of those receiving services under IDEA are basically ignored. Unlike IDEA, which continued to take shape and develop under the auspices of parents and interest groups, challenging the various aspects of NCLB has been left to the individual states (Moores, 2005). (See Table 3.1 for a summary of pertinent legislation.)

TABLE 3.1 Educational Milestones That Have Made an Impact on the Education of Students Who Are Deaf and Hard of Hearing

1954: *Brown v. Board of Education of Topeka* (347 U.S. 483 (1954))
- Held that segregation based on race violated Equal Protection under the 14th Amendment
- Reversed the "Separate but Equal" finding in *Plessey v. Ferguson*
- The Court extended its findings to include disabilities ("unalterable characteristics")
- Established the foundations for the Civil Rights Act of 1964 and subsequent legislation affecting DHHS students
- Provided the legal precedent for efforts for students with special needs to gain equal access to educational opportunities as part of a free and appropriate public education
- Catalyst for parental advocacy for students with special needs (Yell, 2006)

1965: Elementary and Secondary Education Act (ESEA).
- Enacted during the administration of President Lyndon B. Johnson (LBJ)
- Part of the broad sweeping Civil Rights Act of 1964
- LBJ believed that education was the key to social mobility and that too many schools lacked the resources needed to provide the necessary skills to students from disadvantaged backgrounds (McGuinn, 2006, p. 27)
- The ESEA was intended to be primarily a redistributive bill to put a floor under spending in the nation's poorest communities and to lend federal muscle to efforts to innovate and improve educational services
- Title I of the legislation states: "provide financial assistance . . . to expand and improve . . . educational programs by various means...which contribute particularly to meeting the special educational needs of educationally deprived children." (Spring 1976, p. 31)

1973: Vocational Rehabilitation Act (VRA) (Public Law 93–112, Section 504)
- Defines "Handicapped person"
- Defines "appropriate education"
- Prohibits discrimination against students with disabilities in federally funded programs (Vaughn, Bos, Schumm 2003)

1974: Educational Amendments Act (Public Law 93–380)
- Grants federal funds to states for programming for exceptional learners
- Provides the first federal funding of state programs for students who are gifted and talented
- Grants students and families the right of due process in special education placement

---

1975: Education for All Handicapped Children Act (EAHCA) (Public Law 94-142, Part B)
- Known as the Mainstreaming Law
- Requires states to provide a free and appropriate public education for children with disabilities (ages 5 to 18)
- Requires individualized education programs (IEP)
- First defined "least restrictive environment"

(*Continued*)

TABLE 3.1 Educational Milestones That Have Made an Impact on the Education of Students Who Are Deaf and Hard of Hearing (*Continued*)

1983: A Nation at Risk: The Imperative for Educational Reform released

- Cited declining test scores
- Acknowledged the evidence that in U.S. schools there were large socioeconomic and racial achievement gaps
- Concern that even the country's "good" schools were not good enough
- The weak performance of U.S. students compared with students in other industrialized nations
- Highlighted the number of functionally illiterate adults
- Marked the first wave of educational reform in the United States
    1. The goal of the first wave was to raise educational quality by requiring more courses, and more testing of student and teacher performance. States were to assume the leadership in improving existing practices. This wave continues to be the strongest

---

1986: Second Wave Begins

- Based on educators such as Theodore Sizer, John Goodlad, and Ernest Boyer, rather than politicians and business leaders
- This wave stressed the need for basic reform of school practices. Recommendations included:
    1. Students should cover few subjects but study them in depth
    2. Hiring teachers who were more highly trained
    3. Strengthening the role of the principal

1986: Education of the Handicapped Act Amendments (Public Law 99-457)

- Requires states to extend free and appropriate education to children with disabilities (ages 3 to 5)
- Establishes early intervention programs for infants and toddlers with disabilities (ages birth to 2 years)

1988: Marks the third wave of reform

- Recognized that struggling families were unlikely to possess the time and resources required to ensure high-quality education
- Advocated for full-service schools
- Provided a network of social services
    1. Nutrition
    2. Health care
    3. Transportation
    4. Counseling
    5. Parent education (Sadker & Zittleman, 2009)

1989: Initiation of the Standards Movement. President Bush convenes a "National Educational Summit"—The document produced from the Summit—"Education 2000" was modified as "Goals 2000" under the President Clinton administration, and a list of worthy but unrealistically optimistic goals were established. These goals included:

- All children will start school ready to learn (in 2000 only one half of the youth were enrolled in preschool) with many of the programs being poor in quality
- These national goals were never achieved

TABLE 3.1 *(Continued)*

- Even though these goals were never achieved, they put the nation on a course of self-examination, and developing standards of learning that dominated much of the educational literature during the 1990s

As a result content standards were initiated and developed. Many of these early standards were rejected by political leaders.

1990: Americans with Disabilities Act (ADA) (Public Law 101-336)

- Prohibits discrimination against people with disabilities in the private sector
- Protects equal opportunity to employment and public services, accommodations, transportation, and telecommunications
- Defines "disability" to include people with AIDS

1990: Individuals with Disabilities Education Act (IDEA) (Public Law 101-476)

- Renames and replaces P.L. 94-142 (EAHCA)
- Establishes "people first language"
- Extends special education services to include social work, assistive technology, and rehabilitation services
- Extends provisions for due process and confidentiality for students and parents
- Adds two new categories of disability: autism and traumatic brain injury
- Requires states to provide bilingual education programs for students with disabilities
- Requires states to educate students with disabilities for transition to employment and provide transition services
- Requires the development of individualized transition programs for students with disabilities by the time they reach the age of 16

1997: Individuals with Disabilities Education Act (IDEA) (Public Law 105-17)

- Requires that all students with disabilities must continue to receive services, even if they have been expelled from school
- Allows states to extend their use of developmental delay category for students through age 9
- Requires schools to assume greater responsibility for ensuring that students with disabilities have access to the general curriculum
- Allows special education staff working in the mainstream to assist general education students when needed
- Requires a general education teacher to be part of the IEP team
- Requires students with disabilities to take part in statewide and districtwide assessments
- Requires states to offer medication as a voluntary option to parents and educators to resolve differences
- Requires a proactive behavior management plan be included in the students' IEP if a student with disabilities has behavior problems
- Limits the conditions under which attorneys can collect fees under IDEA

2002: No Child Left Behind (NCLB) enacted

- Described by both Democrats and Republications as "the most significant change in federal regulation of public schools in three decades." (Sadker & Zittleman, p. 34)

(Continued)

TABLE 3.1 Educational Milestones That Have Made an Impact on the Education of Students Who Are Deaf and Hard of Hearing (*Continued*)

- NCLB dramatically changed and expanded the federal role in elementary and secondary education policy. The new law represents the consolidation of a reform movement that began in the wake of 1983. (McGuinn, 2006)
- Major provisions of NCLB include:
  1. Annual testing—reading and math assessments are required annually in grades 3 to 8 and once in high school. Each state determines which test is to be used. 2007-08 students also began taking standardized science tests at least once in elementary, middle, and high school
  2. Academic Improvement—states must define academic proficiency for all students and all students must be proficient in reading and math by 2013-2014. States must report Adequate Yearly Progress (AYP) if a school does not meet their AYP for two consecutive years they are labeled as underperforming
  3. Report cards states and school districts must provide the public with report cards of district and school progress
  4. Faculty qualifications—all teachers must be highly qualified—licensed with an academic major in the filed they are teaching
  5. Increased access for Deaf and Hard of Hearing Students (DHHS) to core curricular content due to mandatory testing regulations
  6. DHHS students are held accountable through disaggregated data
  7. Increased attention paid to the creation and implementation of valid accommodations for DHHS
  8. Underscores challenges of tracking progress of DHHS students in district/regional programs and mainstream schools (Cawthon, 2008)

2004: Reauthorization of IDEA—P. L. 108-446, the Individuals with Disabilities Education Improvement Act of 2004. The reauthorization is closely aligned to NCLB and focuses on:

- Academic results
- Early intervention
- Parental choice
- Except for the 1% of students taking alternative assessments, short-term objectives and benchmarks in Individualized Education Programs will be replaced with the NCLB system that measures academic progress toward state standards
- Accountability for academic achievement for children with disabilities must conform to the state systems established under NCLB. (Moores, D., 2005)

2009: Race to The Top Program

- Part the American Recovery and Reinvestment Act of 2009 (P.L. 111-5)
- Awards states grant monies to states that
  1. Create educational environments conducive to innovation
  2. Achieve significant improvement in student academic outcomes
  3. Close achievement gaps
  4. Improve high school graduation rates
  5. Ensure student preparation for success in college and the work force
- Awards funding to states that
  1. Adopt "internationally benchmarked standards" that prepare students for college or the workforce

TABLE 3.1 *(Continued)*

2. Build data systems that more effectively measure student academic achievement
3. Increase teacher and administrative efficacy and establish an equitable distribution of effective school personnel
4. Reverse the decline of the lowest-performing schools

- Provides incentives for states to more effectively track progress of students with special needs, including DHHS
- Provides incentives to states to research and develop effective educational approaches for students with special needs, including DHHS
- Provides states with incentives to increase the number and quality of teachers in hard to staff disciplines, including Deaf Education

Scheetz, N. & Grubbs, S.

What other factors have been instrumental in shaping the lives of individuals who are deaf and hard of hearing? When one takes a historical look at deaf education and the Deaf community, it becomes apparent how residential schools, clubs, and organizations initiated by the Deaf community and fostered primarily through their efforts, have played a significant role in the formation of a Deaf identity. What are some of these organizations? Are they still active today? What role will they play with future generations? The section that follows describes a few of the major organizations that have played, and continue to play, a significant role in the identity and cohesiveness of the Deaf community.

ORGANIZATIONS, CLUBS, AND CULTURAL EVENTS

With shrinking enrollments at schools for the deaf, and technology frequently replacing face-to-face conversations, it is easy to forget that these developments are relatively new and had little, if anything, to do with the lives of previous generations of individuals who were deaf and hard of hearing. Those growing up prior to the 1970s, before the advent of modern technology, relied on schools for the deaf and involvement in clubs and organizations for the Deaf for social networking.

The oldest organization serving the Deaf population is the National Association for the Deaf (NAD; www.nad.org). It developed in the United States when oral language instruction, the Oral Method (teaching individuals who were deaf to speak and instructing them through speech), came to the forefront in the education of deaf children and Deaf teachers and professionals who embraced sign language were being devalued by the educational system. Established in 1880, the NAD's primary mission, since its inception, has been to safeguard the accessibility and civil rights of Americans who are deaf and hard of hearing in a variety of areas, including education, employment, health care, social services, and telecommunications. Today NAD has chapters in 50 states, and although grassroots advocacy remains at the core of this organization, it also provides numerous leadership development opportunities for students who are deaf, including the Junior NAD and the NAD Youth Leadership Camp.

Other organizations that have played an integral role in the development of a Deaf identity have been the National Fraternal Society for the Deaf (NSFD) and the USA Deaf Sports Federation. The NSFD was incorporated in 1907 for the primary purpose of offering insurance policies to persons who were deaf. Its focus has also been to promote the gainful employment and welfare of adult deaf individuals. The USA Deaf Sports Federation (USADSF) is the athletes who are deaf. It was originally established as the American Athletic Association for the Deaf (AASD) in Ohio in 1945, and the change to USADSF (www.usadsf.org) was adopted in 1998. USADSF supports national competitions in both summer and winter sports, including baseball, basketball, bowling, cycling, football, wrestling, cross-country skiing, downhill skiing, ice hockey, snowboarding, and more. It also provides year-round training and competition for developing elite athletes. It assists them in developing physical fitness, sportsmanship, and self-esteem and helps them prepare for the Deaflympics.

One other important organization that merits discussion is the World Federation of the Deaf (WFD). The WFD (www.wfd.org) was established in 1951. It is an international, non-governmental, central organization comprised of national associations of Deaf people. The organization represents approximately 70 million Deaf people in 123 countries worldwide. Its focus remains to improve the status of national sign languages, advocate for better education for Deaf people, improve access to information and services, and improve human rights for Deaf people in developing countries.

The organizations highlighted here have fostered a sense of community and a sense of camaraderie. It is imperative to recognize that Deaf individuals have a long history of bonding together and working for the betterment of the group. Through their shared experiences, their cherished language, and their culture, they have provided support to those who are deaf and those who choose to identify with the Deaf community. (A list of additional organizations is included at the end of this text.)

DIMENSIONS OF DEAFNESS: IDENTITY, ETHNICITY, AND SOCIAL DEVELOPMENT

In the literature, the community of deaf people is frequently referred to as a low-incidence disability group. So stated, this microcosm of society, although small, is representative of the larger hearing community within which it resides. Characterized by individuals with varying degrees of hearing loss, ethnic and family backgrounds, socioeconomic status, and communication preferences, the group represents a diverse segment of society.

Deaf children born to Deaf parents form an early Deaf identity and develop an affiliation with the Deaf community, advocating for the social, linguistic, and cultural attributes of what it means to be Deaf. For others, this identity will be a slow process, developing as the child matures from childhood into adulthood. Among those who are deaf, some will continue to experience life while maintaining a hearing identity and placing a high premium on spoken language, communication, and socialization within the larger hearing community. Still others are beginning to develop a bicultural identity, finding that they are able to navigate between the Deaf and hearing communities with relative ease. The last 30 years have seen an abundance of articles as researchers have begun, and continue, to deconstruct the medical model of deafness as a disability and replace it with a social model of a community characterized by unique and identifiable features (Padden & Humphries, 1989). Further attention is being given to the range of diversity that is evident within the population comprised of deaf individuals.

With the majority of students who are deaf being educated in the mainstream, and the use of cochlear implants increasing, how will this impact and affect their sense of identity as well as their psychological and social development? As they interact with their hearing peers, what types of social relationships will be formed? Will the hearing status of the child determine the quality of these relationships? Will students educated in the mainstream develop a bicultural identity and become bilingual? Will the levels of educational achievement increase in these settings?

These and other questions are pertinent to the field today. As parents, Deaf and hearing professionals, and those involved in daily interactions with children who are deaf continue to raise expectations for them, the field will continue to examine and evaluate future directions to meet these expectations. What can educators do to promote successful adults who are deaf? What can be done to ensure that children who are deaf will view the fact that they are deaf as a positive attribute, thus acknowledging it in the same way they accept the other positive characteristics that shape their unique identities? How can we communicate these concepts to young children who are deaf or hard of hearing?

Communication lies at the heart of our existence; it provides an avenue for sharing information while allowing us to connect with the world around us. It is fundamental to our overall development; the intricacies of how our minds evolve, mature, and flourish; and how the culture we are raised in becomes embodied in the identities of us all. From a very young age, children who are deaf as well as children who can hear begin to form relationships with others. However, unlike their hearing counterparts, many of those who are deaf are faced with socialization challenges that are unique to this population. Frequently these challenges are imposed by barriers to communication.

It is well established that the majority of children who are deaf or severely hard of hearing are born into hearing families. Unlike deaf children born to Deaf parents, who are exposed to ASL early in life, these children enter the world with a preestablished barrier that prevents them from sharing a common language with their parents, neighbors, or community (Mitchell & Karchmer, 2004). As a result, the ease in spoken exchanges is lost as parents try to convey information to their offspring. Unprepared to deal with a diagnosis of hearing loss, communication exchanges may be reduced if not altogether eliminated during the critical, formative years. Even in families that opt for some form of sign communication early in life, as their child enters school they may find they struggle with keeping abreast of their child's language development. As their child's language continues to grow, parents may sense that they are falling farther behind in their mastery of the syntax of the language. Consequently, they find they are unable to provide an adequate role model for their child who is deaf.

Recognizing the importance communication plays in human growth and development, the American Deaf community has long supported the need for children who are deaf to have increased access to, and contact with, Deaf adults who are seen as both skilled communication partners and positive role models. Access to Deaf adults in the context of the home and later in the school is thought to combat the isolation often felt by the student who is deaf and attends traditional public schools. Furthermore, these Deaf role models can also provide a positive example for all students who are deaf regardless of their school placement (Wilkens & Hehir, 2008).

One of the key functions of communication is to serve as a mechanism in the formation of one's identity. How we see ourselves in respect to others, and how others react to us, are critical factors throughout the developmental process. We know that the majority of students who are deaf and hard of hearing are being educated in the mainstream today. A number of them, especially those enrolled in programs located in rural areas, are discovering they are the only student who is deaf in their class and, oftentimes, the only student who is deaf or hard of hearing in their school. Members of the Deaf community have grave concerns about these enrollment trends. Some Deaf community members fear that these children who are deaf will be socially isolated and educated in a completely hearing-oriented world. An additional concern is that the child will accept "the hearing world's judgment and condemnation of the Deaf as medical anomalies—rather than people—who are lacking or incomplete" (Wilkens & Hehir, 2008).

Mainstream environments provide students, both hearing and deaf, with a wide array of academic offerings and extracurricular activities that are sometimes not available at small residential or day schools. Furthermore, there is evidence of improvement in academic achievement for many students educated in mainstream schools (Kluwin & Moores, 1985; Stinson & Antia, 1999). However, concern remains that students who are deaf who receive all their education in this environment are showing signs of social isolation when compared with their peers attending residential schools (Stinson & Antia, 1999; Vostanis, Hayes, DuFeu, & Warren, 1997).

Several studies have focused on social relationships, coping skills, and deaf students' social experiences in mainstream settings. These findings suggest that the experiences these children have can vary widely depending on the characteristics of the school setting and peer community (Christiansen & Lee, 2002; Martin & Bat-Chava, 2003). When barriers exist, thus preventing children who are deaf from establishing relationships with children who can hear, it is primarily attributable to communication difficulties (Martin & Bat-Chava). This is due, in some measure, to unclear speech on the part of the child who is deaf and impatience on the part of the child who can hear (Foster, 1998). Further problems can arise if students who are deaf lack the social skills appropriate for peer interactions.

A study conducted by Cappelli, Daniels, Durieux-Smith, McGrath, and Neuss (1995) assessing the social status of students in a mainstream school reported that 39% of students who were deaf felt that they were rejected by their peers compared with 13% of hearing students feeling that they were rejected. However, Bat-Chava & Deignan (2001) found that children with cochlear implants were able to form close and satisfying relationships with hearing children in spite of the communication challenges.

In a more recent study, Martin & Bat-Chava (2003) examined coping strategies of children who were deaf in mainstream settings. Their findings indicate that the children participating in their study had "few difficulties establishing relationships with their hearing peers, regardless of the severity of their hearing loss or amplification device (cochlear implant or hearing aids)" (Martin & Bat-Chava, 2003, p. 518). They further report that the participants all had good oral communication skills, making social interactions with hearing children easier. When comparing younger children with older children, the study supported previous findings indicating that older children have better peer relationships than younger ones. The authors attribute this to the development of better communication skills that have improved over time.

Additional research conducted by Wald and Knutson (2000) examined the Deaf cultural identity of adolescents with and without cochlear implants. Findings from their study reveal that students who are deaf place an extremely high value on bicultural identities. Furthermore, students surveyed in this study indicated that they would always be deaf but wanted access to both the hearing and Deaf worlds as much as possible. These studies and others continue to highlight the need for further research into the effects mainstreaming is having on the formation of identity and social development of children who are deaf. Although placing children who are deaf in mainstream schools increases opportunities for contact between students who can hear as well as those who are deaf, questions continue to be raised as to the quality of the relationships that are formed between these two groups of students (McIntosh, 2000).

Summary

This chapter has explored some of the changes that have impacted the lives of individuals who are deaf throughout the past 50 years. The etiology of deafness continues to change and is mirrored by the tapestry of diversity that is evident in the population. Although legislation has provided equal access for individuals who are deaf and hard of hearing, it has also mandated where students will receive their education and what they should be able to achieve. Even though positive outcomes can be noted in the educational achievement levels of children who are deaf, the fabric of the Deaf community is changing threads and patterns due to the lack of unity once fostered and developed in residential school settings.

Technology—in terms of cochlear implants, digital hearing aids, and handheld devices—has significantly impacted the way deaf individuals communicate with each other, as well as how they conduct their daily lives. Connecting individuals who are deaf globally has provided opportunities for those in rural areas to form connections with people who are deaf residing in distant locations. In a broader sense, computer technology has begun to level the playing field, providing individuals who are deaf and hearing alike with access to the information superhighway.

All these factors have played, and will continue to play, a vital role in the way deaf individuals interact with society and thus establish a sense of identity and belonging. Furthermore, all these factors are instrumental in determining who we are, what we believe, what we like, and how we view ourselves and others. How we reflect on these interactions is ongoing and impacts our development throughout the course of our lives. From the time we are born we are influenced by those who raise us. Family diversity and dynamics, modes of communication, use of technology, educational setting, and social and personal experiences all affect the development of one's sense of being and belonging.

As increasing numbers of children who are deaf interface with children who can hear on a daily basis, they will be challenged to communicate, socialize, and compete with those who can hear. By continuing to educate the majority of students who are deaf in general education classrooms, daily exposure to ASL by Deaf professionals will be lost, and the unity that was once fostered in schools for the deaf will be changed. What effect will all this have on future generations of individuals who are deaf?

The remaining chapters in this book will focus on several of the issues that have been briefly discussed in these pages. The intent is to provide the reader with a broad overview of the various topics that continue to be of concern to individuals who are deaf, as well as their hearing counterparts, who have a vested interest in this dynamic and diverse population.

4

The Science of Hearing and Hearing Loss

The Acoustics of Speech and the Transmission of Sound

The hearing population is exposed daily to a cacophony of sounds permeating the environment, consciously or unconsciously, with an abundance of information. Although sirens, blaring horns, howling winds, and the sound of alarms warn of impending danger, the sound of the ocean, raindrops hitting a tin roof, and a soft breeze blowing through the pines can be soothing at the end of a stressful day. Sounds alert listeners to the events occurring in their immediate surroundings while also providing them with a channel whereby spoken communication can be exchanged. This link with others provides an avenue for knowledge to be acquired, language to be developed, and feelings to be expressed. Furthermore, this mecca of sound generates a wealth of information and is instrumental in contributing, both directly and indirectly, to the growth and development of the individual.

Before embarking on a discussion of how sound impacts human growth and development, it is beneficial to understand how sound is produced and received. With this foundation we can examine how the hearing mechanism functions, how hearing tests are administered, and how hearing loss is identified. This information provides the foundation for understanding the various degrees and types of hearing loss as well as the terminology associated with the amount of loss one experiences.

THE NATURE OF SOUND

Sound originates when a force initiates vibrations in the air, causing a sound wave to travel through a medium. As the sound wave travels, it may ultimately be received by the hearing mechanism and then transmitted to the brain where it can be interpreted accurately. This process involves four components: a vacillation of some type, a force to generate vibrations, a medium through which sound waves are transported, and a hearing mechanism that has the ability to receive and unerringly perceive the sensation.

Sound waves are comprised of two characteristic phases or density levels: compression and rarefaction. These two phases work in tandem with each other. Think of striking a tuning fork. Once the tuning fork begins to vibrate, sound waves travel outward, the molecules of the medium are forced together, and compression occurs. Then, as the molecules attempt to separate

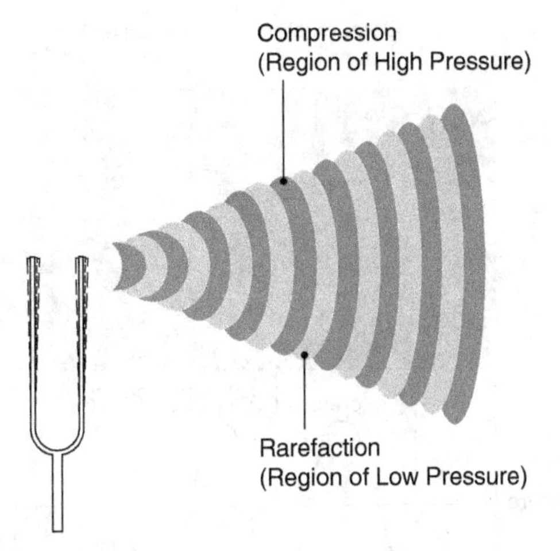

FIGURE 4.1 The wave nature of sound. When objects are made to vibrate they disturb the surrounding air in wavelike fashion, much like a water wave is produced when you toss a stone into a pond. However, Unlike the up-and-down motion of a water wave, a sound wave is a high-pressure (rarefaction) alteration, as illustrated in the sound wave produced by a tuning fork.

Source: Courtesy of Marie A. Scheetz.

from each other, thus regaining their original density level, the rarefaction phase ensues. This process continues as sound-producing sources continue to vibrate, thus creating an ongoing oscillation of alternating compression and rarefaction. This reciprocal movement characterizes the sound wave, originating from the sound source and radiating outward at a constant velocity. This process is illustrated in Figure 4.1.

The transmission of sound can further be illustrated visually by imagining a group of people lined up, waiting to buy their tickets to enter the theatre. The person at the end of the line loses her balance and accidentally pushes the man ahead of her. He, in turn, loses his balance and pushes the man in front of him and so forth, creating a chain reaction. The woman who initially lost her balance eventually regains it and has ceased to make contact with the man in front of her. This is true of all the people in the line. Now, if the same woman continues to lose her balance and the process continually repeats itself, a wave of compression will occur every time someone is pushed, and a wave of rarefaction will take place every time the individuals regain their balance.

Sound is transmitted through the air in basically the same way. The source of the sound causes the air molecules to push against each other, creating compression, at which point they bounce back to their original state of rarefaction, only to be pushed again. This is illustrated in Figure 4.2.

As this process is consistently repeated, sound waves are produced. In essence, sound waves are vibrations in the air and can be measured in units that describe the intensity and frequency of the vibration. Intensity (loudness) is measured by examining the height of the peaks, and frequency (pitch) is measured by examining the distance between adjacent peaks. A complete succession of one compression and rarefaction constitutes a cycle. Therefore, the frequency of a sound wave can be determined by measuring the number of cycles that occur in a second's time. Figure 4.3 illustrates the frequency and amplitude of sound waves.

There is a positive relationship between the physical property of intensity and its psychological correlate that we know as loudness; it is due to the fact that as the intensity of a sound is

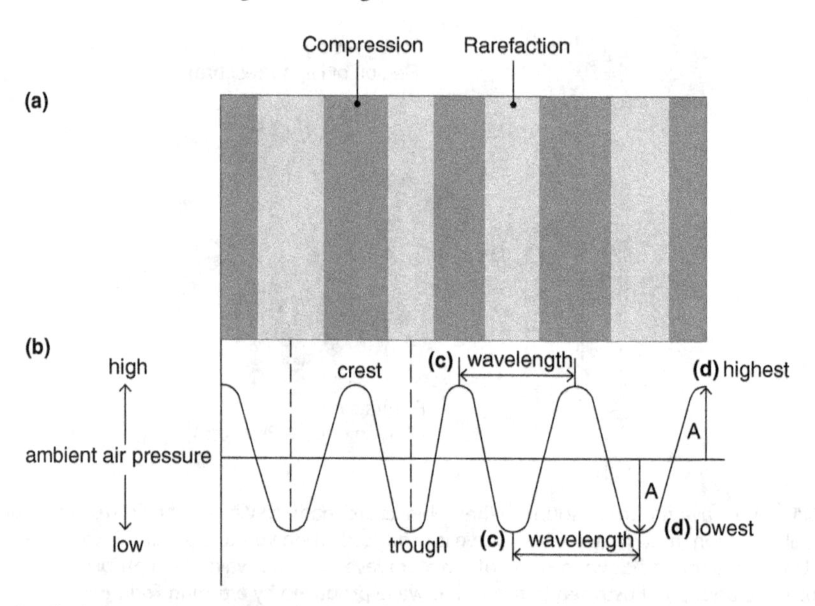

FIGURE 4.2 The compression and rarefaction of a sound wave. The compressions and rarefactions of a sound wave depicted in (a) correspond to the crest and trough, respectively, of a water wave in (b). The peak (or trough to trough) distance shown in (c) is the wavelength of the wave. The highest (or lowest) pressure variation from the ambient (undisturbed) air pressure shown in (d) is the amplitude of the wave.

Source: Courtesy of Marie A. Scheetz.

increased we perceive the sound as becoming louder. Although there are special linear scales for rating loudness, known as SONES, these scales are impractical for measuring what the human ear can hear (Anderson & Shames, 2006). Instead, the intensity or loudness of a sound is measured in decibels (dB), named in honor of Alexander Graham Bell. Zero dB represents the smallest sound a person with normal hearing can perceive. As sounds become louder the number represented in dB becomes larger. The dB scale, which is logarithmic rather than linear, is based on ratios with each 10 dB increment representing a tenfold increase in intensity. Therefore, a 20 dB sound is 100 times more intense than a 10 dB sound, and a 30 dB sound is 1,000 times more intense than a sound at 10 dB (Schirmer, 2001, p. 3). For example, a low whisper produced approximately 5 feet away from a listener occurs at about 10 dB, whereas a running automobile registers at approximately 65 dB. Although conversational speech from a distance of 10 to 20 feet falls within the range of 20 to 55 dB, a sound produced at 125 dB or louder causes pain to the average person (Heward, 2003).

Frequency, like intensity, is a physical property with its perceptual correlate being pitch. As such, frequency has a relationship to pitch in much the same way that intensity is related to loudness (Anderson & Shames, 2006, p. 509). Frequency of a sound is measured in hertz (Hz), or the number of cycles per second, with 1 Hz equaling 1 cycle per second. Longer wavelengths denote low-frequency sounds while shorter wavelengths indicate high-frequency sounds.

Just as there are scales to measure loudness, pitch scales have been developed to illustrate the subjective highness (treble) and lowness (bass) of sounds. When a sound consists of only one frequency, it is referred to as being a pure tone. Examples of pure tones are whistles, tuning

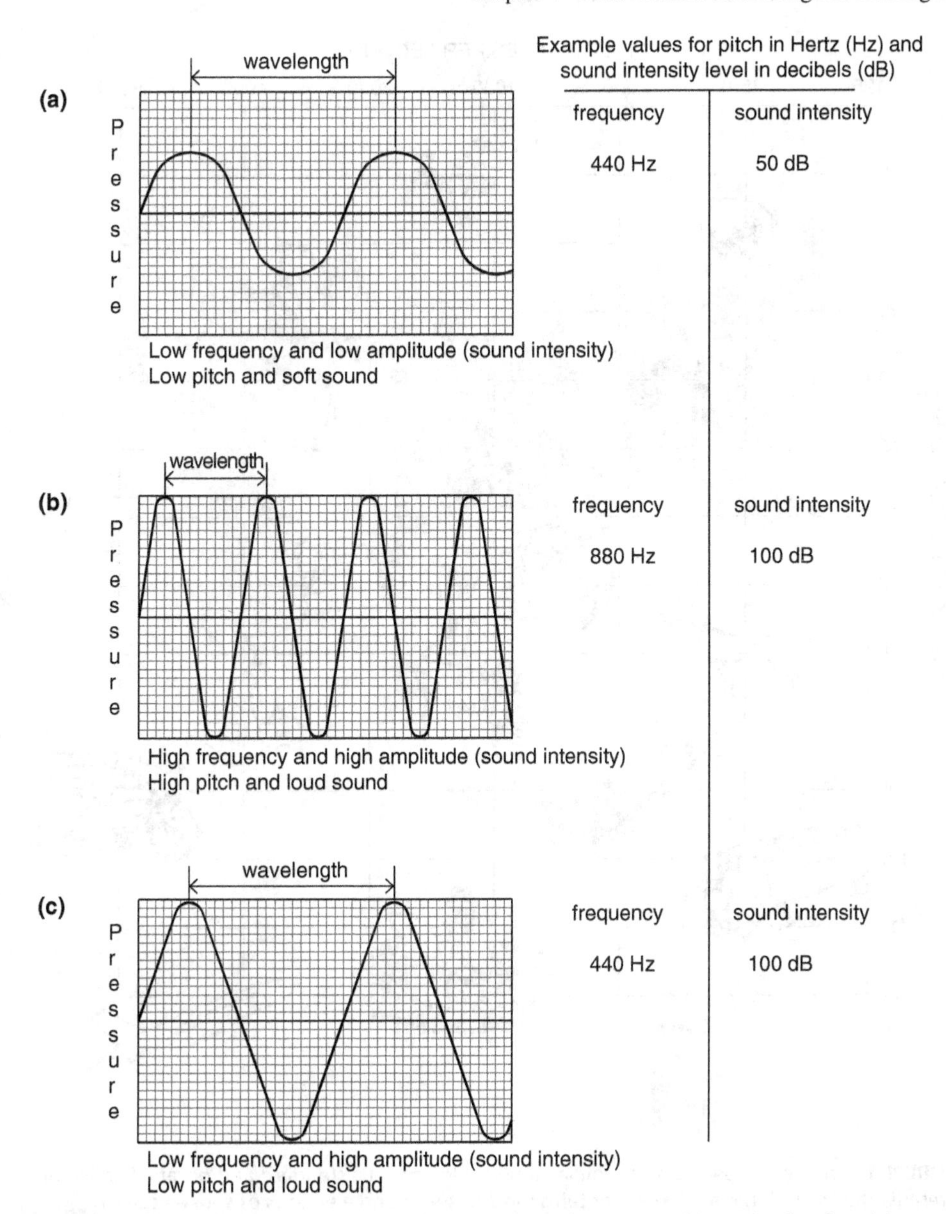

FIGURE 4.3 Differences between frequency/pitch and amplitude/sound intensity (loudness) in sound waves. First, note that a longer wavelength of sound denotes a lower frequency and a shorter wavelength a higher frequency. (a) A sound wave of low frequency and pitch (e.g., 440 Hz) and low amplitude and sound intensity (e.g., 50 dB) compared to the sound wave in (b) in which the frequency and amplitude are doubled (880 Hz and 100 dB, respectively). Compare the wavelengths and peak heights in (a) and (b). In (c) the frequency is the same as (a) (compare wavelengths) and the amplitude is the same as in (b) (compare peak heights). In this manner, one could imagine a sound wave of high frequency and low amplitude (high pitch, soft sound). (For more information on sound measurements in Hertz (Hz) and decibels (dB), see the section pertaining to audiological evaluation.)

Source: Courtesy of Marie A. Scheetz.

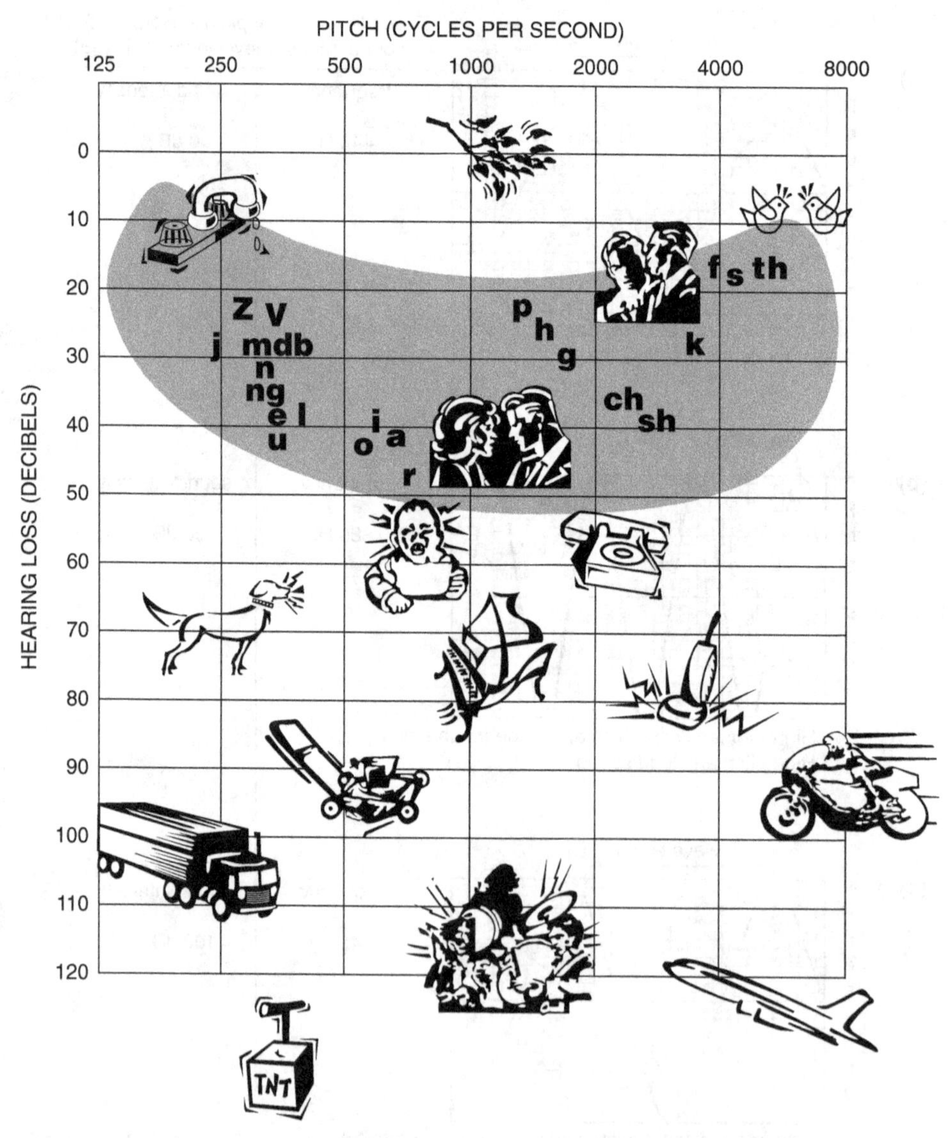

FIGURE 4.4 Frequency spectrum of familiar sounds plotted on a standard audiogram. Shaded area represents the "speech banana" that contains most of the sound elements of spoken speech.

forks, and electronic devices. However, speech and the majority of environmental sounds consist of complex tones, encompassing a wide range of frequencies.

Human hearing falls within the range of approximately 20 to 20,000 Hz. However, within this range, the range considered most important is the one required for hearing spoken language. Although most speech sounds occur between 500 and 2,000 Hz, some speech sounds occur above or below that range. According to Northern and Downs (1991) the /s/ phoneme, as in the word *sit*, is a high-frequency sound typically produced between 4,000 and 8,000 Hz. Figure 4.4 illustrates the frequency range of familiar sounds.

ACOUSTICS OF SPEECH

Speech sounds (vowels and consonants) are transmitted through the air as complex waves that are constantly changing. Although vowels tend to repeat their waveforms over time, the manner in which they are produced is influenced, in part, by the consonants that surround them. Consonants comprise the majority of sounds in the speech spectrum. Each of the consonants varies to some degree in its production (and perception), depending on its position within the word; whether or not it is an initial, medial or ending sound; and the influence of the other phonemes contained within the word. For example, the phoneme /t/ is different in words like *top, hit, letter,* and *mast*. Each of these variations is referred to as an allophone (Anderson & Shames, 2006, p. 510).

Although vowel sounds produce most of the intensity of speech, consonants contribute to most of its intelligibility. Therefore, when an individual with normal hearing within the low-frequency range experiences a high-frequency loss, he or she can frequently hear the vowel sounds but miss many of the consonants. When this occurs the person often complains of being able to hear the sounds but unable to understand the words.

In addition to being able to comprehend both vowel and consonant sounds, the listener attends to the prosody of the message. Prosody includes the rhythm, tempo, quality, intonation, pitch, loudness, stress, and duration of the speech sounds. Those who experience a hearing loss may find that they are unable to comprehend the message not only because they cannot understand the words (vowels and consonants) but because they are unable to decipher the prosodic elements of speech.

THE HEARING MECHANISM

The first part of this chapter provided a brief synopsis of the nature of sound, how it is produced, and the elements of speech the listener is unconsciously or sometimes consciously attending to when engaging in a conversation or listening to a speaker. Once the sounds are received by the listener, how are they received and processed by the auditory system? How is the ear structured, and how does it transmit sound to the brain where sound is eventually deciphered and comprehended? What happens if one of the parts of the ear does not function properly? Furthermore, what additional factors contribute to an individual's ability to receive warning sounds, ideas, information, and, most important, spoken communication?

STRUCTURE AND FUNCTION OF THE EAR

The ear is usually described in terms of three distinct divisions: the outer, middle, and inner ear. Each of these parts serves an integral function, from gathering sound waves from the environment, to converting them into mechanical energy, and to transporting them to the brain, where they are translated into meaningful information. Figure 4.5 provides an illustration of the structure of the auditory apparatus.

The Outer Ear

The external or outer portion of the ear is composed of the auricle, or pinna, and the external auditory meatus, or ear canal. The auricle is the visible flaplike portion of the hearing mechanism and is connected to the side of the head. Its primary function is to receive sound waves and direct them into the external auditory meatus. The canal between the pinna and the tympanic membrane is referred to as the external ear canal.

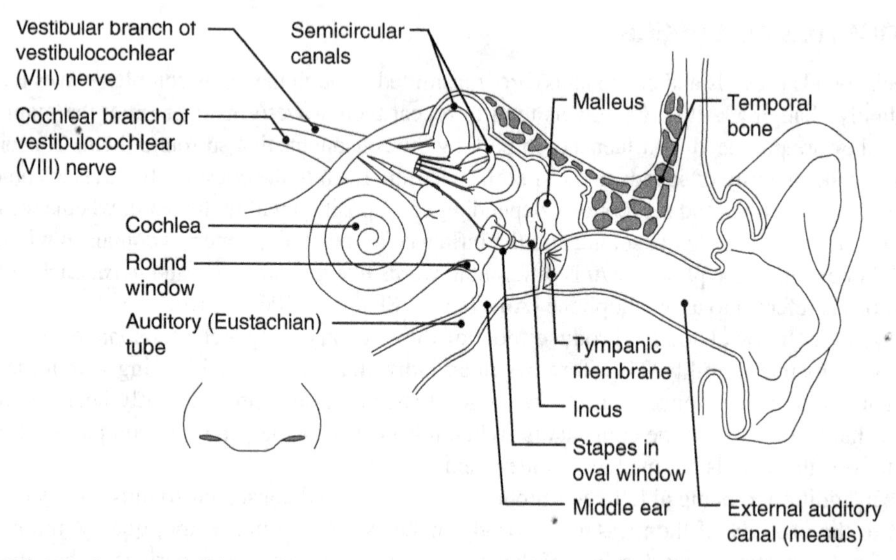

FIGURE 4.5 Structure of the auditory apparatus: the left ear seen through the left side of the skull. The three divisions of the ear—external, middle, and internal—are portrayed.

Source: Courtesy of Marie A. Scheetz.

The pinna is created by pieces of cartilage in the form of ridges and decompressions. Averaging about 3.5 inches in height and approximately 1.5 inches wide, each individual's auricle is unique in the way that it is formed. Its purpose is to collect sound while enhancing the sound pressure of certain frequencies. In addition to increasing some high-frequency sounds, it is also useful in assisting the listener in identifying the sources of high-frequency sounds that are located overhead, such as those produced by flying insects (Plante & Beeson, 2008).

The external ear canal is cylindrical in shape, approximately 1 inch long, and about 0.4 inch in diameter. It enters the skull at a slight angle and contains hair follicles and wax-producing glands. The waxy substance, cerumen, serves to protect the tympanic membrane from foreign substances. The outer part of the canal is larger at the auricular orifice and is formed with cartilage. As the canal approaches the tympanic membrane (eardrum), the inner part of the canal becomes smaller and is framed by hard bone. Thus, through the length and shape of the ear canal, sound pressure is enhanced. Functioning together with the pinna, the ear canal can enhance sounds that are produced in the mid- and high-frequency region of the sound spectrum.

The Middle Ear

The tympanic membrane, or eardrum, stretched across the opening of the external canal, forms the external boundary of the middle ear. Almost all the sound energy entering the canal pushes on the eardrum. Thin and flexible by design, the eardrum's circular shape measures about 1 cm in diameter, is a little less than ½ inch thick, and is strong enough to withstand changes in pressure when humans dive 100 or more feet below the surface of the ocean (Plante & Beeson, 2008, p. 248).

The tympanic cavity is irregularly shaped, has a vertical dimension of approximately 15 mm, and varies in width from 2 mm to 4 mm. Located within the cavity are several moving parts and the Eustachian tube, a ventilating tube that connects the cavity to the pharynx, which work together to boost the pressure created by the sound energy that arrives at the tympanic membrane. This cavity is housed within the petrous portion of the temporal bone and can be viewed in two sections. The topmost portion extends upward beyond the superior border of the tympanic membrane and is referred to as the attic or the epitympanic recess. Because the tympanic antrum communicates with the mastoid air cells, the two portions have indirect communication. The portion of the cavity that lies medially to the tympanic membrane is referred to as the tympanic cavity proper; it is formed of bone covered by thin mucosa similar to the lining of the nasal cavities.

Housed within the middle ear cavity between the tympanic membrane and the oval window, marking the entrance to the inner ear, is the ossicular chain. Comprised of the three tiniest bones in the body—the malleus (hammer), incus (anvil), and stapes (stirrup)—the ossicles span the entire middle ear cavity. The malleus, the largest of the bones, is about 9 mm long, and its long arm is attached on one side to the middle, connective tissue fibers of the tympanic membrane. Its other side connects to the incus. The incus is the second ossicle and is about 7 mm in size. The head of the incus and head of the malleus are covered by tissue that holds them together so they move together. The third ossicle is the stapes. Resembling the bottom of a stirrup, the footplate of the stapes is oval and is about 3 mm in length and 1 mm in width (Plante & Beeson, 2008, p. 248). The footplate is inserted against the oval window. The ossicular chain appears to serve two main purposes: first, to supply a vehicle for transporting sound vibrations to the inner ear fluids and, second, to provide a buffer to protect the inner ear from excessively strong vibrations.

Within the middle ear the ossicles are attached to two small muscles: the tensor tympani and the stapedius; they are the smallest striated muscles in the body. The tensor tympani muscle pulls the malleus inward toward the center of the head. The muscle is named for its function, as it tenses or stiffens the tympanum or eardrum. It contracts when we chew, swallow, and yawn, and it is responsive to tactile stimulation of the skin of the face. When the second muscle, the stapedius, contracts, it pulls the stapes outward. In essence, these muscles serve a dual purpose. First, they enhance the movement of the tympanic membrane and the ossicular chain when the signal is weak; second, they enable us to hear important sounds, such as speech, in noisy situations. Traditionally it was thought that these muscles were designed to inhibit the movement within the middle ear when intense stimulation was received, such as the sound of jet engines, loud thunder, or intense industrial noises. Although they may help protect the ear from these intense sounds, their primary role is to work together with the ossicular chain to supply a vehicle for transporting sound vibrations to the inner ear.

The Eustachian tube, located in the middle ear, provides a secondary safety device that-serves as an air pressure equalizer and provides a means of ventilating this cavity. The Eustachian tube also connects the air-filled middle ear with the mouth cavity. When changes in air pressure occur, the Eustachian tube expands, thus permitting the middle ear to compensate for changes in outside air pressure.

The round window and the oval window mark the boundary between the middle ear and the beginning of the inner ear. Both of these windows serve an integral function in the transmission of sound from the environment as it travels on its path to the auditory center housed in the brain. A schematic diagram of the middle ear can be viewed in Figure 4.6.

The Inner Ear

The inner ear serves a very important role in the hearing process. As it converts energy into a code that can be interpreted by the brain, it functions in much the same way as the retina of the

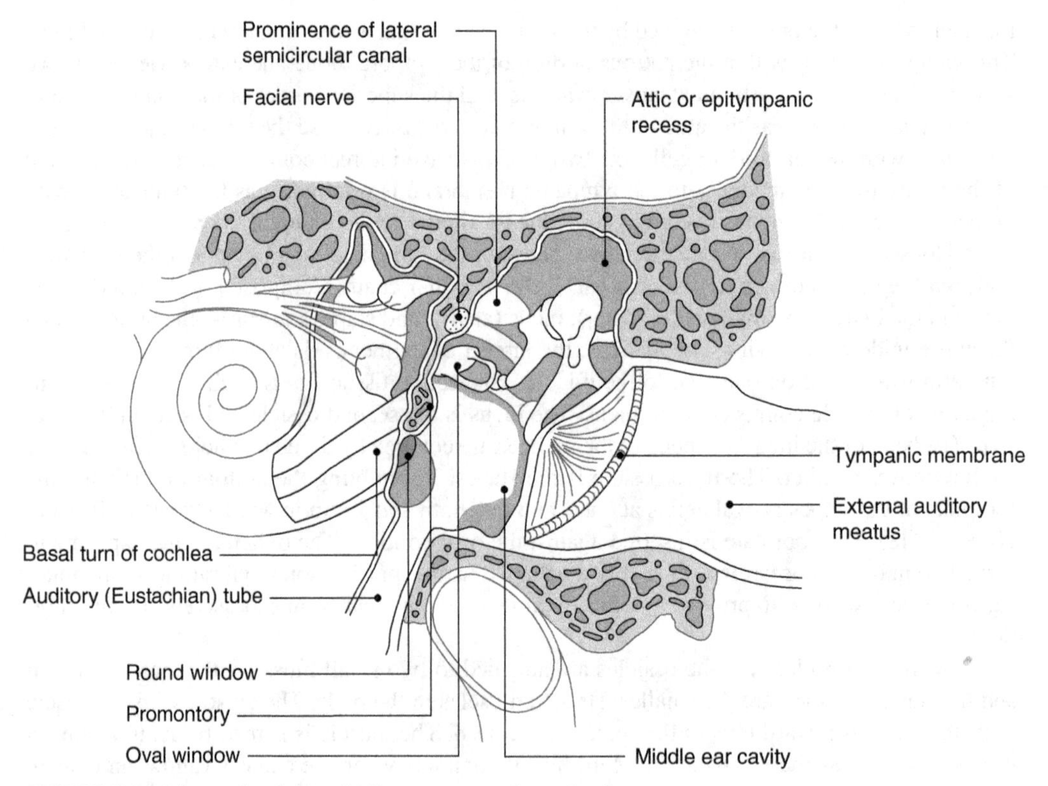

FIGURE 4.6 Schematic of the middle ear as seen from the front.

Source: Courtesy of Marie A. Scheetz.

eye, the taste buds, and the olfactory receptors of the nose. Within the ear, the process of conversion is called transduction. The inner ear is comprised of three separate transduction systems: (a) the vestibule, (b) the semicircular canals, and (c) the cochlea. Because of its appearance, the inner ear is frequently referred to as a labyrinth due to its resemblance to a winding and twisting cave. It can be divided into two cavity systems. The vestibular portion houses the sensory organ required for establishing one's balance and equilibrium. The cochlear portion provides the framework for the essential organ of hearing. The cochlear portion also functions as a transducer, which converts the mechanical energy created by the middle ear into an electrochemical signal, which can then be sent to the brain for processing. The two organs of the inner ear share the same bony labyrinth and the same fluid system. Figure 4.7 provides a detailed view of the inner ear.

The entire outer shell of the inner ear is referred to as the bony labyrinth, and the inner membranous portion is called the membranous labyrinth. The entire inner ear is filled with fluid. The membranous labyrinth is protected from the bony labyrinth by a fluid, perilymph, which is actually spinal fluid supplied from the ventricles of the brain. Endolymph, which is similar to perilymph but very viscous and somewhat different in chemical composition, is the fluid that is found within the membranous labyrinth and is entirely separate from the perilymphatic system.

The vestibular portion of the inner ear that is responsible for equilibrium is often referred to as the vestibular apparatus. Within this vestibule lie the utricle and the saccule, both of which

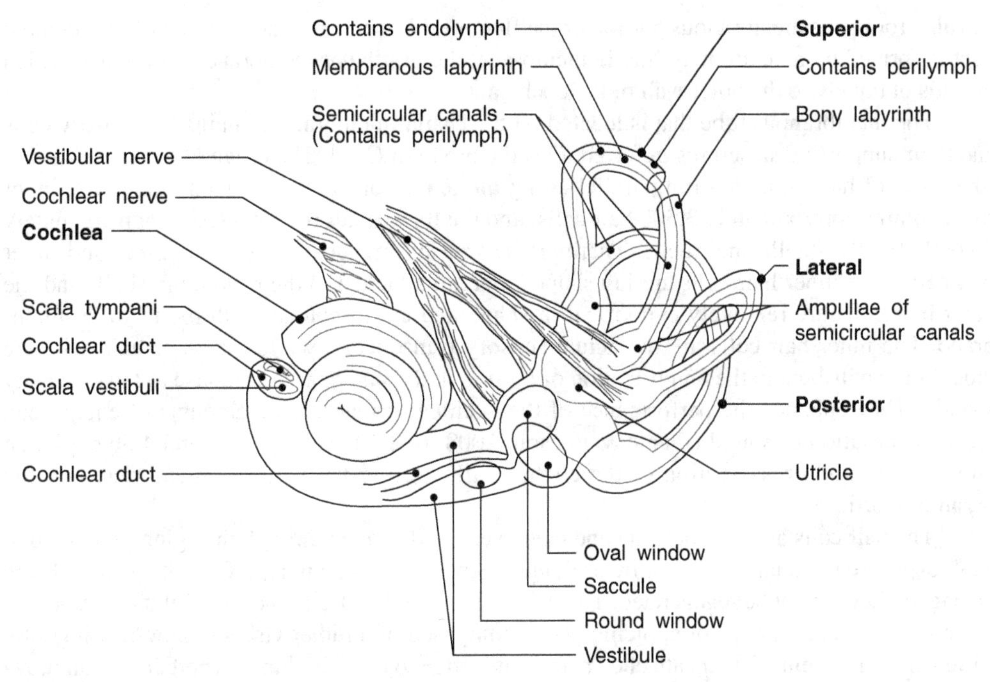

FIGURE 4.7 Details of the inner ear.

Source: Courtesy of Marie A. Scheetz.

function as sensors for the pull of gravity and acceleration. The central portion of the vestibule communicates with three semicicircular canals. The semicircular canal systems provide us with information about head position and help us to maintain a fix on visual targets when we are moving. This bony structure also provides for the continuation of the cochlea, the snail-like shell within the inner ear that contains the transducers for hearing.

The three semicircular canals, the anterior and posterior vertical canals, and the horizontal or lateral canal open into the vestibule through five orifices located at right angles to each other and forming the sense organ for turning in space. The cochlea, which is a continuation of the vestibule, consists of a base followed by 2¾ turns. The canal supports approximately 12,000 hair cells and is approximately 36 mm long, ending blindly at the apex; its basal end is nearest to the middle ear, and the apical end is the farthest from it.

The canal is partly divided into two galleries, or scalae—the upper portion is the scala vestibule and the lower portion is the scala tympani. The two chambers are separated by a spiral shelf of bone, the osseous spiral lamina. The osseous spiral lamina consists of two layers of bone, each of which is continuous with structures that form the cochlear duct of the membranous labyrinth. The division of these two galleries is completed by a fibrous flexible membrane: the basilar membrane that stretches across from the lower edge of the bony shelf to the spiral ligament that attaches it to the outer wall.

The shape of the basilar membrane influences how sound energy is analyzed by the cochlea. The membrane is relatively narrow at the base, the end near the stapes. It is about ten times wider at the apex. The basilar membrane and the shelf both terminate approximately 2 mm short of the end of the gallery. Thus, the basilar membrane completes the roof of the scali tympani and also forms the membranous portion of the floor of the cochlear duct. The roof of the cochlear duct is formed by an extremely fragile membrane, the vestibular membrane of Reissner, which extends obliquely to the outer wall of the cochlea.

The membranous tube that is located on the basilar membrane contains the sensory cells and their supporting structures, referred to as the organ of Corti. The organ of Corti consists of four rows of hair cells that run parallel along the length of the basilar membrane. The inner row contains approximately 3,500 hair cells, and the three outer rows consist of approximately 20,000 slightly smaller hair cells. There are several differences between the inner and outer hair cells. The inner hair cells are jug shaped and are attached to the rigid bony shelf, and the outer hair cells are relatively cylindrical in shape and are in contact with the tectorial membrane. The inner hair cells are the actual sensory transducers, while the outer hair cells are thought to contribute to the amplification of motion in the inner ear in response to low-intensity sounds. They enhance the performance of the cochlea so that minute amounts of energy can create a sensation of sound (Plante & Beeson, 2008, p. 257). Figures 4.8a and 4.8b depict an enlargement and cross-section of the cochlea, illustrating the tectorial membrane and the organ of Corti.

The hair cells are very delicate and can be easily damaged through the aging process, disease, exposure to certain drugs, or by prolonged exposure to loud noises. Once the hair cells are damaged, they cannot be regenerated. The hair cells are embedded in the tectorial membrane that extends over them. The tectorial membrane is composed of a rather viscous, slow-flowing jelly stiffened by a system of fibers attached at the outer edge to the solid limbus (border); it can move up and down in a somewhat stiff fashion. The tectorial membrane also attaches itself loosely to

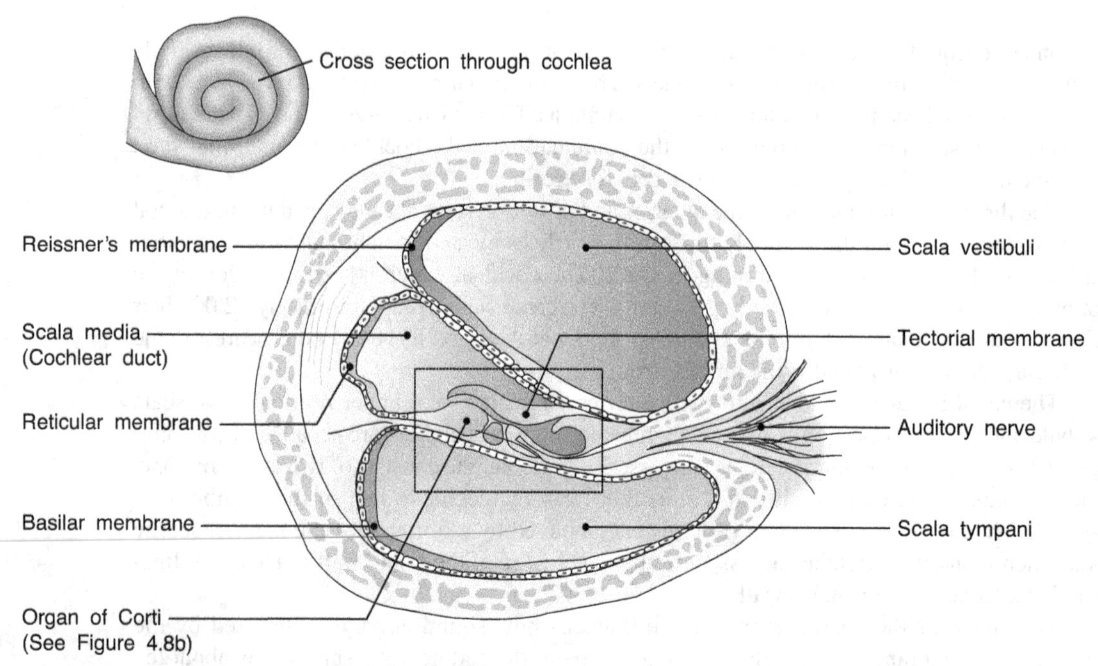

FIGURE 4.8a A cross-section through the cochlea.

Source: Courtesy of Marie A. Scheetz.

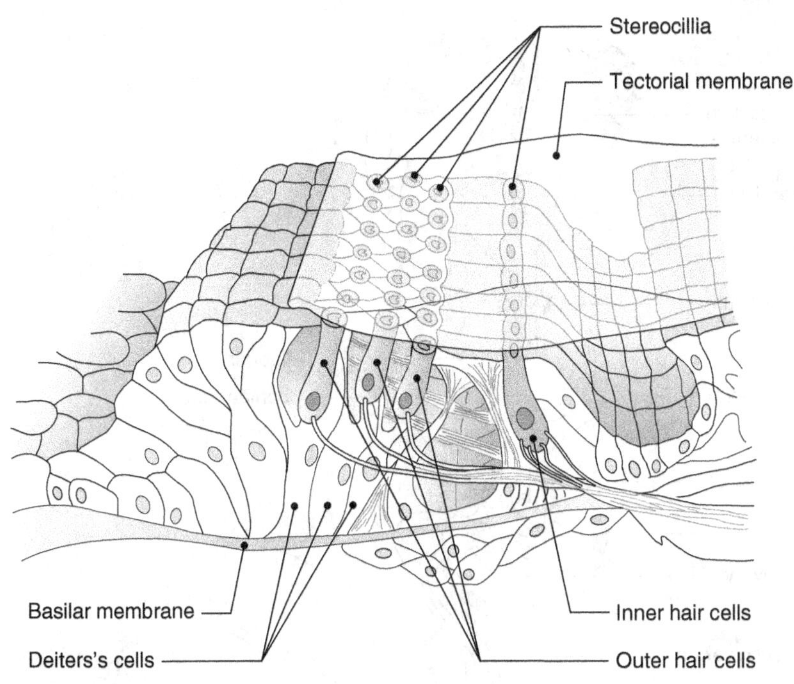

FIGURE 4.8b Organ of Corti.

Source: Courtesy of Marie A. Scheetz.

the organ of Corti before attaching again more firmly to the limbus. The organ of Corti and the tectorial membrane slide past each other slightly as they move up and down together. This movement bends the hair cells, setting off nerve impulses in the nerve fibers.

The hair cells housed in the central core of the cochlea unite with the nerve fibers to form the auditory nerve, the acoustic branch of the eighth cranial nerve (VIII). This auditory nerve passes through a channel in the temporal bone and sends impulses to the auditory center of the cerebral cortex located in the temporal lobes of the brain. The auditory pathway is illustrated in Figure 4.9.

AUDITORY CONNECTIONS IN THE BRAIN

The auditory center for hearing is housed in the brain, not in the ears. Each ear communicates with the central nervous system through ascending and descending connections. The central nervous system is organized so that information about individual tones projects to specific places in the brain. As auditory stimuli are received from the right and left ears, the input is mixed together in the brain stem. This allows the listener to identify, as well as detect, the location of incoming sounds.

THE PHYSIOLOGY OF HEARING

Sound is transmitted to the human ear via air and bone conduction. However, the majority of the sounds we attend to are airborne since the mechanism of air conduction is more sensitive than the mechanism of bone conduction. Sound waves traveling through the air are received by the pinna

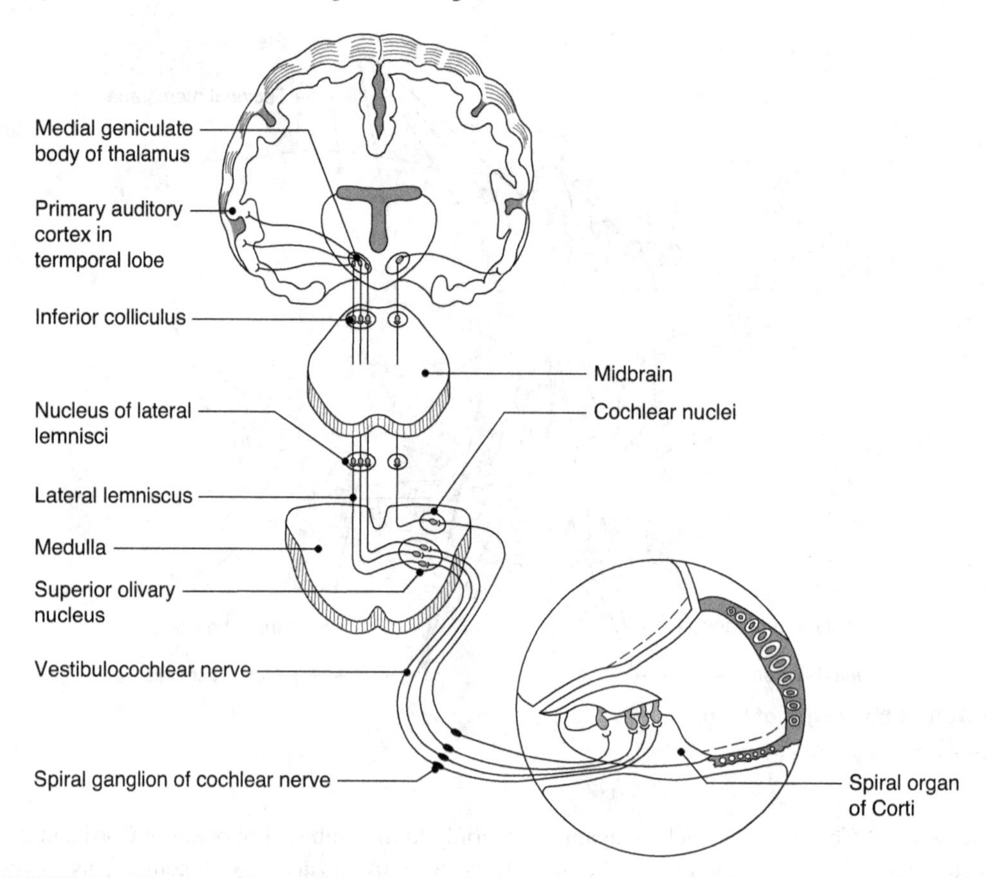

FIGURE 4.9 Diagram of the auditory pathway from the organ of Corti to the brain: a simplified illustration of a view from the left ear.
Source: Courtesy of Marie A. Scheetz.

and directed into the external auditory meatus where they impinge on the tympanic membrane. The tympanic membrane is set into vibration by the moving air particles that are adjacent to it.

As the tympanic membrane begins to vibrate, the malleus, whose handle is embedded in the eardrum, sets the ossicular chain into vibration. As the ossicular chain continues to vibrate, the stapes generates movement within the oval window, which produces a pressure wave in the perilymph of the vestibule. In addition to transmitting sound, the ossicles regulate the energy collected by the tympanic membrane into a movement of greater force with less excursion, or range of movement, thus matching the impedance of sound waves in air to that in fluid. In the event an extremely loud sound is produced, the stapedius and tensor muscles function as a damper for the vibrations; thus the chain provides protection for the inner ear.

As the footplate of the stapes produces pressure on the inner ear, the round and oval windows respond to provide relief from the increased pressure. The interaction of the two windows is complex but can be described simply. When the footplate is pushed into the vestibule, the round window is bulged outward toward the middle ear cavity. The reciprocal action of these two windows compensates for the compressibility of the perilymph and the movement of the ossicular chain.

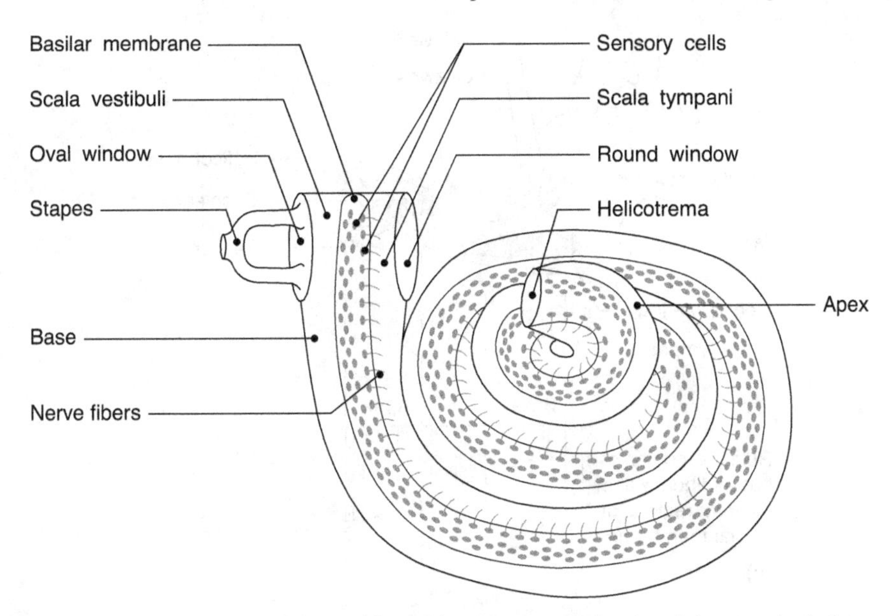

FIGURE 4.10 The components of the cochlea with respect to the oval and the round windows. Within this hard shell, a flexible membrane containing nerve fibers moves in response to fluid displacement, transmitting electrical signals to the auditory nerve.

Source: Courtesy of Marie A. Scheetz.

The fluid motion from the oval window to the round window is transmitted through the cochlear duct. As the perilymph of the scala vestibule is compressed, the vestibular membrane, or membrane of Reissner, bulges into the cochlear duct, causing movement of the endolymph and creating movement of the basilar membrane. As the basilar membrane is displaced, the tectorial membrane creates a "shearing" action on the hair cells that initiates nerve impulses. (See Figure 4.10) These impulses are carried by nerve fibers to the auditory portion of the eighth cranial nerve and then to the auditory center of the brain.

Sound can also be transmitted through bone conduction. Because the inner ear is encased in the temporal bone, vibrations of this bone will directly influence the movement of the fluid within the inner ear. As a result, those sounds transmitted by bone conduction are somewhat distorted. The nerve fibers compose a series of ascending and descending fibers that transmit the nerve impulses and "fine-tune" the signals. (See Figure 4.11.) Once the auditory signal reaches the auditory cortex (brain), interpretation occurs and meaning is given to the transmitted signal. (Refer back to Figure 4.9.)

• Bone conduction utilizes two modes of vibration: inertial, or translator motion, and compressional motion. In inertial motion the bones resist acceleration caused by an external force. In turn, in compressional motion the surface is pressed upon and becomes smaller. When a low-frequency sound is produced, the force and movement of the ossicular chain excites the hair cells, and the skull as a whole moves in response to the stimulation. However, when a high-frequency stimulus is received, the skull does not move as a whole but, rather, vibrates so that opposite surfaces move in an out-of-phase relationship. The back and front of the skull move outward as the sides of the skull move inward. This movement produces a compression of the

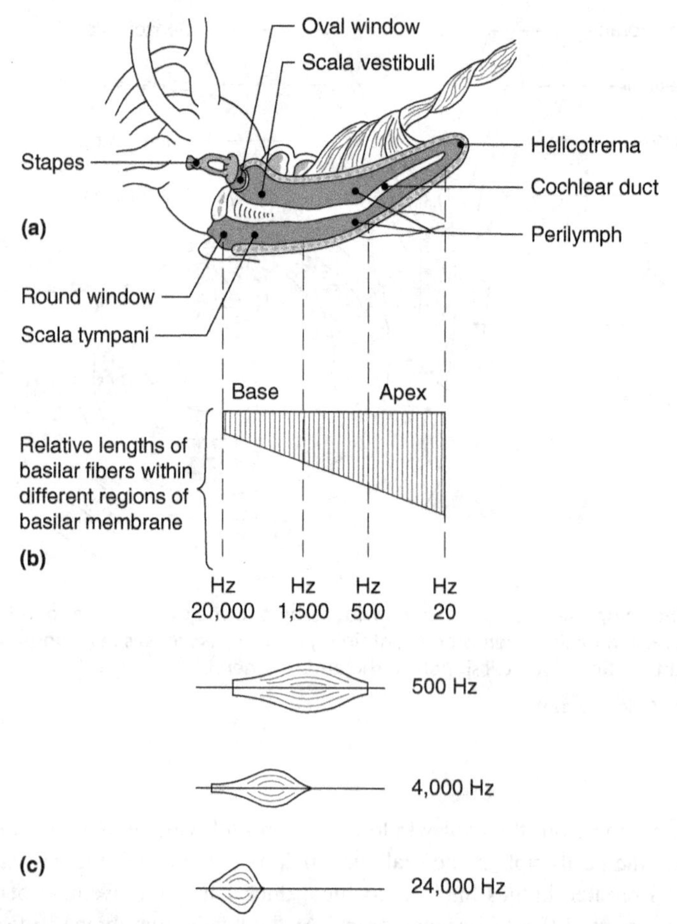

FIGURE 4.11 The basilar membrane reflecting resonance and the activation of hair cells found in the cochlea. (a) The cochlea is illustrated in a linear fashion, enabling the viewer to observe how sound is transmitted. Low-frequency sound waves (below the level of hearing) are routed around the helicotrema without exciting the hair cells. Higher frequency sounds create pressure waves that permeate through the cochlear duct and basilar membrane and arrive at the scala tympani. This creates vibrations in the basilar membrane in response to certain frequencies. (b) Reflects the varying length of basilar fibers found within different areas of the membrane. (c) High-frequency sounds create maximum excitation of the hair cells near the oval window, and low-frequency sounds excite hair cells near the cochlear apex.

Source: Courtesy of Marie A. Scheetz.

cochlea. As the fluid within the cochlea is compressed, the movement that takes place activates the nerve impulses.

One is not ordinarily conscious of sounds being transmitted through bone conduction as most of the sounds we are attuned to are airborne. However, when the head is in contact with a solid surface and the bones of the skull receive vibrations, one becomes more aware of the functioning of the bone-conduction mechanism. A summary of the structures for the ear and their functional roles is presented in Table 4.1.

TABLE 4.1 Summary of the Structures of the Ear and Their Functional Roles

Structure	Functional Role
External (outer) ear	**Collects and absorbs sound waves**
Pinna (auricle)	Receives sound waves
External auditory canal (meatus)	Transmits sound waves toward the tympanic membrane
Tympanic membrane	When sound waves come in contact with the tympanic membrane, they cause it to vibrate, thus setting the ossicular chain into motion
Middle ear	**Converts sound waves into mechanical vibrations**
Auditory ossicles	Transmit sound waves from the tympanic membrane to the oval window
Auditory tube (Eustachian tube)	Provides a mechanism to equalize pressure on both sides of the tympanic membrane
Inner ear	**Involved in the transduction of mechanical and hydrodynamic energy into neural impulses**
Vestibular apparatus	Concerned with equilibrium
Utricle	Static equilibrium
Saccule	Static equilibrium
Semicircular canals	Dynamic equilibrium
Cochlea	Consists of a series of fluids, channels, and membranes; responsible for transmitting sound waves to the organ of Corti (the organ of hearing) where nerve impulses are transmitted to the VIII (eighth) cranial nerve where neural impulses are transmitted to the auditory center of the brain

PREVALENCE AND ETIOLOGY OF AUDITORY DYSFUNCTION

Terminology

HEARING LOSS. Within the medical profession those who experience difficulty receiving stimuli through the auditory channel have been referred to as having a *hearing loss*. This broad term refers to anyone who is hard of hearing as well as senior citizens who have lost their auditory acuity due to the aging process. Under the broad umbrella of hearing loss are categories that further classify the degree of hearing loss and the effect it has on the individual's ability to function auditorily within his or her environment.

When determining how many individuals have a hearing loss, the statistics vary tremendously depending on the definition of *deaf*. The National Institute on Deafness and Other Communication Disorders (NIDCD) reports that approximately 36 million Americans, most of whom are adults, report difficulty hearing, and approximately 2 to 3 out of every 1,000 children in the United States are born deaf or hard of hearing (NIDCD, 2010), which impairs their ability to communicate and may require some level of habilitation. Ross, Brackett, and Maxon (1991) further report that there are 16 to 30 times more children who are hard of hearing than children who are deaf and that the hearing loss experienced by these individuals can significantly impact their ability to access the educational curriculum. The National Center for Health Statistics indicates the number of people who are profoundly deaf and residing in the United States at more than 400,000, and those functioning as hard of hearing as numbering over 20 million or about 8% of the total population (Bacon, 2009). According to the Gallaudet Research Institute (GRI) based on statistics provided by the National Health Interview Survey (NHIS) or the Survey of Income and Program Participation (SIPP):

- About 2 to 4 of every 1,000 people in the United States are "functionally deaf." However, more than half of them became deaf relatively late in life; fewer than 1 out of every 1,000 people in the United States becomes deaf before 18 years of age.
- If people with a severe hearing impairment are included in the statistic with those who are deaf, then the number becomes 4 to 10 times higher. That would mean anywhere between 9 and 22 out of every 1,000 experience a severe hearing impairment or are deaf. Keep in mind that at least 50% of these people reported their hearing loss after 64 years of age.
- Furthermore, if everyone who experiences any kind of "trouble" with their hearing is included, then anywhere from 37 to 140 people out of every 1,000 residing in the United States report some type of loss. The majority of these individuals are at least 65 years of age. (GRI, 2009)

In the past the term *hearing impaired* has been used to describe individuals with varying degrees of hearing loss (Scheetz, 2004). Even today the U.S. Census Bureau identifies those who experience difficulty hearing as having a hearing impairment. They further categorize these individuals as having difficulty hearing normal conversation (what most people would call hard of hearing) and unable to hear normal conversation (what most people would call deaf) (Gallaudet Research Institute, 2009). Although some individuals who are hard of hearing and deaf continue to use the term *hearing impaired* today to describe their hearing loss, others who are deaf may find the use of the term offensive. These individuals frequently prefer to be referred to as deaf or hard of hearing.

DEGREES OF HEARING LOSS. When describing hearing loss, attention is usually given to the age of onset at which the loss occurred, the type of loss the individual has, and the impact this has on spoken language development and communication. Individuals who lose their hearing prior to the age of 3 years are referred to as prelingually deaf, and those who lose their hearing after their auditorily based speech and language patterns have been established are identified as being postlingually deaf. Typically categories are used to describe the degree and severity of the hearing

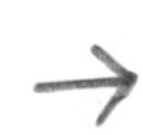

loss. For adults, those with a 26 to 40 dB loss are referred to as having a mild loss, a 41 to 55 dB loss is classified as a moderate loss, a 56 to 70 dB loss is considered to be moderately severe, a severe loss is categorized as a 71 to 90 dB loss, and a profound loss is classified as a 91+dB loss.

When screening children, the classification system changes somewhat, recognizing that children who experience even a slight loss of hearing sensitivity can be significantly impacted while in the process of acquiring language (DeBonis & Donohue, 2008). The following categories are used to describe the degree and severity of their hearing loss. Children in the −10 to 15 dB range are referred to as functioning within the normal range. Those with a 16 to 25 dB HL are referred to as having a slight hearing loss. A mild hearing loss is designated as 26 to 40 dB, and a moderate hearing loss is considered to be 41 to 55 dB. A moderately severe hearing loss occurs within the 56 to 70 dB range, and a severe hearing loss is indicated by 71 to 90 dB. Those experiencing a 91+dB hearing loss are said to have a profound loss.

It is important to note that many professionals working in the field of audiology today posit that the term *mild hearing loss* can be confusing and misleading when applied to children. Although the child's audiogram may reflect a hearing loss that occurs in the mild range, the effect of the loss in real-life environments can be tremendous. It is critical that audiologists and other professionals within the field educate parents and classroom teachers to the additional factors that will impact language development and communication needs for each of these children (DeBonis & Donohue, 2008).

Children are one group of individuals who receives special consideration when a hearing loss is identified. On the other end of the continuum are those individuals who lose their hearing later in life and are referred to as the deafened population or late-deafened adults. Although the deafened adult's language needs vary considerably from those of the young child who experiences a significant loss, when viewed from a medical perspective all share common characteristics relative to the degree of hearing loss. Table 4.2 illustrates the various categories of hearing loss and the implications for spoken communication.

TABLE 4.2 Categories of Hearing Loss and Implications

Degree of Hearing Loss	Label	Implications
−10 to 15 dB	Normal	No impact on communication.
16 to 25 dB	Slight	If the environment is quiet there is usually no difficulty recognizing and understanding speech; however in noisy environments speech can be difficult to understand.
26 to 40 dB	Mild	When surrounded with a quiet environment and familiarity with the topic and limited vocabulary, communication can be established. However, speech produced faintly or at a distance can become difficult to hear. Typically placed in regular education program; preferential seating is important; may benefit from a speech reading program.
41 to 55	Moderate	Has the ability to understand conversational speech at a distance of 3 to 5 feet. Can benefit from a hearing aid, auditory training, and speech therapy; preferential seating is beneficial. Group activities can be challenging.
56 to 70	Moderately severe	Conversation will not be heard unless it is loud. The person will benefit from all of the above and should also receive enhanced language instruction. An individual who experiences this degree of loss may produce speech that is not completely intelligible.
71 to 90	Severe	May identify environmental noises and loud sounds. May be able to distinguish vowels but not consonants; special education classes designed for deaf children may be beneficial. Speech is not always intelligible.
91+dB	Profound	Does not rely on hearing for primary means of communication; may hear some loud sounds; special education services are beneficial. Speech may be difficult to understand or may not be developed.

Source: Based on Keith (1996); Turnbull, Turnbull, Shank, Smith, & Leal (2002).

HARD OF HEARING. Audiologists use the term *hard of hearing* to identify those individuals who exhibit a slight to moderate hearing loss. A person who experiences a loss of this nature may benefit from the use of hearing aids, assistive listening devices, and other forms of amplification. By incorporating communication strategies, some individuals who are hard of hearing are able to access the mainstream of the larger hearing society and interact with those who can hear with relative ease. However, other individuals who also identify with being hard of hearing can find the task of engaging in free and easy conversation extremely challenging, if not altogether daunting, due to the type of hearing loss the person possesses. Even though both of these people might self-identify as being hard of hearing because the term is broad and encompasses a wide range of abilities and limitations, the word's connotation is as varied as the hearing profiles of the individuals who identify with the term. Although some individuals encounter high-frequency losses, and are thereby prevented from hearing high-frequency sounds, such as a whistle, doorbell, or a bird chirping, others experience losses within the range of hearing that contribute to the ability or inability to hear and understand speech. Even a mild loss can prevent a person from conversing with men, women, and children who are soft spoken or have voices that fall within the frequency where they have experienced a loss. Although they may comprehend some of the sounds within specific words, enough of the vowels or consonants may be inaudible to prohibit comprehension. For example, those with a high-frequency loss might miss the /th/ and /s/ phonemes, as in the word *thistle,* and individuals with low-frequency losses might miss the /b/ and /d/ phonemes, as in *bad*. Those who experience high-frequency losses typically have difficulty understanding women's voices, and those who have a low-frequency loss generally experience more difficulty understanding men's speech (Schirmer, 2001). Losses of this nature are oftentimes further exacerbated when one attempts to engage in a conversation on the telephone, leaving the person with a hearing loss feeling inept and frustrated.

DEAF. The term *deaf* is used to identify individuals who experience a hearing loss so severe that speech cannot be understood through the ear alone, with or without hearing aids. In essence these individuals cannot process linguistic information through hearing with or without amplification. Although they may hear some loud sounds, they do not rely on their auditory mechanism as their primary channel of communication.

ETIOLOGY OF AUDITORY DYSFUNCTION

When discussing the various types and causes of hearing disorders, one can begin by categorizing them into groups according to the age at onset of the hearing loss and the anatomical location of the dysfunction. Those dysfunctions that are present at birth are congenital losses, and those occurring after birth are acquired losses.

The area of the ear in which the impairment occurs designates the type of loss possessed by the individual. Conductive losses are those in which the dysfunction occurs in the outer or middle ear with the inner ear functioning normally. In *sensorineural loss,* one's hearing loss occurs due to pathology in the inner ear or the auditory nerve.

Conductive Hearing Loss

Conductive losses refer to any obstruction in the conduction (transmission) of sound from the external ear to the inner ear. In a conductive loss the problem lies with the individual being unable to conduct sound to the remainder of the hearing mechanism. Causes of conductive losses include certain congenital anomalies, childhood diseases, ear infections, and physical injuries to the ear.

One of the leading causes of conductive losses in children is otitis media, a middle ear infection. Such infections frequently affect the Eustachian tube, causing middle ear pressure to be less than adequate. This, combined with an excessive buildup of fluid in the cavity, often causes otitis media to be a very painful experience for the child.

Some other causes that contribute to a conductive hearing loss include missing or malformed pinnas; obstructions and tumors found in the external ear canal; and atresia, or an occluded auditory canal. Additional causes include impaired movement of the tympanic membrane; an anomaly in the middle ear evidenced by missing, malfunctioning, or restricted movement of the ossicles; and otosclerosis, in which the typical movements of the three bones of the ossicular chain are prohibited. The latter affects women more than men and is frequently accompanied by tinnitus (a sensation of ringing or humming in the ears).

The prescribed treatment for conductive losses may be medical or surgical. Those experiencing a blockage in the ear canal can usually have the obstruction removed. For those who have a type of otitis media, antibiotic therapy can be prescribed. Those experiencing difficulty with the tympanic membrane can undergo a myringoplasty, a skin graft to repair the damaged area, or a tympanoplasty in which hearing is restored by repair or reconstruction of the damaged parts contained in the middle ear. A stapedectomy (a surgical technique) may be employed when the dysfunction occurs in the ossicular chain. Use of this procedure allows the bones to become mobile again, thus increasing the individual's ability to hear.

Sensorineural Hearing Loss

Sensorineural losses, unlike conductive losses, occur when the dysfunction is located in the cochlea, or along the nerve pathway from the inner ear to the brain stem. A pure sensory disorder has its origin in the cochlea, whereas a neural disorder stems primarily from pathology of the cochlear nerve. Caused by exposure to drugs that are ototoxic, aging of the auditory system, autoimmune ear disease, or noise exposure (Paul & Whitelaw, 2011), this type of hearing loss can be characterized by an individual's inability to perceive sounds at varying frequencies with the same level of intensity. Very frequently, the ability to hear high frequencies is lost, except in the case of Meniere's disease, when the individual's ability to hear low sounds is more greatly affected.

Recent technological advances make it possible to pinpoint the etiology of the hearing loss and determine the cause of the sensorineural loss: the cochlea or the eighth cranial nerve. One example of a sensorineural loss is a recently identified disorder referred to as auditory neuropathy/dys-synchrony (AN/AD). Individuals with AN/AD have cochleas that are functioning properly. However, the auditory nerve is unable to relay electrical signals to the brain in a synchronous manner, resulting in information being delivered to the auditory center of the brain in an inconsistent fashion. Variation in AN/AD is considerable among those experiencing it; when it occurs it can affect word recognition skills and make it difficult for individuals to have complete functional use of their residual hearing (Paul & Whitelaw, 2011).

Sensorineural losses cannot be cured by prescription drugs or by medical interventions. The loss is typically permanent and, in some instances, progressive over time. Individuals with this type of hearing loss tend to speak with an excessively loud voice, even in situations in which that degree of volume is not required; they do not possess the ability to hear their own voices in order to monitor them, experience difficulty with speech discrimination, and can generally receive sounds produced at lower frequencies.

When people experience a sensorineural loss they may be aware that sounds are being produced during a typical conversation but have difficulty in differentiating which words are being spoken to them. In addition, those experiencing this type of loss do not receive protection from loud sounds as evidenced in a conductive loss. As a result, although faintly produced high-frequency sounds may not be heard, other sounds that are very intense can be received and are powerful as well as painful. Therefore, the range of hearing for people with this type of loss is somewhat limited and narrow. The loudness of sounds tends to occur rapidly and "recruitment" follows. Recruitment is defined as the abnormally rapid growth in the sensation of loudness (Katz, 2009). Characteristic of this condition is the individual who is complaining one minute that he cannot hear and in the next breath is accusing others of shouting at him.

Persons experiencing sensorineural losses may also share the sensation of tinnitus (buzzing in the ears), commonly found among those with conductive hearing losses. Individuals usually complain of a buzzing or ringing sound that may be apparent in either ear or not localized at all. The ringing sound may be confused with external sounds, such as a doorbell or telephone.

As mentioned above, it is well documented that certain drugs can damage the cochlea and the eighth cranial nerve, thus causing a sensorineural loss. The most common drugs being used are aminoglycosides, such as streptomycin and gentamicin. Other causes include fractures, vascular occlusion, and inflammatory lesions that may be viral (e.g., mumps). Those diseases that involve the nerve cells that relay impulses to the temporal lobe cortex may also produce defects in hearing. In addition, intense noises from industrial sources as well as loud music, such as that experienced by iPod users, are capable of creating permanent damage (Martin & Clark, 2009).

Although the majority of babies born with a hearing impairment have incurred a sensorineural loss, this type of loss can occur at any time in a person's life. Sensorineural losses can be attributed to the effects of the aging process; however, there is evidence that the prevalence of hearing loss in individuals under the age of 18 is increasing due to the high levels of output from sound sources such as toy phones, musical instruments, stereo systems, iPods, firecrackers, and toy guns (Martin & Clark, 2009). The causes for a sensorineural loss can be classified as congenital or acquired (adventitious).

CONGENITAL LOSSES. Congenital losses are present at birth; however, of the cases identified approximately 50% or less are attributed to genetic causes (DeBonis & Donohue, 2008). It is important to note that not all genetic disorders are congenital and not all congenital disorders are genetic. According to Plante and Beeson (2008), syndromes such as mucopolysaccharidosis (MPS), a genetically inherited metabolic disorder, are present at birth, even though the children with MPS are healthy and show no signs of hearing loss. However, the genetic effect of this disorder becomes evident with age as the child begins to experience a progressive hearing loss.

Due primarily to the Human Genome Project, more than 200 kinds of genetic deafness have been identified, although the exact location of the genes is known for only some of them (Moores, 2001). Congenital hereditary hearing loss occurs as a result of mutations in these genes. Approximately two thirds of genetic hearing losses occur as the only abnormality, and one third occur in association with additional abnormalities or as part of a syndrome (Plante & Beeson, 2008, p. 268). The three major types of congenital hereditary deafness are autosomal dominant disorders, autosomal recessive disorders, and X-linked disorders. Some of the most common types of genetic disorders associated with hearing loss are listed in Table 4.3.

Genetically Inherited Hearing Loss. Genetic material in the human body is contained within the deoxyribonucleic acid (DNA) found in the cells of the body in the form of chromosomes. Within each human cell are 22 pairs of autosomal chromosomes and 1 pair of sex chromosomes. At the time of conception the child receives one member of each pair of chromosomes from the father and one from the mother. All the autosomal chromosomes exist in pairs, with the exception

TABLE 4.3 Genetic Disorders Associated with Hearing Loss

Disorder	Clinical Signs
AUTOSOMAL DOMINANT DISORDERS	
Waardenburg's syndrome	Pigment abnormalities including a white forelock and different-colored irises; unilateral or bilateral sensorineural hearing loss.
Alport's syndrome	Nephritis; ocular lesions; progressive hearing loss.
Stickler syndrome	Ocular anomalies; cleft palate; progressive hearing loss.
Treacher Collins syndrome	Facial malformations including depressed cheek bones, deformed pinna, receding chin; conductive or mixed hearing loss.
Branchio-oto-renal syndrome	Ear malformation; renal anomalies, mixed hearing loss.
Neurofibromatosis	Tumor disorder; variable audiological findings.
AUTOSOMAL RECESSIVE DISORDERS	
Usher's Syndrome	Retinitis pigmentosa; congenital sensorineural hearing loss.
Friedrich's ataxia	Nervous system disorder; ocular abnormalities; abnormal movement; progressive sensorineural hearing loss.
Hurler's syndrome	Growth failure; mental retardation; progressive hearing loss.
X-LINKED DISORDERS	
Hunter's syndrome	Growth failure; mental retardation; mixed or conductive hearing loss.
Norrie's syndrome	Progressive visual impairment; mental retardation; progressive sensorineural hearing loss.
Alport's syndrome	Renal disorder; ocular abnormalities; progressive sensorineural hearing loss.

Source: Reproduced by permission of Pearson Education, Inc.

of the sex chromosomes. Furthermore, each pair of genes has a specific location on a specific pair of chromosomes.

Autosomal Dominant Disorders. When genes for hearing loss are inherited in an autosomal dominant manner, only one copy of the affected gene (inherited from either parent) is required for hearing loss to occur in the child who inherits the gene. In essence, this means that when one parent exhibits a hearing loss each offspring has a 50% chance of inheriting the gene for hearing loss. It does not mean that half of the children of a parent with an autosomal dominant gene will be affected but, rather, that each child has a 50% chance of being affected. Approximately 20% of genetic hearing loss is the result of dominant inheritance (Morton, 1991). Figure 4.12 illustrates this genetic configuration.

Autosomal Recessive Disorders. The majority of hearing loss that is inherited is attributed to an autsomal recessive genetic pattern. This accounts for approximately 80% of genetic hearing loss (Shaver, 1988). In these cases there is no evidence of hearing loss in either of the parents. Rather, the parents are carriers of the gene that they pass on to their child. In essence, each parent carries one affected and one nonaffected gene in the pair, so both parents have normal hearing. However, if their child receives both copies of the affected gene—one from each parent—the child will inherit a hearing loss. Figure 4.13 illustrates this configuration. Note that when both parents carry the recessive

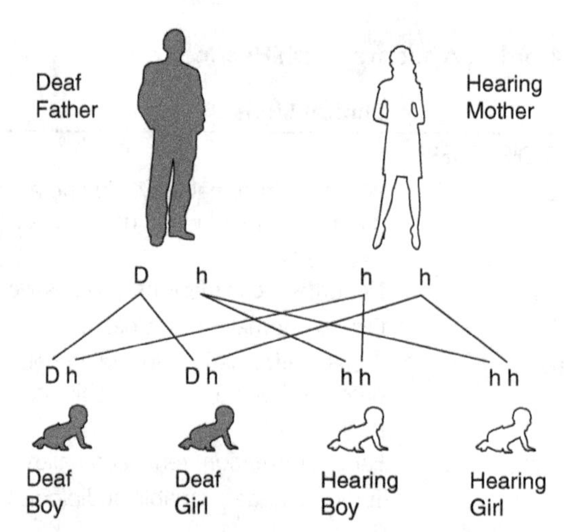

FIGURE 4.12 A single parent with a dominant gene causing deafness. When one parent has a single dominant gene causing deafness (D) and one counterpart normal gene (h), as portrayed in the father here, each of his children will have a 50% chance of inheriting this gene and being deaf. This is also true if the mother has the dominant gene resulting in deafness and the father does not.

Source: Courtesy of Marie A. Scheetz.

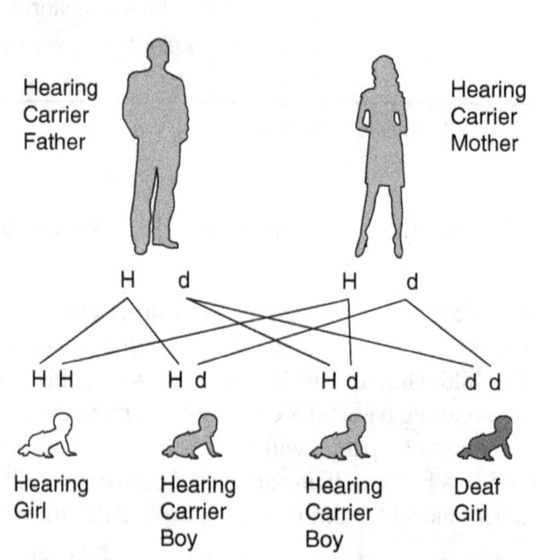

FIGURE 4.13 Both parents with recessive forms of deafness. If both parents are hearing but each carries the recessive form of deafness (d), each time they have a child they will have a 25% chance of having a son or daughter who is deaf. Likewise, they will have a 25% chance of having a hearing son or daughter who does not carry the gene; however, they have a 50% chance of having a hearing carrier son or daughter.

Source: Courtesy of Marie A. Scheetz.

gene each child that is conceived has a 25% chance of having a hearing loss (DeBonis & Donohue, 2008). Research indicates that to date, 22 autosomal-recessive genes for hearing loss have been identified and nearly all of them cause severe to profound loss (Sunstrom, Van Laer, Van Camp, & Smith, 1999).

X-Linked Disorders. Sex-linked congenital deafness is related to the X chromosome. Females inherit an X chromosome from each parent, and males inherit an X chromosome from their mother and a Y chromosome from their father. A female with a recessive gene on her X chromosome will not exhibit a hearing loss. However, each son will have a 50% chance of inheriting the trait, and each daughter will have a 50% chance of becoming a carrier. In the event that the father has an X-linked gene for hearing loss and his mate is not a carrier, he must pass his X chromosome to his daughters, and therefore all of his daughters will become carriers; in the event he has sons, they will all have normal hearing because they inherit only the Y chromosome from their father. Figure 4.14 illustrates X-linked recessive deafness. Approximately 2 to 3% of hearing loss is attributed to the X-linked transmission, making it the least common method of inheriting a genetic hearing loss (Plante & Beeson, 2008, p. 271).

ACQUIRED LOSSES. Acquired or adventitious hearing losses are those that are caused by exogenous (outside the genes) factors such as disease, toxicity, or trauma. They develop after a baby is born and can occur anytime within an individual's life span. When a fetus is exposed to some infections, the result can be a progressive hearing loss that will manifest itself during childhood. Acquired losses include cytomegalovirus (CMV), which is present at birth but can be progressive; meningitis; infections caused by the TORCHES complex; Meniere's disease; premature births; and hearing loss due to the aging process.

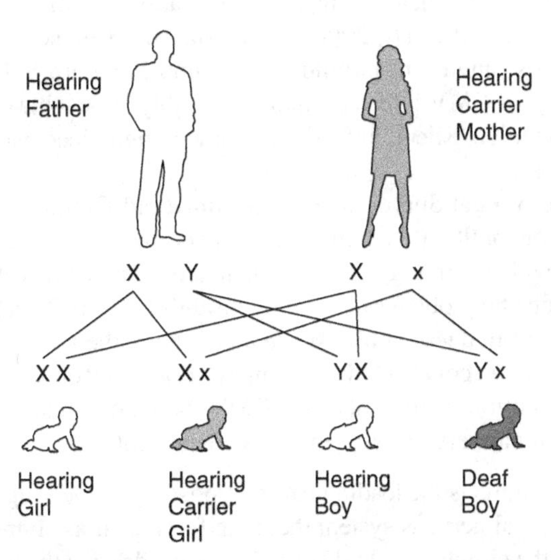

FIGURE 4.14 X-linked recessive deafness. In X-linked recessive deafness, a hearing carrier mother carries a gene on the X chromosome (x) that can cause deafness. If this gene is passed to her son, he will be deaf. If this gene is passed to her daughter, she will in turn be a carrier. As a result, a hearing carrier mother who has a son will have a 50% chance of him being deaf. If she has a daughter, she will have a 50% chance of being a carrier.

Source: Courtesy of Marie A. Scheetz.

Maternal Rubella. Rubella, also referred to as German measles, is a common viral disease that is oftentimes benign in adults and children. However, when contracted by pregnant women during the first trimester, the virus attacks the developing fetus, frequently causing hearing loss, visual impairment, cardiovascular defects, and a variety of other serious disorders. In 1964–1965 a rubella epidemic swept through the United States and Canada. As a result the incidence of hearing loss in children increased significantly and accounted for more than 50% of students enrolled in special education programs in the 1970s and 1980s. Due to the nature of the disease, many of these students had additional disabilities. In 1969 a rubella vaccine was developed and administered throughout the United States. Since that time, the majority of women have been vaccinated against this disease, and although the incidence has declined significantly, it continues to be a cause of hearing loss.

Cytomegalovirus. Although maternal rubella was one of the leading causes of deafness in the 1960s, cytomegalovirus (CMV) has been identified as a major environmental cause of deafness in newborn babies. Both rubella and CMV are members of a group of infectious agents know as TORCHES (toxoplasmosis, rubella, cytomegalovirus, herpes simplex, and syphilis) (Heward, 2003, p. 374).

CMV is a common virus that can remain in the body in an inactive state for the entirety of a person's lifetime. Most people who are infected with it experience minor symptoms, such as respiratory infections that soon disappear. However, unless symptoms are present the individual may not be aware of contracting it.

CMV can be transmitted to the fetus, through the placenta of the mother, during the time of birth as the infant travels down the birth canal or after birth if the virus is present in the breast milk. Approximately 1% of newborns, or about 40,000 infants each year, are born infected with CMV, and 10% of those may later develop various conditions, including mental retardation, visual impairment, and most often hearing impairment (National Institute on Deafness and Other Communication Disorders [NIDCD], 2006). Furthermore, of those 40,000, about 4,000 will experience a hearing loss ranging from mild to profound in nature (NIDCD). NIDCD further reports that the majority of CMV-infected infants—roughly 90%—have no symptoms at birth. Referred to as children with a "silent" infection, it may go unnoticed and manifest itself later in the form of a hearing loss.

According to the Annual Survey of Hearing Impaired Children and Youth (Schildroth, 1994), the following concomitant disabilities have been reported for children experiencing a hearing loss identified with an etiology of CMV: mental retardation in 19% of the children, cerebral palsy in 13%, orthopedic problems or learning disabilities in 10%, behavior problems in 9%, and visual impairment or blindness in 6%. When considering the major causes of deafness, it is evident that only rubella has contributed to as many serious secondary disabilities. Currently, there is no known prevention or treatment for CMV. Screening tests, although available, are rarely done on expectant mothers unless symptoms are present.

Meningitis. Meningitis is the leading cause of postlingual hearing loss. It is a bacterial or viral infection of the central nervous system that manifests itself as an inflammation of the coverings of the brain and the circulating fluid around it. It can destroy the acoustic apparatus of the inner ear, as well as other organs in the body. Children whose deafness is caused by meningitis generally have a profound hearing loss and may experience problems with balance as well as other disabilities. Recent estimates indicate that the percentage of individuals who experience a unilateral severe sensorineural hearing loss due to bacterial meningitis is approximately 21.6% (Barclay & Nghiem, 2006). However, it is important to note that currently those who lose their hearing because of this infection tend to have severe neurological impairments in addition to deafness (Moores, 2001).

Prematurity or Birth Complications. Approximately 11% of all births are at fewer than 37 weeks gestation or a birth weight of 5 pounds, 8 ounces or less, and are referred to as preterm. According to Wilson-Costello, Friedman, Minich, Fanaroff, and Hack (2005), low birth weight resulting from preterm delivery is a strong predictor of developmental problems including hearing loss; however, because low birth weight is more common among children who are deaf than among the general population, it is difficult to precisely evaluate the effects of prematurity on hearing loss.

Other High Risk Factors for Hearing Loss

A number of medical conditions can lead to hearing loss. Each of these can give rise to various types and severity, and two of these conditions merit special consideration: persistent pulmonary hypertension of the newborn (PPHN) and fetal alcohol syndrome (FAS), both of which have been linked to bilateral sensorineural hearing loss.

PERSISTENT PULMONARY HYPERTENSION OF THE NEWBORN. Also referred to as persistent fetal circulation, persistent pulmonary hypertension of the newborn (PPHN) is a physical abnormality of the blood vessels connected to the heart that results in deficient oxygenation of the blood, or severe hypoxemia. Reports indicate that 20% to 40% of infants diagnosed with PPHN have a bilateral, progressive, and sensorineural hearing loss with variability in degree and the possibility of delayed onset (Levitt, Watchko, Bennett, & Folsom, 1987; Naulty, Weiss, & Herer, 1986; Sell, Gaines, Gluckman, & Williams, 1985; Walton & Hendricks-Munoz, 1991). Babies that experience deficient oxygenation of the blood are frequently put on ventilators and given drug therapy. It is believed that the combined effects of these medical procedures, used to keep the babies alive, contribute to the hearing loss.

FETAL ALCOHOL SYNDROME (FAS). The most common preventable cause of birth defects today is fetal alcohol syndrome (FAS). The Centers for Disease Control and Prevention (CDC, 2010) reports that for every 1,000 live births approximately 0.2 to 1.5 babies are born with fetal alcohol syndrome. FAS results from women drinking alcohol during pregnancy. The amount of consumption, the trimester, or trimesters when the alcohol is consumed will influence the severity of the consequent disorders. FAS is characterized by a constellation of physical, behavioral, and cognitive abnormalities (Plante & Beeson, 2008). Although only a few investigations have been conducted regarding hearing status in this population, they suggest a high incidence of recurrent otitis media and a possibly higher than average incidence of bilateral sensorineural hearing loss (Church & Gerkin, 1988; Streissguth, Clarren, & Jones, 1985).

Causes of Hearing Loss in Adults

Approximately 36 million Americans, most of whom are adults, report difficulty with their hearing (NIDCD, 2010). The most common causes of hearing loss in adulthood are attributed to prolonged exposure to noise, ototoxic drugs, the aging process, Meniere's disease, and diseases of the central auditory system.

NOISE EXPOSURE. Occasionally, almost everyone is exposed to loud sounds that may contribute to temporary hearing loss. This can occur when attending live concerts, fireworks displays, or frequenting firing ranges. However, repeated exposure to loud sounds, such as industrial noise, aircraft, amplified music, or hazardous noise levels associated with power tools, snowmobiles, and other recreational activities, may also contribute to permanent hearing loss. According to the NIDCD (2010), an estimated 26 million Americans between the ages of 20 and 69 have high-frequency hearing loss due to loud sounds or noise at work or during leisure activities. This type of loss is due to individuals being exposed to dangerously high sound levels on a regular basis and can be attributed to a "threshold shift" that is initially observed around 4,000 Hz. When this occurs, tones that are produced in the 4,000 Hz frequency region will be more difficult to hear after noise exposure than before. This is due to damaged sensory cells in the cochlea, resulting in sensorineural hearing loss. Individuals who lose their hearing due to repeated exposure to hazardous noise levels may have difficulty understanding speech in noisy environments and in rooms with high levels of reverberation (Plante & Beeson, 2008, p. 305).

OTOTOXIC DRUGS. Ototoxic drugs are often used for treatment of life-threatening diseases, such as cancer, and can have an adverse effect on hearing. These drugs can cause damage to the inner ear, resulting in a sensorineural hearing loss. Individuals on drug therapies may become more sensitive to the hazardous effects of noise damage compared to people who are not receiving such therapies.

THE AGING PROCESS. The term *presbycusis* is used to describe the deterioration of hearing that is associated with the aging process. It can be attributed to a lifetime of environmental noise exposure, disease processes, drug effects, and a genetic predisposition that leads to hearing loss in adults. The proportion of individuals who lose their hearing due to presbycusis increases with age. A special report prepared for the the U.S. Census Bureau in 2005 estimates that 37% of adults who experience hearing loss are 65 years old or older (He, Sengupta, Velkoff, & DeBarros, 2005). As one ages, changes begin to occur in the basal end of the cochlea, the end that is responsible for high-frequency sounds. Therefore, those suffering from presbycusis often indicate that they can hear low-frequency sounds and report that they can hear people talking but cannot understand what is being said. This is because consonants, which so frequrently play a critical role in understanding spoken words, are inaudible.

MENIERE'S DISEASE. Another form of sensorineural impairment, confined to the cochlea, is Meniere's disease. Throughout the United States approximately 615,000 individuals have been diagnosed with this disease, with about 45,500 additional cases being diagnosed annually (NIDCD, 2010). Although the exact cause of Meniere's disease is unknown, it is thought to be primarily caused by an increased buildup of inner ear fluid, endolymph, within the membraneous labyrinth. Although Meniere's disease generally affects only one ear, causing severe recruitment to occur, one third of those with the disease will develop it in both ears. It is characterized by violent attacks of vertigo (dizziness), periods of loud tinnitus (ringing in the ears), and abnormalities in hearing. In addition, the deafness experienced is quite severe, the symptoms disappear at times, and the disease goes into remission. Even though it typically occurs between ages 40 and 60, it has been diagnosed in children younger than 10 and adults older than 90 (Minor, Schlessel & Carey, 2004).

DISEASES OF THE CENTRAL AUDITORY SYSTEM. Hearing loss can occur due to damage that occurs outside of the ear itself. Problems may occur after the nerve impulse enters the brain stem or within the auditory center housed in the cerebral cortex. Hearing anomalies related to the brain stem or the cerebral cortex are referred to as central auditory disorders. This type of hearing loss can be caused by multiple sclerosis, strokes, cortical and brain stem tumors, trauma-induced brain damage, or blood incompatibilities caused by the Rh factor. When a lesion is present in the brain, the blood supply to the cochlea can be disturbed, thereby resulting in damage to the hair cells. This, in turn, can create difficulties with speech processing, especially if the person engaged in listening is located in an environment with background noise. This can be further compounded if reverberation is present, visual cues are not available, or the person is speaking at a rapid rate. Individuals with this type of hearing disorder have a normally functioning ear and are able to transmit sounds through the auditory channel with no amplification. However, once the sound travels beyond the acoustic nerve, the message becomes scrambled and cannot be accurately processed.

Summary

The focus of this chapter has been to acquaint the reader with the nature of sound; the process and mechanism of hearing; and the prevalence, types, and causes of hearing loss. Although the intent has been to provide an overview of the topics, it is hoped that one can begin to see the complexities involved in the transmission of sound and one's ability to receive and perceive meaning from it.

The auditory channel is only one way that we connect with our environment and those that reside in it. However, it does provide a communication conduit between those who can hear and the large body of information conveyed through spoken words expressed both explicitly and implicitly. How hearing loss impacts language, social, cultural, and educational development is as unique as the individual who experiences the loss. Individuals who comprise the deaf and hard-of-hearing population exhibit as much diversity as those who form the fabric of the larger hearing population. The purpose of the chapters that follow is to explore this diversity within the confines of the larger hearing society.

5

Family Dynamics

Response to Diagnosis, Interpersonal Relationships, and Impact on the Family Unit

Family units represent a unique and complex segment of society. Comprised of individuals from varying socioeconomic backgrounds, they mirror the ethnic identities and cultural values of the communities they represent. The structure of the traditional, nuclear, one-income family unit of the past has undergone tremendous change throughout the last few decades. Impacted by the economic climate, the majority of adults are required to work, thus forcing parents to relinquish the care of their children to relatives or professional caregivers for part, if not most, of the day.

Child care facilities provide services for infants and children from nuclear families as well as those who have felt the impact of separation and divorce. Statistics indicate that divorce rates have risen to over 50% in the United States, and as a result approximately 25% of American children are living in single-parent households (Clark, 1995), about 5% are stepchildren within blended families, and approximately 3% of young children are being adopted (Kreider, 2003). In addition, with a growing acceptance of same-sex couples, there is an influx in the number of children being born or adopted into families reflecting this lifestyle. Statistics reveal that over 150,000 gay and lesbian couples now raising children with 65,000 same-sex couples raising adopted children (Romero, Baumle, Badgett, & Gates, 2007). All these dynamics have had a profound impact on the changing nature of family life.

With poverty on the rise, it continues to leave a negative imprint on everyone it touches. Permeating families, the effects of poverty are far reaching and long lasting. According to the National Center for Children in Poverty (Chau, Thampi, & Wight, 2010). In 2009 the documented poverty rate for children under the age of 17 was 15.3 million. Of those affected, approximately 24% (6.1 million) were children under the age of 6, and 19% (9.2 million) were between the ages of 6 and 17. Furthermore, the poverty rate for African American children under the age of 6 was 41%, and the poverty rate for Hispanic American children under the same age was 21.5%. Poverty becomes a stark reality for many single-parent families, affecting 42% of children under the age of 17.

Socioeconomic status is only one descriptor used to characterize American society; another is diversity. Across the United States evidence of widespread ethnic and cultural diversity is apparent. In 2009, the foreign-born population constituted of approximately 38.5 million of the U.S. population, and the percentage is on the rise (Grieco & Trevelyan, 2010). This is particularly evident in certain areas of the country, such as Dade County, Florida, and Queens County, New York, where approximately half of all residents are foreign born (Schmidley, 2003, as cited in Rhoades, Price, & Perigoe, 2004). Many of these families speak languages other than English, embrace different cultural beliefs, and have their own preconceived ideas regarding child-rearing practices. Regardless of the ethnic origins, socioeconomic status, or constellation of the family structure, each family unit represents a microcosm that embraces life's experiences with its own preconceived ideas and expectations.

ANTICIPATION, EXPECTATIONS, AND RESPONSES TO THE BIRTH OF A BABY

From the couple who has been trying to start a family to the young teenage girl who is in high school, the word *pregnant* can have a very different meaning. For some, it brings out elation and excitement, and for others a sense of fear and dread. Although some pregnancies are very much desired, others are unexpected and oftentimes unwanted.

Some pregnancies are met with a great deal of anticipation as siblings await the arrival of their new sister or brother, and frequently extended family members are as excited as the expectant parents for the baby to arrive. Regardless of the family unit, socioeconomic background, or ethnic heritage, almost all those awaiting the birth of a child anticipate that the new baby will be healthy, arrive perfectly formed, and be equipped with all the physical and mental attributes that comprise a perfectly functioning infant. Occasionally, the possibility of a less-than-perfect child being born enters the parents' minds. However, that idea is generally pushed aside by more pleasant thoughts surrounding the parents' image of the "ideal" child.

What happens when a child is born, and the infant does not arrive with all these attributes? In particular, what happens when parents receive the diagnosis that their child is deaf? How they respond to the diagnosis is determined, in part, by their hearing status, their background knowledge of what it means to be deaf, and the professionals who provide them with the initial information. One hearing mother's account of how she responded to the initial diagnosis epitomizes what many other parents have expressed.

HEARING PARENTS' RESPONSE TO THE DIAGNOSIS

The Life of Riley

Terri Patterson 6/10/09

When I was carrying Riley and frantically trying to get Molly, then 2 yrs old potty trained, I remember always having conversations with God about however He may think I could handle anything, please don't choose that for me. Strange, looking back, I never had those feelings with Molly, but I did with Riley. It was an easy pregnancy and childbirth went without any problems (but, plenty of pain!).

Let me back up. . . . Molly had her hearing screened when she was born at Northside Hospital in 1996, because of family history. My husband's brother's third child failed the newborn hearing screening in Arizona 6 months before Molly was born. So, Molly was able to receive a screening. When Riley was born at Cobb Hospital, they did not yet have the equipment or capability to screen Riley in 2000 since Georgia had not yet passed UNHSI. So, they recommended we call and set up an outpatient screening for Riley. As good parents, we made the appointment and didn't think much about it as we sang to him and played music picked specifically for him. The appointment was for 2 months out. During that time, Matt (my husband) and I would go back and forth suggesting that, "I don't think he heard that" and testing him. We had all sorts of excuses; I figured I was just being dramatic. I was ready to just cancel the appointment, but Matt encouraged me to just do it, for peace of mind.

So, let's skip forward to Riley's appointment, Matt and Molly played out in the waiting room, while I held Riley in my arms and rocked him to sleep so the electrodes could be secured. As we sat in the dark room, I watched the screen in front of the audiologist, not understanding anything. But, I still remember the exact moment that I looked at the audiologist and said, "That's not right, is it?" She turned and shook her head, "No."

As the floor dropped out from under me, I remember nodding when she asked if I would prefer for her to go get Matt from the waiting room . . . my eyes blurred through the shock and tears as another assistant ushered Molly down the hall with the promise of toys. I don't remember much from that point on, but knew Matt knew from the moment he saw my face. So, we left with lots of sheets of information and some names of ENTs to follow up with and inconceivable grief. At home the phone began ringing with friends and family waiting to hear good news of needless worrying. I couldn't talk. . . . I just wanted to run away . . . so we packed up and started driving (we were always ones for spontaneous trips). We ended up in Alabama in a hotel room with a toddler and a 2 month old baby . . . not conducive to sleep and peace . . . and the added fact that any time we did calm down that next thought of what Riley "would never be able to do" kept popping into our heads. . . ." Who will marry him and take the time to learn to communicate with him?" "Will my father ever learn sign language?" "Will everyone feel sorry for us and back away?" Silly to think of that now, but very real back then.

One of the first things I did was call my sister-in-law and apologize for never thinking my nephew's hearing impairment was that big of a deal, they made it look easy, and I apologized for ever thinking, "It could be so much worse," because believe me, this time . . . it couldn't, or at least I couldn't see it that way. So . . . we went back home, we scheduled our follow up appointment and called to set up early intervention services. People started showing up at our house, I had to sign papers, we had to fight with our insurance company for referrals . . . the ENT office was phenomenal in helping us, as I screamed into the phone in their waiting room, hysterical. Riley was diagnosed with a bilateral severe to profound sensorineural hearing loss. We were referred so that we could get the hearing aids set up and begin our journey.

Riley was aided by 3 months of age; we were set up with a wonderful Service Coordinator, who is a dear friend and colleague 9 years later. We started receiving GA PINES services and we began trying to find our way through the confusing maze of deciding on a mode and method of communication to fit our family. Wow, that was a confusing thing, we wanted to know, nudge, nudge, what would be the most successful, trying to get some kind of insider information from the professionals around us . . . to no avail. So, we researched and researched and asked questions and made phone calls. We decided that we would try Auditory-Verbal Therapy first . . . it seemed the most challenging for Riley (since he couldn't hear much of anything, even aided), thinking that since we are verbal people that that would be our first choice for Riley. Then, if it didn't work, we would just keep adding cues or sign language, if that is what he needed. The thought of learning a whole new language and taking care of a new baby and a toddler seemed overwhelming, so we decided we would save that for later. He began AVT at 6 months of age, we weren't as strict as we were supposed to be, so there was guilt for me in the beginning, but I thought I had to do what the professionals told me to do. I almost felt a disconnect sometimes to Riley, like I was handing him over to people who knew him better. The change for me came when my wonderful Service Coordinator helped me realize that Riley was our baby and this was our family, so the professionals needed to fit with us, not the other way around. So, we did decide to continue with AVT, but found a therapist that fit us better . . . guilt was gone and it became fun.

As we started AVT we started hearing about Cochlear Implants, so again, we researched, we asked questions and made phone calls. This might be something wonderful for Riley; we learned that we needed to understand all of the risks and work that would be involved, with no guarantee of success. We decided we wanted to try and pursued that route. After a lot of talking to the surgeons in town that do this surgery, other families who have been through this, other adults who have been through the surgery and the companies that make Cochlear Implants . . . we did it. Riley was 13 months when he had his first implant. (I say first because when he was 7 we began hearing about bilateral implants and two years later Riley received an implant in his other ear . . . but that is another story.)

We worked hard, we still work hard and the ironic thing is when we curse the technology because of silly glitches, we have to remind ourselves how much it has enriched our lives and expanded Riley's. We continued therapy until he "graduated" at the end of Pre-Kindergarten. He worked very hard, at therapy and at home. We have always tried to be involved with other families at conferences and workshops. Cochlear Implants have been a good fit for us. Our first shot ended up being a good fit. Was it easy? NO. Are we grateful for all of the amazing people along the way that really pushed and empowered us? YOU BET. Does it work like this every time for every child? NO. But, there is a fit out there for every family; with unbiased support and resources available to families . . . they can find the right fit for their child and their family.

Do we question whether we did the right thing . . . again? YOU BET. But, we get through it the best we can day to day . . . and the memories from our past do still haunt us. That moment in that dark room gazing at that computer screen never fails to put a knot back in my stomach and bring tears to my eyes, but I look forward and know . . . Riley can do and be anything he wants to and because of his life he has only made ours richer. So, now, when he decides to be a "normal" difficult 10 year old boy . . . his hearing loss is the least of our problems! (Used with permission, Terri Patterson, 2009)

Hearing loss is being identified at an early age today, largely due to the increase in neonatal screenings. Through these screenings, the door is opened for early intervention, and although the benefits of this can be great, the initial impact the diagnosis can have on the parents can be both frightening and devastating.

Fitzpatrick, Graham, Durieux-Smith, Angus, and Coyle (2007) conducted a survey with parents to determine the parents' perspectives on being told that their child, at an early age, had a significant hearing loss. Some mothers indicated they were grateful to have been so informed, but others were relieved they did not receive the information until their child was much older. One mother involved in the study stated,

> "she was finally diagnosed [when] she was 25 days old so I think it was hard. . . . I mean it's beneficial to know as early as possible but it's just hard on feelings. I didn't really enjoy (baby) because I was so sorry and frustrated. . . . I think I didn't enjoy the new baby like other mothers do 100% . . . it was hard. . . . Now . . . we understand, oh, she's just our baby, well she's hearing-impaired but she's still our baby." (Fitzpatrick et. al., 2007)

Another mother shared her experience of not finding out about her child's hearing loss until the child was over a year old. She expressed the following views:

> "And to be completely honest, I had a lovely year at home with him, in that quiet land of a happy baby, no idea . . . because, I imagine if somebody had told me at day one or day five . . . that something was wrong, you would have just gone off the deep end. I imagine, because you pretty much do that anyway, but later. But at least then you have, you know, the child is your child and. . . . If somebody said it at day five, and you've barely sort of recovered from having the baby, never mind someone telling you that there's something wrong with the baby." (Fitzpatrick et. al., 2007, p. 101)

Other views emerged from the study that merit mention here. Some parents felt a great deal of regret and reflected with sadness as they recounted the fact that their child's diagnosis was not made earlier; they definitely felt they had spent a lot of time trying to close the developmental gap that would never have occurred if a diagnosis had been made sooner:

> "[W]e feel like we've been doing tons of catch up. . . . and you know when we look back on her first birthday, and we see her and we're singing happy birthday, and realize she was never hearing any of that. I think wow, you know, you look at those videos, I can't watch them really, I have a hard time." (Fitzpatrick et al., 2007, p. 101)

Other parents were very thankful that their child's hearing loss was identified at an early age, as is evident in their comments. One mother commented that she felt it was better to receive an early diagnosis. Although she stated it was traumatic for them when they found out she indicated that, looking back, she was glad that they knew. She commented on how beneficial it had been for her child to be fitted early with hearing aids:

> "[H]e's grown up with them, so that's a part of who he is. You know, if he would have gotten hearing aids at three years, it would have taken, it took adjustment back then but I think it would have taken more adjustment because I would have known him as a child who I would consider, you know, to be normally developing including the hearing, but that was basically part of who he was almost from the beginning." (Fitzpatrick et al., 2007, p. 102)

The literature reflects an abundance of articles describing the grief hearing parents experience when they discover their child is deaf. Parents frequently blame each other or themselves for the child's deafness. Accusations may be converted into multidimensional feelings that are expressed in the form of anger, guilt, or hurt. Frequently parents turn to their own parents for help, only to realize they have no answers for them. Drawing from the much larger hearing society for advice, they may receive sympathy from those who view being deaf as a serious disability that should be eradicated. Oftentimes, they begin to search for ways to help their child become "normal" as they continue to struggle with the diagnosis and attempt to comprehend what the disability entails. As they are faced with the task of determining a communication mode and later locating a beneficial educational setting, parents frequently experience a great deal of tension and stress. This can create a tremendous amount of strain in the marital relationship, often contributing to separation or divorce.

During the period when it is critical to establish a healthy maternal relationship with the child, the mother may still be coping with all the ramifications of hearing loss. As a result, the bond between the mother and the child who is deaf may become strained. Early in life children become very sensitive to the tension in their environment are very quick to pick up on the unsettled climate. Subsequently, in lieu of a warm, nurturing environment, the child may be cared for in a mechanical fashion as the parents come to grips with the diagnosis.

DEAF PARENTS' RESPONSE TO THE DIAGNOSIS

When deaf babies are born into homes where the parents are deaf, the diagnosis is usually viewed in a very different manner. If the parents have established a Deaf identity, they welcome the child into a community that views being deaf as another descriptor of their overall persona, rather than a disability. This is apparent in the literature when the discussion focuses on whether Deaf women want to have children who are hearing or deaf. Najarian (2006) investigated the mothering experiences of college-educated Deaf women. During her study she conducted interviews with a group of Deaf mothers to determine how they viewed their experiences raising children and what types of challenges they had faced as Deaf mothers functioning in a hearing society.

As the women progressed through their pregnancy, Najarian (2006) sought to determine if the mothers specifically wanted their child to be born hearing or deaf. Many of the women's responses were very insightful and strikingly indicative of the Deaf community. One mother described her feelings when she thought her child could hear:

> "When my son was born, I thought he was hearing. So, we were heart broken. I thought, 'Oh, my God, what do we do with a hearing child?' (She laughs). I was born deaf. Our children helped us to understand how my husband became deaf. With my two children it was a progressive hearing loss. Their hearing loss is different from many deaf people. My husband didn't really understand how he became deaf. His parents told him he became deaf when he was four from nerve deafness. But that helped my husband understand it was the same. . . . It is normal for parents to want to have children that are the same as them. If I had blue eyes, I would want my children to have the same. My parents are deaf. I have a wonderful relationship with them. I want that. It's important that they're healthy." (Najarian, 2006, p. 109)

All parents want to produce offspring who are healthy, who manifest similar characteristics reflective of their personal attributes, and who can engage in social communication exchanges with them. When this occurs the foundation is laid for the establishment of close parent–child relationships that can be further nourished throughout the course of the child's lifetime.

Equating having a child with blue eyes with having a child who is deaf indicates how deafness is considered a physical attribute, rather than a disability. Wanting a child who is healthy, one with whom you can communicate and establish an early bond, is valued equally by Deaf parents and hearing parents. This is reflected in another Deaf woman's comments when the doctor diagnosed her baby as deaf.

> "When Kate was born, my husband and I were thrilled. We were surprised and happy. I felt good because it would be easy to communicate as a family. The doctor offered to give Kate a cochlear implant. I said, 'No,' because the family is Deaf. We prefer that. But, I told him, we will get her hearing aids because she's hard of hearing. It would help to improve her lip reading." (Najarian, 2006, p. 115)

Communication, acceptance, and providing children with the tools they need to navigate between hearing and Deaf individuals were critical to all these mothers, all of whom wanted their children to be happy, healthy, and establish their own identities. As one mother stated in response to being asked if she and her husband preferred to have a deaf child: "We were willing to accept it either way. If she's deaf, we know what to do because we were too. If she was hearing, we would also accept her. We don't care as long as she's healthy. That's important. When she was born, we were happy to have her" (Najarian, 2006, p. 110).

All parents, regardless of their hearing status, continually echo similar sentiments. They want their child to be healthy, happy, and able to communicate with them. Furthermore, they want their children to develop a sense of independence and self-worth. Consequently, within the family unit parents endeavor to foster a sense of interconnectedness that promotes the development of competent children. Young children being raised in homes that emulate open communication and creative problem-solving techniques are provided with a foundation for problem-solving strategies that they can draw from as they enter their teen years. By watching their parents incorporate and model these skills, they are privy to tools that will assist them when they are confronted with complex internal and external social situations later in life (Luckner & Velaski, 2004).

In essence, these children are being raised within a healthy family. Concurrent to communication and creative problem solving, additional characteristics are evident in homes that epitomize environments where optimum growth and development can occur. What are some of these characteristics? What attributes distinguish healthy families from those who are dysfunctional? What dispositions are portrayed in these families that are not discernable in others?

CHARACTERISTICS OF HEALTHY FAMILIES

An extensive body of research addresses the nature of the healthy personality that, in turn, contributes to the healthy family unit. The healthy family unit consists of parents who possess the qualities of a healthy personality and are depicted as mature and emotionally secure individuals who are cognizant of who they are and are secure in their relationships with others and with interfacing with the world around them. They embrace a forward-looking philosophy and are motivated by long-range goals and plans as well as a sense of directedness (Allport, 1965).

Healthy parents are further described as individuals who become actively engaged in the learning process and espouse creativity and spontaneity. Daily, they embrace the importance of living fully while making optimum use of the experiences in their environment. They welcome contact with varying segments of society and strive toward becoming self-actualized people (Rogers, 1961).

Abraham Maslow (1954) shares Carl Rogers's view that self-actualization is at the core of the healthy personality. By meeting a series of needs, beginning with our very basic physiological needs, we ascend up the hierarchy to the level of esteem needs. Therefore, as our basic needs are met, we eventually progress to the levels of belonging and love needs, which subsequently allow the individual to concentrate on a sense of self-esteem. Maslow states that these individuals are not concerned with making up for deficits; rather, they are in a state of being whereby they can experience optimum growth and maturation.

Parents play a vital role in the family unit and provide one of the most critical elements in child development. Through their love, nurturing, and communication, they provide the structure and scaffolding for their children to grow and mature into healthy young adults. Daily, they are faced with success and challenges as they traverse life events. What do hearing parents, in particular, do to ensure their child who is deaf will be provided with the same opportunities as a child who can hear? What factors contribute to the development of healthy children who are deaf and, in turn, healthy families?

FACTORS THAT CONTRIBUTE TO HEALTHY FAMILIES WITH CHILDREN WHO ARE DEAF

A plethora of research has explored the changes in family dynamics that occur when a child is diagnosed with a profound hearing loss. Many of these articles have focused on a pathological viewpoint of deafness and have described strategies to deal with the emotions of grief, depression, and feelings of overall loss. More recently, a paradigm shift has occurred within the field of special education and deaf education. Subsequently, professionals have shifted their perspective to examine the internal strengths and external resources that parents use to foster optimum growth and development within their children and within the family (Luckner & Velaski, 2004).

Furthermore, studies have been conducted to identify the characteristics that can be used to describe healthy families with children who are deaf.

In a study conducted by Luckner and Velaski (2004), teachers in one western state were each asked to nominate a family who emulated the characteristics personified by a healthy family and had a child who was deaf. The families were then contacted; if they agreed to participate in the study, the researchers interviewed them by following a semistructured format. Participants were asked a series of eight open-ended questions. Two of them merit particular attention: first, why they felt they had been described as a healthy family and, second, how they would describe the challenges they faced raising children who are deaf. Following their responses they were then asked to share any advice they would give to other families who also have children who are deaf.

Those participating in the study identified five factors they felt contributed to the overall dynamics of a healthy family unit. These factors included "commitment to the family, learning to sign with their child, support from extended family, friends and members of the community, support from the professionals working at the educational program their child was attending, and high expectations for their child with a hearing loss" (Luckner & Velaski, 2004, pp. 328–329).

Parental comments in response to the questions were particularly telling. Several parents reported that they held the concept of family in very high regard. They indicated that receiving support from all family members and being able to spend time together were essential. The majority also stressed the importance of communication, stating that it is the key for providing children who are deaf with access to their world and their surroundings.

When describing challenges they faced raising their children, topics that emerged included locating a good educational program, learning to sign, helping people understand deafness, and providing an environment in which their child could establish and develop friendships. One family reported finances as presenting a considerable problem, while another family identified communication in terms of learning sign language as one of the biggest challenges they faced (Luckner & Velaski, 2004, pp. 329–330).

When asked to offer advice for other families with children who are deaf, six overall suggestions were provided: become an advocate for your child, familiarize yourself with your rights and identify resources, maintain high expectations for your child, learn sign language, become involved in your child's education, and provide love and encouragement for your child on a daily basis. One mother summed up her feelings nicely by stating, "Know that your children are not broken and need to be fixed. They are still able to learn and be successful, so don't hold them back." Another reiterated similar thoughts by stating, "These children are not 'disabled'; they are 'able to rise to great heights' with support, encouragement, and lots of love" (Luckner & Velaski, 2004, p. 331). When these guidelines are followed, children who are deaf are provided with the foundation and support to develop and mature into independent and successful Deaf adults. Evidence of this is apparent in earlier research that was conducted by Luckner and Stewart (2003).

Interested in determining factors that contribute to successful adults who are deaf, Luckner and Stewart (2003) conducted interviews with 14 adults who were deaf. Nominated by their peers as being successful, they wanted to ascertain what the individuals felt had contributed to their success. Those individuals participating in the study were asked ten questions pertaining to their family support, education, personality traits, and social life. Following these responses participants were asked to provide recommendations to parents, teachers, and future employers.

When the interviewees were asked why they thought they had become successful, their responses were very consistent: "The study participants reported that they worked hard and that they received ongoing support from their families" (Luckner & Stewart, 2003). When asked to describe how their families contributed to their success, several mentioned that a wide variety of family members served as their primary source of inspiration and that they were always included in different activities. One person stated, "My parents were really good at treating me equal" (Luckner & Stewart). Additional themes that emerged from the study included the importance of self-determination, effective communication skills, and the critical role of family support. This study reinforces previous findings that stress the importance of family interaction and support, effective communication skills, and motivation and self-determination on the part of the individual. Being treated as an equal and being invited to participate in conversations and activities are essential to our well-being. It is critical that we maintain our focus on the whole child, recognizing what the child who is deaf can do, while engaging him or her in meaningful activities. Communication is vital to the development of all children, both hearing and deaf.

COMMUNICATION: CONNECTING AND INTERACTING WITH OTHERS AND SOCIETY

Communication provides one of the lifelines contributing to the emotional well-being of healthy individuals. From infancy through adulthood we are exposed to a wealth of ideas, information, and knowledge, thus impacting how we form perceptions, gather insights, and develop our thought processes. In essence, our ability to communicate with those around us contributes to our emotional, social, and cognitive well-being.

The early communication link formed between mother and child provides one of the earliest bonds that will strengthen and grow as the child matures and develops. These early interactions provide an avenue whereby the child will be exposed to an infinite onslaught of words that will later afford the toddler opportunities to engage in familial and social interactions. The quality of these exchanges will be a contributing factor in language development and will later impact the child's ability to unlock the complexities of his or her parents' native language. This early communication link also becomes one of the primary pipelines for cognitive growth to occur while allowing for the expression of one's emotions. Later, these emotions will be shaped to meet the expectations generated by society.

Through recurrent interactions, those who can hear are exposed to a wealth of information both through direct contact and incidental learning; facts are shared, views are exchanged, and conversations are overheard. Frequently, we form opinions and generate new ideas without being cognizant of the origins of these thoughts. What constitutes a solid communication base? What factors are required to promote the development of effective communication skills? What types of exchanges are deemed necessary to ensure optimum language, cognitive, social, and emotional growth will occur? What types of early language activities are required for this to take place? What impact does being deaf have on these developmental processes?

The Building Blocks for Communication

Language provides the building blocks for communication. Emerging in infancy, it has the potential to flourish throughout one's lifetime. Language originates in the home and is influenced by the cultural and ethnic backgrounds of the family unit. It further provides a conduit allowing individuals to connect with others, gather ideas, and establish a sense of identity. In essence, learning how to communicate may be one of the most important and impressive accomplishments of infancy (Traci & Koester, 2003).

During the first few weeks of life, babies begin to attend to and imitate facial expressions. They become very adept at distinguishing facial expressions and can equate them with emotions such as happiness, sadness, and surprise (Meltzoff & Moore, 1977). By the third month of life they have all the emotional expressions in place and begin to make judgments about how to respond when placed in a variety of situations (Walden, 1993).

From these early interactions, infants develop attending behaviors, and by 6 months of age they begin to show an interest in sounds and respond to voices. By their first birthday they can speak one or two words clearly and follow simple requests, and by 18 to 24 months of age they have a vocabulary of between 200 and 300 words. At this stage in their development children are expressing themselves in two-word statements. By age 5 their vocabularies have expanded to approximately 2,000 words, and they are capable of producing lengthy sentences that contain information that pertains to the past and future (Bernstein & Tiegerman-Farber, 2009). Vocabulary growth and development continue to occur at a rapid pace throughout the school years, with the average high school student acquiring a vocabulary of more than 30,000 words by the time of graduation (Nagy & Herman, 1987).

All parents want their children to experience these milestones, and parents who have children who are deaf are no different. Faced with barriers to spoken communication, parents and primary caregivers must determine how they will communicate with their children in order to provide them with the same opportunities afforded to those who can hear. Recognizing that they provide the initial language role model for their children, they search for strategies to enhance language learning, fully aware that it will become the starting point for mastering literacy. In their search they consider mode of communication—whether their children will use sign or speech or a combination of both as their primary means of expressing themselves—type of amplification, and what their overall goals are for their children.

Selecting a Mode of Communication: Factors Families Consider

Annually, approximately 5,000 families experience the birth of an infant who is deaf (Thompson et al., 2001). While coming to terms with the diagnosis of deafness, professionals frequently encourage primary caregivers to select a communication method that, essentially, will eventually play a contributing role in their child's identity and how he or she views being deaf. When parents select a mode of communication, they search for a means to engage in meaningful exchanges with their child; however, the mode they select will also inadvertently convey what being deaf means to them. Therefore, what might initially appear to be a simple decision on the surface can become a very complex and overall daunting task with considerable and significant far-reaching ramifications. In reality, when they select a communication mode, they also make a statement regarding their acceptance of their child's deafness and whether they want their child to develop a Deaf identity, a hearing identity, or both.

Several factors contribute to the decision-making process. These include, but are not limited to, the caregivers' background knowledge and understanding of what it means to have a significant hearing loss, plus the initial viewpoints they hear from professionals to the field of deaf education. Other factors include the caregivers' perceptions of assistive technology, the quality and availability of support services, and their feelings of self-efficacy (DesJardin, Eisenberg, & Hodapp, 2006; Eleweke & Rodda, 2000). Based on a study conducted by Eleweke and Rodda, parents were strongly influenced by the information professionals provided to them regarding hearing loss, especially during the period immediately after the hearing loss was diagnosed. Their data further indicated that parents' perceptions of hearing aids and other assistive listening devices also influenced their choice of a communication approach.

Research indicates that the mother is frequently the primary individual who determines the mode of communication that will be used in the home (Kluwin & Gaustad, 1991). Oftentimes, she is also the individual who engages the child in activities that will promote language development. Studies conducted by DesJardin et al. (2006) reveal that mothers who are self-efficacious feel more competent interacting with their child in activities that promote language development. They tend to spend more quality time immersing the child in a variety of activities that draw on higher level language strategies and are more persistent in their attempt to promote growth and development. Conversely, mothers who are not self-efficacious are more likely to employ more lower language strategies and experience lower quality interactions with their child.

These early language experiences have been shown to make a profound impact on the child and what he or she learns on a daily basis (DesJardin et al., 2006). It is well established that language provides an avenue for lifelong learning; it also serves an integral function as children begin to develop the basic skills for social functioning. As parents engage their children in effective back-and-forth exchanges, they are laying the foundation for their child's acquisition of language while supporting the structure for both social and academic development (Freeman, Dieterich, & Rak, 2002).

As children get older these linguistic interactions become even more critical for social and emotional development. It is through this sharing of information that social norms are communicated, behavioral rules are conveyed, and explanations are provided for observed and imminent social-emotional events. When this information is effectively conveyed it allows for a more rapid and detailed transmission of social information both implicitly and explicitly. Several studies have indicated that children have a tendency to develop impulsive behaviors when this type of communication is lacking; oftentimes, they have a poorer self-image, display more disruptive behavior, and have an external locus of control (Marschark, 1993).

SIBLING RELATIONSHIPS

A plethora of research validates the critical role parents play in child development. However, parents are only one part of the family unit. The family has been described as a powerful system that is divided into subsystems where family relationships are formed that are both interdependent and mutually interactive. According to Minuchin (1974), if a change occurs in one part of the system it can have a dynamic affect on all the other subsystems. Siblings comprise one of these subsystems, and siblings who can hear have been studied extensively by researchers. Several of these studies have highlighted the importance of sibling relationships in child development (Garcia, Shaw, Winslow, & Yaggi, 2000) as well as how these permanent and longitudinal relationships affect their social and cognitive skills as well as their self-concepts (Azmitia & Hesser, 1993; Weaver, Coleman, & Ganong, 2003).

After the birth of a younger sibling, firstborn children may experience a variety of feelings. Although some may feel that their parents love them less than before and are more enamored with the newborn (Dunn, 1985; Dunn & Kendrick, 1982), others may be excited about the new child viewing him or her as a potential playmate, confidante, and friend (Cicirelli, 1995; Lamb & Sutton-Smith, 1982). Parents may opt to delegate new responsibilities to older siblings, thus encouraging them to become more independent. Some children accept these responsibilities eagerly and are willing to help care for the younger child, but others may feel that they are being slighted and become more clingy and demanding as they vie for their parents' attention.

Once the newborn has been assimilated into the family unit, each individual generally assumes a myriad of new roles and responsibilities. The interactions that will follow have the potential to impact and contribute to the emotional well-being of each family member. Research indicates that older brothers and sisters can serve as positive role models, companions, and playmates for their younger siblings (Cicirelli, 1995; McHale, Whiteman, Kim, & Crouter, 2007). Studies also reveal that the temperament of each child can influence the degree of companionship, support, rapport, competitiveness, or rivalry outwardly expressed in these relationships (Brody & Stoneman, 1993; Cicirelli, 1995). Furthermore, studies that have examined parental practices, traditions, and morals related to ethnic and cultural backgrounds indicate that all these factors play a role in family dynamics and the forming of sibling relationships (McHale et al., 2007).

Although copious studies have been conducted on hearing families regarding the emotional well-being of siblings within the constellation of the family unit, very few published studies pertain to siblings of children who are deaf or hard of hearing (Bat-Chava & Martin, 2002). General research on children with disabilities and their siblings indicates that the child without a disability may display a wide array of reactions to having a child with a disability in the family. For some the disability elicits a heightened sense of responsibility, new insights, understanding, and enlightened perspectives on interactions and bonding (Crnic & Leconte, 1986; Dyson, 1998). These children exhibit greater tolerance for differences; they are well adjusted and demonstrate maturity, empathy, and a sense of pride in the accomplishments of the child with a disability (Powell & Ogle, 1985).

Other studies reveal a more negative perspective. One body of research has examined some of the social concerns siblings without a disability have when they have a younger sister or brother who has a disability. Some worry about the social stigma of being with a sibling who has a disability (Boyce & Barnett, 1993; McHale et al., 2007; Nixon & Cummings, 1999). They recognize that they may have to contend with how their peers will react toward their brother or sister during social interactions within the classroom, community, and other school-related events. Subsequently, they may have fears that their sibling will be treated differently or badly (McHale et al.).

Research pertinent to family interactions reveals that it is very difficult to predict the effect, if any, a child with a disability can have on sibling relationships. This is due, in part, to numerous static factors such as age, sex, birth order, age spacing, family size, and type and severity of the disability (Verte, Hebbrecht, & Roeyers, 2006). This has led researchers to examine the more dynamic aspects of the family system, such as parental preferential treatment (Bat-Chava & Martin, 2002; McGuire, Dunn, & Plomin, 1995; McHale & Pawletko, 1992; Woolfe, 2001), temperament of the sibling (Dunn & McGuire, 1992), how the parents cope with stress (Dyson, 1996; Roeyers & Mycke, 1995), and parental expectations and communication used by the parents (Kaminsky & Dewey, 2001; Pollard & Rendon, 1999; Prizant, Meyer, & Lobato, 1997; Van Eldik, Veerman, Treffers, & Verhulst, 2000).

Sibling Relationships: Interactions Between Children Who Are Deaf and Those Who Can Hear

Although a paucity of research focuses on how siblings, deaf and hearing, feel about each other, those published findings reveal varying results. Several of the existing studies that address the psychological adjustment of both groups of siblings generally base their findings on extensive case studies or on reports provided by parents. Very rarely have the siblings been interviewed (Israelite, 1986). However, upon review of the available studies, it becomes apparent that the emotional issues and relationships cited in these studies are similar to those exhibited by siblings of children with other disabilities and children with no disabilities (Atkins, 1982; Israelite; Schwirian, 1976).

Research conducted by Raghuraman (2008) explored the emotional well-being of older siblings of children who are deaf and hard of hearing and older siblings of children with typical hearing. Through a series of interviews and questionnaires, three main findings emerged. First, she determined that children who have a disability do not have a negative effect on sibling relationships. This is contrary to previous research conducted by Atkins (1987), Dyson, Edgar, and Crnic (1989), and Lobato, Barbour, Hall, and Miller (1987).

Second, the parents and siblings surveyed in the study appeared to share similar perceptions regarding sibling relationships, with the exception of interpersonal concerns. Parents expressed concerns indicating they felt that their hearing children wanted to spend more time with them and less time with their sister or brother who had the hearing loss. Furthermore, parents perceived that the hearing siblings felt they were being ignored by their parents and that the child with the hearing loss dictated what the family could do. However, the older siblings did not seem to feel as strongly as the parents did regarding these concerns (Raghuraman, 2008). Third, with respect to temperament, parental perceptions indicated older siblings seemed to experience greater difficulties dealing with their younger siblings who had a less severe hearing loss, being more tolerant and accepting of those with more severe losses.

Verte, Hebbrecht, and Roeyers (2006) have also compared siblings of children who are deaf with siblings of children with typical hearing. Their investigation first examined the quality of sibling relationships and the psychological adjustment siblings experience when a sister or brother becomes part of the family unit. Second, they wanted to determine how the quality of the relationship is related to the development of the siblings. Was there any evidence of differences for siblings of a child who is deaf or hard of hearing when compared to siblings of typically hearing children? Third, they wanted to compare the perceptions of social competence in siblings as expressed by both the parents and the siblings.

Based on the premise that positive sibling relationships are associated with less loneliness, anxiety, and behavior problems, they wanted to determine if there were any significant differences between the two groups of children. Their findings indicated that there were no significant differences in the quality of the sibling relationships. This further confirms previous studies indicating siblings of a child with a disability tend to exhibit very positive feelings toward their brother or sister who has a disability (Bagenholm & Gillberg, 1991; Kaminsky & Dewey, 2001; Roeyers & Mycke, 1995). Results of this study further indicated only a few differences between the siblings in both groups in the domain of social competence (Verte, Iverson, & Castrataro, 2006). Findings suggested younger children between the ages of 6 and 10 felt they were less competent than those between 11 and 16 years of age. Keeping in mind that peer relationships become increasingly important as children age, the increased number of contacts with peers can become a contributing factor to why siblings feel more competent as they become older.

SELF-ESTEEM: A REFLECTION OF ONE'S SELF-IMAGE

Social competence, family cohesion, and communication exchanges all play critical roles in enhancing one's quality of life. Another important attribute frequently cited in the literature is self-esteem. Self-esteem can be viewed as a reflection of the individual's self-worth or self-image. Several factors have been identified as having a direct bearing on how one develops positive self-esteem. These include early parent–child interactions as children begin to form their perceptions of who they are; recognizing that the individual is loved for himself or herself (Luterman & Ross, 1991); being the recipient of affection; experiencing harmony in the home; becoming an active participant in family activities; and being respected for individual differences (Santrock, 1999).

Desselle and Pearlmutter (1997) have investigated the effect that parents' communication methods have on the self-esteem of their children who are deaf. Hearing parents of adolescents who are deaf ranging in age between 13 and 19, and all fluent in ASL, were administered a communication inventory while their children responded to a questionnaire related to self-esteem. Findings revealed that the mode of communication utilized by the parents can contribute to their deaf adolescent's level of self-esteem. Parents who communicated through ASL and used Total Communication conveyed a sense of acceptance of their child's deafness, thus influencing the child's feelings of self-worth in a positive way. Their results further indicated that when parents had mastered only a few signs or communicated primarily through speech, and their children were required to rely on speech reading, for the majority of their conversations they, in turn, expressed lower levels of self-esteem.

Research conducted by Woolfe (2001) examined a group of children who were deaf to determine if their levels of self-esteem were influenced by the hearing status of both of their parents as well as their siblings. Forty-five children between the ages of 10 and 14 participated in the study. Ten children had parents and siblings who were deaf, 4 with parents who were deaf and siblings who could hear, 11 with hearing parents and siblings who were deaf, and 20 with hearing parents and hearing siblings. All the children completed the Battle "Self Esteem" Inventory and the Family Systems Test.

Results of Woolfe's study (2001) indicate that deaf children of deaf parents have higher self-esteem scores than deaf children of hearing parents. This pattern was consistent regardless of whether the sibling was deaf or hearing. This finding is consistent with previous research conducted by Bat-Chava (1993). Qualitative interviews conducted as part of the study revealed that ease of communication and understanding between parents and siblings were important and salient factors in the deaf child's world. Furthermore, the lower self-esteem ratings exhibited by children who were deaf whose parents could hear were seen in children if communication and understanding on the part of the child was viewed to be of poor quality (Woolfe). These findings reiterate previous findings of Rodda (1966) and Gregory (1976).

Interviews conducted by Woolfe (2001), Corker (1996), and others have shed additional insights into the impact parental interactions, communication mode, and the quality of family relationships have on the feelings of self-esteem of the child who is deaf. Oftentimes, when a diagnosis of deafness is made parents are so overcome by their own feelings of grief that they fail to see the impact their emotions are having on their child. One deaf man described his feelings when his parents were told he was deaf:

> "He repeated the same kinds of tests that my mother and father had tried and eventually announced that I was deaf. My parents were broken apart. My mother and father were crying—I'd never seen them do that before. . . . I remember feeling that awful sinking feeling inside because I didn't know what I had done. . . . I didn't understand. I thought I was responsible for their tears and I was very worried." (Corker, 1996, p. 69)

Woolfe (2001) reiterates some of the feelings deaf children of deaf parents and deaf siblings expressed regarding their perceptions of communication and their feelings of self-esteem:

> "We are all close, never left out. . . . If I have problems I always tell my Mum and Dad who often understand my view."
>
> "I understand all of my Mum and Dad's conversations."

> "My brother is Deaf and I like him, he is always showing me different things and tells me how to cope with problems. I feel he is like my future as he is Deaf too." (Wolfe, 2001, p. 8).

These are contrasted by the feelings of children who are deaf who have hearing parents and hearing siblings:

> "I don't understand my parents' conversations, I feel left out. My family often talk amongst themselves; it's making me worried and frustrated."
>
> "I have a nice family, my parents do not sign. My family are all hearing. . . . I don't understand what they say. I just daydream."
>
> "My brother won't let me join his friends because he is embarrassed. He has his own friends, my friends are Deaf. My brother won't learn to sign, my Mum is trying to teach him." (Wolfe, 2001, p. 10)

Summary

Parents provide the cornerstone for child development. Serving as the initial caregivers for infants, they instill in them feelings of trust, love, and acceptance. Later, they provide the extended network that will support their children through a lifetime of growth and enrichment as their offspring emerge into independent young adults. Family units are comprised of extended family members, siblings, and significant others from various ethnic and socioeconomic backgrounds. They can be characterized as dynamic, multifaceted, unique, and diverse segments of society who serve a vital role in the transmission of cultural ideals, beliefs, and values. Striving for a sense of equilibrium, they are forced to deal with a multitude of uncertainties when a child who is deaf enters the family unit. For parents who are Deaf, the child is usually welcomed with joy and anticipation of what the future holds for them. For parents who can hear, their limited background knowledge and basic understanding of what it means to raise a child who is deaf can initially be viewed as a frightening and overwhelming undertaking.

From the beginning, parents face an onslaught of decisions regarding hearing-aid technology, communication methods, and issues surrounding cultural identities. The choices they make will play a contributing role in the child's development, his or her self-concept, and, in essence, their impact on virtually every member of the family. As parents convey unconditional love and acceptance, and treat each child as an equal, respected, and valued member of the family, healthy personalities are able to take root and begin to develop.

The choices parents will make are as varied as the individuals who will make them. For some, electing to use sign language with their children will be a good fit. For others an auditory verbal approach will open the door to successful communication. Although some will seek out Deaf role models for their children, thereby encouraging a bilingual/bicultural identity, others will devote hours to speech development and rely on hearing members of society for role models for their children. However, by accepting the child as a whole child, and by recognizing the potential that lies within, the stage is set for each individual to embrace life and engage in all the experiences life has to offer.

6

Language Acquisition
Acquiring the Building Blocks for Communication

Language is central to our existence. Defined as a socially shared code, it provides a mechanism whereby individuals can connect with others, engage in the exchange of information, think, and express ideas. It further functions as an avenue for emotions to be conveyed and identities to be revealed. Language serves an integral role in psychosocial development while creating inroads into the rich vernacular that surrounds us. We can use language to communicate by speaking, signing, or writing. Regardless of the form it takes it must be shared to be considered language. What are the components of language? How does language develop in children who can hear? How does it develop in children who are prelinguistically deaf? What modes of communication do children and adults who are deaf and hard of hearing use?

THE COMPONENTS OF LANGUAGE

All languages are comprised of complex rules that govern how words are used, how sentences are formed, and, thereby, how meaning is conveyed. These rules provide users of the same language with the tools to understand or comprehend what is being expressed while also providing them with correct linguistic structure so they can formulate ideas that will be understood by others. Children and adults are considered to be linguistically competent when they possess an implicit knowledge of the rules regarding language use. With these rules in place, individuals can create an infinite number of sentences and can manipulate words in a variety of ways, be cognizant of what they are saying, and recognize when they are and are not making sense (Bernstein & Tiegerman-Farber, 2009). According to Bloom and Lahey (1978), language can be divided into three major components: form, content, and use.

Form refers to the surface structure of the language and is represented in phonology, morphology, and syntax. In essence, it reflects the grammatical features of the language.

Content refers to the semantics of the language, describing the meaning of words. Through semantics, languages have the capacity to refer to content and expand upon the implied meanings of words.

Use refers to pragmatics, the communicative function or intent of the words. It describes how words are used to deliver information, make requests, and convey ideas within various situational contexts.

Form

Based on Bloom and Lahey's (1978) conceptual framework, form refers to the linguistic elements that connect sounds and symbols with meaning. By following the rules that govern sounds and their various combinations (phonology), adhering to the rules that govern the internal organization of words (morphology), and abiding by the rules that specify word order (syntax), a variety of sentence types can be expressed.

PHONOLOGY. Phonology refers to the system of rules that govern sound production in a language. Furthermore, each language can be characterized by the specific phonemes, or speech sounds, that distinguish it as a language. A phoneme is defined as the smallest linguistic unit of speech that signals a difference in meaning. Phonemes consist of vowels and consonants; when one or both of these components are altered, the meaning of the word changes. Words, such as *cat* and *hat,* differ in initial sound only, *pet* and *put* in medial sounds, and *ear* and *eat* in final sounds. Therefore, by definition, in these words, the /c/, /h/, /e/, /u/, /r/, and /t/ are all different phonemes.

Two rules govern phoneme use. The first is the distributional rule, which describes how sounds can be placed in various word positions. The second is the sequencing rule, which dictates which sounds can be used together within the same syllable (Bernstein & Tiegerman-Farber, 2009).

MORPHOLOGY. Morphology is the second component of language. It studies the structure of words and word formation. It examines the smallest linguistic units that have meaning and those that represent a grammatical function. Some words can be viewed as a single unit, and others can be divided into smaller units. The smallest unit of a word is a morpheme (Valli & Lucas, 2000).

Morphemes that can stand alone as words are referred to as free morphemes. Words such as *girl, cute, house,* and *please* are examples of words that cannot be divided into smaller parts and still have meaning. However, morphemes can be added to words to reflect plurality or tense. When used in this manner they are referred to as bound or inflectional morphemes. For example, the *s* or the *ed* in *girls* or *talked,* respectively, performs a grammatical function, thus altering the meaning of the word. Although the *s* and *ed* are the smallest units of the word, in isolation they have no meaning and therefore cannot function as free morphemes.

Bound morphemes function as affixes. When added to the beginning of words they are referred to as prefixes, as in *unemployed.* When they occur at the end of the word, they are identified as suffixes, as in *employable.* In addition, they can be used to change one word into another, thus creating new words. For example, the word *happy* can be changed into *happiness* by adding *ness;* when this occurs, the word reflects a different part of speech and is referred to as a derivational morpheme (Bernstein & Tiegerman-Farber, 2009).

SYNTAX. Syntax refers to word order designating how words must be arranged and organized within sentences; it studies phrases, clauses, and sentence types. Moreover, it allows language users the flexibility to combine words into phrases, to combine phrases into sentences, and to transform one sentence type into another. In essence, it provides a mechanism for generating an almost infinite number of sentences from a finite set of words. It assists in the orchestration of sentences by establishing parameters for appropriate word order (correct use of the parts of speech) and phraseology.

When we are familiar with syntactic rules we are alerted to the fact that sentences have different structure and/or meanings. This is illustrated in the following sentences:

The dog chased Faye and Megghan.

Did the dog chase Faye and Megghan?

The dog was chased by Faye and Megghan.

Megghan and Faye were chased by the dog.

Megghan chased the dog and Faye.

These rules also alert us to sentences that are not grammatically correct, such as these:

Dog the Faye chased Megghan and.

Was chased Faye Megghan dog and by the.

Syntax allows for the development of simple and complex sentences. It provides the structure for word use and the flexibility to convey a multitude of thoughts and ideas.

Content

From a linguistic standpoint the term *content* refers to the component of language that involves meaning. It allows for the formation of language maps while providing us with information about objects, events, people, and the relationships among them. Included in content are the rules that govern semantics, the subsystem of language that addresses words and their meanings, as well as the links that bind them together (Bernstein & Tiegerman-Farber, 2009).

SEMANTICS. Semantics focuses on the meaning of words (lexicon), phrases, and sentences. It directs its attention to how words are used to describe objects, people, and situations, and how they can further be used to refer to animate as well as inanimate objects. Semantics relies on the mental word dictionaries of language users. It recognizes the fact that children's comprehension of words varies appreciably from that of adults, and that breakdowns in the transmission of messages can lie in the connotation as well as the denotation of the word choice. For example, a young child's mental image of the word *monster* might equate with a character on *Sesame Street.* In turn, overhearing an adult refer to a "monstrous house," the description of size would quite possibly be lost as the child's content map would register a mental image of the furry characters, thus assuming that monsters lived in the house.

Use

When referring to the use component of language, linguists pay particular attention to the rules that dictate how language is used in a variety of social contexts. These rules are referred to as pragmatics. Pragmatics encompasses the rules that determine the reason(s) for communicating, referred to as communicative functions or intentions, and that govern the choice of codes to be used when communicating (Bloom & Lahey, 1978).

PRAGMATICS. Pragmatics addresses how language is used to communicate in social contexts. It examines the rules that set the stage for the exchange of language, and it focuses on the reasons why individuals converse with each other. In addition, the pragmatic aspect of language examines how those involved in dialogues initiate and take turns during a conversation. Pragmatics influences the word choices we elect to use and how we use these words to interact with our friends, co-workers, and subordinates. For example, although it might be acceptable to address a friend with "Hey, dude!" that same phrase would be considered an inappropriate greeting to use in professional settings. Gaining mastery of pragmatics is instrumental in granting children entry into and maintaining their place in their peer group. The study of pragmatics further probes how those engaged in discourse remain active participants in a conversation once it has been initiated, how they change topics, and how they end conversations (Hall, Oyer, & Haas, 2001).

Pragmatics delves into the realm of discourse and analyzes how speakers organize their thoughts into coherent conversations. Furthermore, it takes into consideration the speaker's word choice, the recipient's knowledge base, and the choice of words that are selected to convey the message. Although some conversations involve the exchange of information between individuals, one knowledgeable regarding the subject matter while the other is not, other exchanges involve participants with equal knowledge bases. Familiarity with context will determine how much background information is needed for comprehension to occur.

Pragmatics differs from semantics. Although semantics examines what words mean, pragmatics reflects on the intent of the content. In addition, it observes the rules speakers must follow as they initiate and maintain a dialogue, and how they learn how to make appropriate comments once they begin conversing with someone. Individuals who posses all these skills are deemed effective communicators.

STAGES OF LANGUAGE DEVELOPMENT

The foundation for language learning originates in infancy. From the first weeks of life babies begin to attend to and imitate facial expressions. Furthermore, they quickly become adept at distinguishing emotions such as happiness, sadness, and surprise (Meltzoff & Moore, 1977). By the third month of life, they have all the major emotional expressions in place and begin to make judgments about how to respond when placed in a variety of situations (Walden, 1993).

From these early interactions, infants develop attending behaviors. Between 3 to 6 months of age they begin to show an interest in sounds and respond to voices. Throughout this same period, babies engage in babbling. In the beginning, they produce single units consisting of combined, loosely formed consonants and vowels such as *goo* and *ah* (Marschark, Lang, & Albertini, 2002). Between 6 and 8 months of age vocal play emerges with an increase in the variety of sounds that the child produces. At this same time, hearing infants begin to produce well-formed syllables that signal the onset of repetitive babbling. From the early *bababa* and *gagaga*, the foundation is laid for spoken language development, for as infants begin to produce these sounds, they elicit responses from their parents that signal the beginning of language-based, parent–child interactions (p. 93).

Between 8 and 12 months of age, variegated babbling appears, consisting of strings of alternating consonants and vowels (e.g., *babigabadidu*) that corresponds with the intonation patterns of adult language (Werker & Tees, 1984). During this same period echolalia appears, characterized by a parrotlike imitation of another's speech including tonal qualities and gestures (McLaughlin, 1998). By 12 months of age jargon emerges, consisting of strings of syllables that mirror the stress patterns of adult speech (Bernstein & Tiegerman-Farber, 2009).

From these early beginnings the foundation is laid for the development of both expressive and receptive language skills. By the time young children are 12 months of age they typically have an expressive vocabulary of 1 or more words; this increases to a 4- to 6-word vocabulary by 15 months, a 20-word vocabulary at 18 months, and a 200- to 300-word vocabulary at 24 months. Generally speaking, children's receptive vocabularies exceed their expressive vocabularies. It has been noted that when children have an expressive vocabulary of 10 words they are usually able to comprehend at least 50 words (Bernstein & Tiegerman-Farber, 2009, p. 36). Needless to say, children's vocabularies grow at an astonishing rate. Owens (2001) estimates that children add approximately 5 words to their vocabularies every day between the ages of 18 months and 6 years. Furthermore, it is interesting to note that children's initial expressive vocabularies have been found to be very similar, in spite of differences in environment and their upbringing (Pan & Gleason, 2001).

Children's vocabularies continue to increase as they enter school and begin their educational journey. By 6 years of age, the child possesses an expressive vocabulary of 2,600 words and a receptive vocabulary of between 20,000 and 24,000 words (Owens, 2005). As children progress from elementary school through high school they expand their basic word definitions to include a broader understanding of abstract vocabulary, metaphors, idioms, and proverbs. By fourth grade children have acquired and are able to comprehend more abstract vocabulary items (Miller & Gildea, 1987), and by sixth grade their receptive vocabularies have grown to 50,000 items.

As children progress through school they rely on this word base to gather knowledge, perform academic tasks, and engage in social discourse. When they initially enter the classroom it is generally assumed they are "language ready." Spending the majority of their day in language-rich settings, they are required to draw upon these skills to comprehend the academic aspects of what is being taught. Within a very short time it becomes apparent to them that their command of both spoken and later written language is critical if they want to be successful. Furthermore, they realize that they are also expected to be familiar with the rules for social interaction so they can participate in classroom exchanges.

Throughout these early school years important linguistic growth occurs. Perhaps the most significant advances are made in the area of language use, or pragmatics. During this time children learn how to become good communication partners, how to make indirect requests, and how to process language that is exchanged in the classroom. Development of pragmatics involves more than the mastery of syntactic structures. It entails developing a familiarity with sociolinguistic rules that are related to language use within a variety of communication settings. These rules involve the act of speech; however, they also govern the discourse structures in which speech acts are embedded (Haynes & Shulman, 1998).

From an early age children become adept at incorporating different registers as they address their friends, parents, siblings, and authority figures. (*Register* refers to formal or informal word choices used in direct address, as well as simple versus complex sentence structures.) They quickly learn that speech can be used to administer directives as well as to elicit responses. By the time children are 8 years old they incorporate different registers when addressing infants, their parents, and other adults. They seem to recognize that they must reduce the length and complexity of their sentences when speaking to infants. Furthermore, although they may interact with their parents using short conversational narratives peppered with occasional whining and more demanding requests, they are also capable of interacting with adults in a more polite and formal manner (Owens, 2005).

As children progress from kindergarten through third grade their metalinguistic skills begin to develop, and during this time they begin to think and talk about language. According to VanKleek (1984), as this evolves, children begin to recognize that language is an arbitrary and conventional code, that it is a system of units and rules, and that this system can be used for communication. Throughout middle and late childhood, children use these skills to analyze how words are used. This provides them with insights into the world of abstractions and affords them the opportunity to understand that words can represent inanimate objects and thus have no direct bearing on their personal experiences.

The transition from childhood to adolescence can be observed in classrooms where students are expected to translate their "word knowledge" into "world knowledge" (Wiig & Secord, 1992). At this juncture new words and concepts are added to the lexicon, and old words assume new and subtle meanings. Double-functioning words such as *cold* and *bright* assume a psychological as well as a physical meaning, thus reflecting the development of advanced language skills (Asch & Nerlove, 1960).

Throughout high school, students are exposed to technical terms, abstract concepts, and words that have multiple meanings, as well as words that serve multiple functions. Thus, at the time of graduation, these individuals have been exposed to, and have learned the meaning of, at least 80,000 different words (Nippold, 1998b). This period is further marked by adolescents who are capable of producing complex sentences, use communication for purposes such as persuasion and negotiation, and engage in some metalinguistic discussions (Nippold, 1994; Whitmore, 2000).

During this developmental period, adolescents master more sophisticated communication strategies. They are able to take the perspective of the other listener and are capable of recognizing and correcting inept communication acts. The ability to use language in the conversational domain becomes even more critical as children move into adolescence (Nippold, 2000; Whitmire, 2000). During this time, conversations become a pivotal point in social development as preteens and teens seek peer acceptance and build friendships. These conversations are interspersed with idioms, puns, and sarcasm, as well as slang and "in-group language." The ability of adolescents to discern the appropriate uses of this slang is a contributing factor in group membership and peer acceptance (Nippold, 1998a). As teens near young adulthood their language abilities continue to mature and they are able to incorporate more sophisticated linguistic and pragmatic skills.

Language learning spans one's lifetime. Beginning in infancy, and continuing over the duration of only a few short years, most children develop a rich and complex linguistic system. This system is acquired with little apparent effort and with no formal instruction. From this starting point, children quickly progress from expressing simple semantic relationships using two-word utterances to formulating and expressing more sophisticated concepts in multiword sentences (Rose, McAnally, & Quigley, 2004).

Throughout early childhood, shared environmental influences play a significant role in language development (Spinath, Price, Dale, & Plomin, 2004). The quality of the interactions that occur between children and their primary caregivers, fostered through direct and indirect learning experiences, provide children with early language role models, thus fostering language development. Then, through a process of imitating and modeling they acquire a command of spoken language and learn how to engage in verbal exchanges with others. In time, these verbal exchanges evolve into conversational fluency, a precursor to mastering comprehension of printed materials. When children possess fluency in their native language they can later be taught how to transfer their mastery of sentence formation, vocabulary, and world knowledge into decoding printed text, an essential skill needed throughout life.

From these early language experiences children are provided with vocabulary to use as a mechanism for conveying their basic needs to others. Later, as their linguistic abilities become more sophisticated and their understanding of communication rules are deepened, they possess the fundamental skills needed to engage in the verbal sharing of thoughts and ideas with others.

Subsequently, as individuals form additional interconnections and engage in spoken exchanges, linguistic skills are enriched and their knowledge base is enhanced.

For those who can hear, this is initially accomplished automatically by being privy to the ambience of spoken language. However, when infants are born deaf or lose their hearing prior to age 2, the challenge of mastering the intrinsic complexities required for successful communication to transpire through an auditory/verbal language can become a daunting, if not altogether impossible, task. Throughout the past several decades the potential for children who are deaf to develop and communicate through spoken language has improved tremendously. This is attributed to two major factors: technology and teaching/learning methods (Blamey, 2003). Although the majority of hearing parents elect speech as their primary mode of communication for their children who are deaf, others prefer using ASL or a form of manual communication.

What are the various communication approaches used today? What impact does mode of communication have on language development? How does it affect spoken word acquisition and later complex written forms of expression and recognition? Furthermore, what bearing does it have on vocabulary growth and development in their children who are deaf or experience difficulty hearing speech?

MODES OF COMMUNICATION

The term *communication* can be defined as a process in which two entities enter into an exchange of information to transmit thoughts, messages, or ideas. Conveyed in various ways, it may take the form of speech, text, signs, symbols, or gestures. Described as an interactive process, it requires a sender who formulates or encodes a message and a receiver who comprehends or decodes the message (Owens, 1990). Successful communication ultimately occurs when those involved in the exchange are actively engaged and attuned to the needs of the other. By attending to body language, intonation patterns, stress, and speech/sign rate, the listener can ascertain the emotions and attitudes conveyed by the speaker/signer.

Parents and caregivers are ultimately responsible for determining which language and what mode or modes of communication they will use to converse with family members. Within hearing families, the parents' native language is generally used without giving it much, if any, thought. However, when a child who is deaf becomes part of the family unit, parents are faced with the monumental task of determining how they will communicate with a child who cannot hear. Some rely on professionals for help, and others seek the opinions of family members and friends or search the Internet for suggestions.

As parents begin the journey in search of the most beneficial mode of communication to use with their child, they frequently encounter professionals with divergent viewpoints. Although some professionals promote an oral approach, others foster a visual approach and will provide parents with a wide array of choices including using ASL or one of the manually coded sign systems. Still others will encourage the use of a multimodal communication approach and will discuss options such as sign-supported speech (SSS), Total Communication, or Cued Speech. What is an oral approach? What is a visual approach and what does it mean to use ASL as a language to communicate? What is involved in a multimodal communication approach, and how does one incorporate sign-supported speech while talking? What is Cued Speech, and when would one use it? Figure 6.1 provides a synopsis of the three major approaches to communication. They move along a continuum from an oral approach to an approach that relies on multiple modalities to convey information and connect with others.

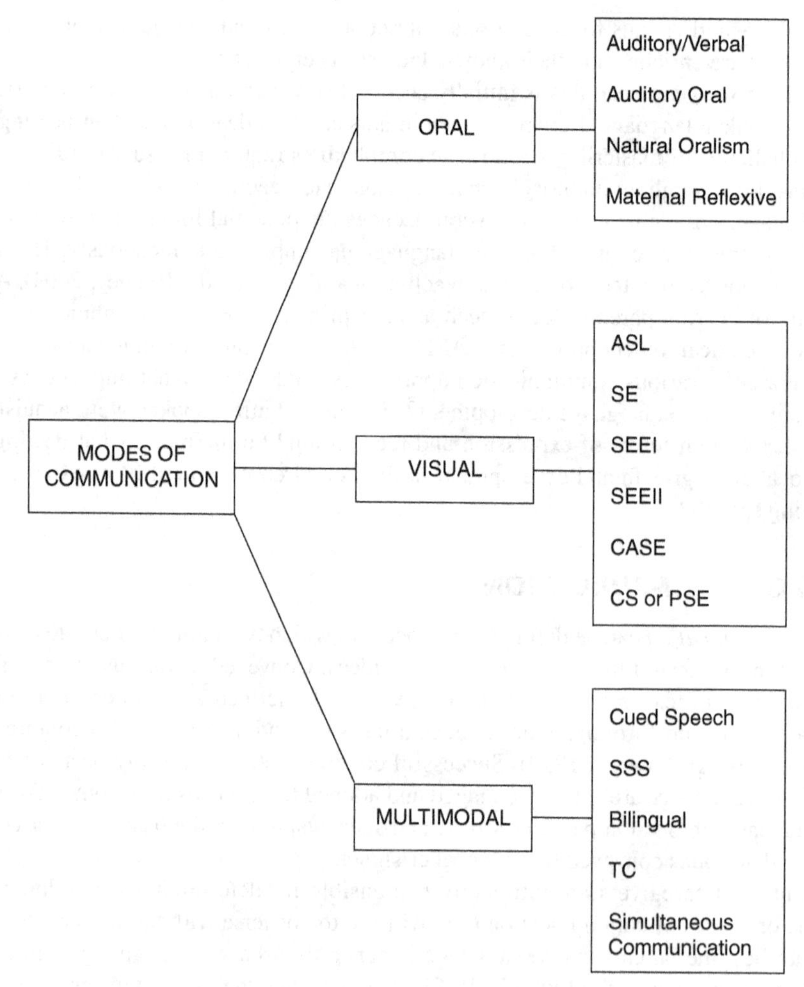

FIGURE 6.1 Communication modes: oral, visual, multimodal.

Oral Methods: Acquiring Spoken Language

Oral methods have a rich history of contributing to the communication and education of children who are deaf and hard of hearing. Broadly defined, they encompass those methods that focus on the "production and reception of spoken language without the support of a visual-manual language or an artificially developed communication system" (Beattie, 2006). Throughout the history of deaf education, oral methods have been described under the auspices of a multitude of names. (For a detailed list of oral methods, names, characteristics, and features, see Beattie.)

Contemporary oral methods practiced today include auditory-verbal therapy, the auditory oral approach, natural oralism/natural auralism, and the maternal reflective method. Although each of these approaches is unique in nature, the similarities all of them share are far more prevalent than their differences.

AUDITORY-VERBAL. Estabrooks (1994) defines auditory-verbal (AV) therapy as an approach that relies on the application and management of technology along with strategies, procedures, and techniques that focus on teaching children who are deaf or hard of hearing and how they can communicate through speech. Early in the therapy sessions, emphasis is placed on listening while restricting the child's access to lipreading (Andrews, Leigh, & Weiner, 2004). Auditory-verbal therapy stresses the importance of early identification, the consistent use of binaural amplification, strong parental involvement, and integration into family, academic, and social activities (Andrews et al., 2004).

Those who engage in AV therapy emphasize that parents play a primary role in the learning process. By teaching parents how to provide beneficial listening environments that promote listening and auditory learning, they become instrumental in the therapeutic process. Therapists invest time instructing parents on how to structure sequential activities that will foster enhanced audition, cognition, communication, language, and speech (Boucher Jones, 2001).

Those who embrace an AV approach attribute its success to the comprehensive nature of the activities. Contemporary AV therapies are based on the belief that as children begin to understand the value of sound they will later intuitively understand the function hearing serves as they develop emotionally, physically, psychologically, and socially (Beattie, 2006). The ultimate goal is to provide children with the strategies and techniques so they can utilize their residual hearing to the fullest extent possible. This will enable them to actively engage in spoken exchanges that transpire among family members and friends. Furthermore, these techniques will assist them as they interact within their neighborhood schools and within their communities.

AUDITORY-ORAL. Contemporary auditory-oral (AO) approaches share many of the tenets found in the AV approach. Both support the importance of early identification, a high level of parental involvement, advanced technology to facilitate auditory input, and interaction with highly qualified AO professionals. Proponents of the original AO approach placed emphasis on strategies that simultanously promoted the use of residual hearing and techniques that fostered lipreading. Thus, children were encouraged to develop their spoken language skills by using both auditory and visual cues. However, today equal attention is no longer given to the visual channel. Even though lipreading is not restricted as in the AV approach, it is no longer a focal point for therapy (Beattie, 2006).

Other differences merit discussion. Although supporters of the AV approach acknowledge educational success occurs when children are placed in their neighborhood schools in included classrooms, those fostering an AO approach believe that success can be measured in a wide variety of educational settings. Recognizing that students who are deaf and hard of hearing may benefit from a resource room or from partial mainstreaming, they further support the concept that children may attend a variety of educational settings before graduating from high school. In addition, the method of teaching language differs between the two approaches. AV therapeutic methods focus on normal developmental sequences, whereas AO techniques may be delivered in either a structured fashion or by using a more natural approach (Beattie, 2006).

NATURAL ORALISM/NATURAL AURALISM. The roots of natural oralism/natural auralism (NA) can be traced to the 1980s in Britain. Originally referred to as *natural oralism* (Harrison, 1980), it later became known as *natural auralism,* with emphasis placed on hearing and listening. Contemporary practitioners refer to it as the "oral/aural" or "auditory/oral" approach/method (Watson, 1998, as cited in Beattie, 2006).

According to Lewis (1996) emphasis is placed on the use of residual hearing while facilitating natural language development. Regardless of the degree of hearing loss, parents are instructed to talk with their child using age-appropriate language, never encouraging the child to imitate or respond vocally to any of their comments. However, parents are also told to respond positively to any and all attempted vocalizations produced by the child (Wells, 1986, as cited in Beattie, 2006).

Sharing like features with AV and AO, the oral/aural approach emphasizes the need for early intervention, the use of current technology, and the need to emphasize how to make maximum use of residual hearing. However, a unique feature of the NA approach encourages children to be active participants in the communication process without being corrected on their speech production. Furthermore, the child should be presented with a variety of topics, including those that are controversial and creative in nature. This will afford them the opportunity to increase their language base and draw on context clues that they have previously acquired.

MATERNAL REFLECTIVE METHOD. The maternal reflective method (MR) and the natural oralism/natural auralism approaches share several features. Both stress the importance of promoting spoken language skills, value the importance of emphasizing the use of residual hearing, recognize the importance of audiological support, and believe that language develops through a conversational approach (Powers et al., 1999, as cited in Beattie, 2006).

However, two distinguishing features separate the MR approach from the others. The first can be found in the attention given to exposing children to text from the very beginning stages. A second distinguishing feature involves reflection. Although other approaches mention reflection as part of their approach, the MR method is the only one that describes the procedure for completing this task. To accomplish the reflective piece, students are asked to write down the conversation and then analyze it while paying particular attention to the grammar, register, style, and form presented in the document.

These four oral approaches represent options parents have when selecting a viable means they can use to communicate with their child who is deaf or hard of hearing. Although the majority of hearing parents elect to embrace an aural/oral approach, others opt to use a visual/manual approach and learn ASL, or rely on one of the sign systems. ASL is a language that can be used in place of spoken English. In contrast, the sign systems are all visual representations of the English language and are designed to be used simultaneously with speech. These systems include the broad umbrella term Manually Coded English under which are found the Rochester Method, Seeing Essential English (SEE I), Signing Exact English (SEE II), and Signed English (SE). (See Table 6.1 for a summary and comparison of the oral modes of communication.)

Visual Modes of Communication

AMERICAN SIGN LANGUAGE. As you will recall from Chapter 2, ASL is a visual, gestural, rule-governed language that was created by and for deaf individuals living in the United States. Like other languages, it provides a systematic means for communicating thoughts, ideas, and feelings through the use of conventional symbols (Schein, 1984). Unlike spoken languages that rely on audition for transmission, ASL uses the visual representation of concepts utilizing three-dimensional space to transmit information (Borden, 1996).

Although many people have formed the misconception that ASL is merely English conveyed on the hands, a manual code for representing English, linguistic research has demonstrated that it is comparable in complexity and expressiveness to spoken languages (Smith, Lentz, & Mikos, 1988). ASL is not a form of English, and it is not universal. Consisting of its own grammar and syntax, it is comprised of precise hand shapes and movements as well as nonmanual

TABLE 6.1 Oral Methods of Communication

Auditory-Verbal	Auditory-Oral	Natural Oralism/Natural Auralism	Maternal Reflective Method
• A unisensory approach to communication and language. • Audition is considered the most important sense. • Emphasis is placed on listening to environmental sounds and voices on a continual basis (Estabrooks, 1994). • Visual cues are removed during directed listening therapy sessions, eliminating the opportunity for speechreading.	• A multisensory approach to communication. • Listening, speechreading, gestures, print, and environmental cues are all utilized to promote speech recognition. • Parents are encouraged to promote listening skills in natural settings where routine communication takes place.	• Originated in Britain. • Focus is on residual hearing while facilitating natural language development. • Encourages children to actively engage in the communication process without correcting their speech.	• Stresses the importance of utilizing residual hearing. • Believes language develops through a conversational approach. • Encourages students to reflect on various aspects of communication including grammar and register.

features. The shape and movements of the hands comprise the manual features of the language while the movement of the cheeks, lips, tongue, eyes, eyebrows, shoulders, and body shifts reflect the nonmanual features (Paul, 2009).

Because ASL is a rule-governed language, signers must adhere to the finite set of rules that delineate how the signs are formed, sequenced, and executed (Paul, 2009, p. 221). As versatile as any spoken language, ASL provides signers with a complete language whereby they can convey complex ideas, discuss abstract thoughts, and share everything from the most mundane content to the most beautifully expressed poetry and prose. Characteristic of other languages, new vocabulary is continually evolving in response to cultural and technological changes (Smith et al., 1988, p. 3)

The grammar of ASL is not based on sound; rather, it relies on "images made by fingers, hands, and arms—images that are linguistically shaped by movements of the eyebrows, lips and cheeks, by the hunching and thrusting of the shoulders, by the signer's posture" to communicate with those who share a common language (Schein & Stewart, 1995). Messages are conveyed within the signing space, an area that includes the space from the waist to the top of the head. Although the majority of signs are produced within an area referred to as the normal or general signing space—6 to 8 inches above the head and out from the shoulders—the area reserved for fingerspelling is much smaller. (Figure 6.2 provides an illustration of the space used to communicate using signs and fingerspelling.) By adhering to this area, the viewer has the opportunity to maintain eye contact while at the same time observing the speaker's hands and upper torso, thus attending to the signs and nonmanual signals being presented.

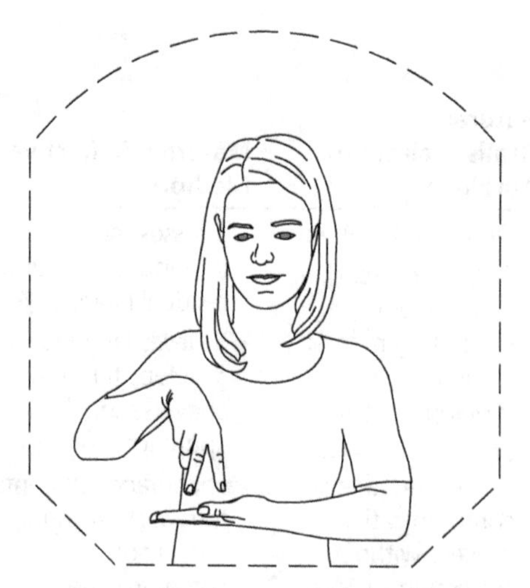
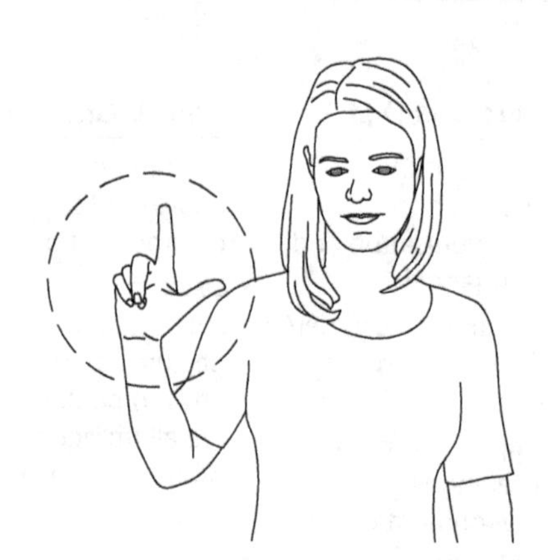

FIGURE 6.2 Signing and fingerspelling space.

Source: Courtesy of Marie A. Scheetz.

Sign space plays an integral role in ASL. It provides the backdrop for thoughts, ideas, and concepts to be expressed. It also affords the signer the opportunity to describe relationships, incorporate directional verbs, and utilize time indicators. Spoken languages follow a linear order, sound by sound, word by word, whereas ASL is produced visually with signs, simultaneously communicating additional information (i.e., number, adverbials, questions versus statements, and other grammatical information). This simultaneous additional information is conveyed through the signs, spatial relationships, sign movements, and nonmanual signals. As a result, signed messages require a two-part process on the part of signers. First, signers initiating a message must possess the ability to mentally construct a visual image of what they want to convey. Second, they must be able to accurately present concepts visually to ensure that recipients of the message are provided with the information that is intended.

Although ASL was developed by American Deaf people to communicate with each other, the standardization of the language did not begin until 1817 when the first school for the deaf opened in the United States. Under the leadership of Laurent Clerc, a deaf instructor originally from France, and Thomas Hopkins Gallaudet, the language passed from one generation to the next primarily through children who were deaf attending residential schools specifically designed for them. Due to the early influence of the teachings of Laurent Clerc, approximately 60% of the signs found in ASL are of French origin (Vernon & Andrews, 1990).

Even though the history of using sign language is well documented, it was not until the seminal work of Bill Stokoe in the 1960s that ASL was recognized as a bona fide language. Through his research he determined that signs could be viewed as having independent parts and that ASL could be expressed in a written format by transferring each part into its respective symbol.

MANUALLY CODED ENGLISH SIGN SYSTEMS. As previously emphasized, ASL has been developed by Deaf people and is widely used in the Deaf community. It is used for social exchanges of information and, with few exceptions, is not used by hearing teachers for instructional purposes in included or mainstream settings. This is due, in part, to the philosophy that students who are deaf and hard of hearing should be provided with a visual representation of

English. Originating in the 1970s, manually coded English sign systems were developed to assist students with the acquisition of spoken and written English.

Although schools may adopt a manual communication philosophy, it is generally housed within the confines of a signed English base. For the past several decades, the field of deaf education has been dominated by teachers who can hear. Embracing English as their first language, they have searched for ways to bridge the communication gap between those who are fluent in ASL and those who communicate through a form of English, regardless of whether it is spoken or written. Due to the vast grammatical differences that exist between the two languages (ASL and English), English-based signing systems have been developed to help bridge this gap. These systems are referred to as manually coded English.

Systems are not languages but, rather, are visual representations of the English language. In essence, they follow English word order, use contrived signs, and are designed to reflect the structure and vocabulary of English (Baker-Shenk & Cokely, 1980). These sign codes include the Rochester Method, Signed English (SE), Seeing Essential English (SEE I), Signing Exact English (See II), and Conceptually Accurate Signed English (CASE) (Humphrey & Alcorn, 1995). A brief description of these systems is included below.

Rochester Method. The Rochester Method was originally called "The Great Innovation." It is a system consisting solely of fingerspelling. One handshape is incorporated for each letter in the alphabet. (See Figure 6.3 for the Manual Alphabet.) Fingerspelling, or dactylogy, was formally introduced into the public school system in 1878. During that time, Zenus F. Westervelt was the superintendent of the School for the Deaf in Rochester, New York. Westervelt was a staunch oralist. However, during his tenure at the school, he became keenly aware of the students' deficiencies in English, especially when they expressed themselves through writing. As a result he looked for alternative methods to help ameliorate this problem.

Fingerspelling is a manual representation of the language that is spoken. Therefore, it has no separate syntax, morphology, phonology, or semantics; rather, it is dependent on the linguistic structure of the language it is representing (Wilbur, 1987). As words are spoken, they are spelled out letter by letter. The reader has the opportunity to view each letter as words are produced. Fingerspelling was designed to be used simultaneously with speech. However, for a person to spell at a conversational speed, he or she would be required to spell 12 letters per second. According to Bornstein (1974):

> "A comfortable rate of speed for adults transmitting to experienced readers is about 300 letters per minute or, using five letters for an average word, 60 words a minute (Bornstein, 1974). Moreover, it is doubtful that this rate would be comfortable for very long, for example, much more than 15 minutes. Using 150 words per minute as an average rate of speech, this fingerspelling rate is about 40 percent of the rate of speech or a 1:2½ ratio." (p. 331)

Signed English. The origins of Signed English can be traced to the mid 1970s and the work of Harry Bornstein and his associates. It grew out of a need to provide children who are deaf with a visual model of the English language. Although initially developed for use with preschool children, it later was used in the elementary school setting. Signed English is an English-based sign system designed to be used simultaneously with speech. Within this system two types of visual representations are used: approximately 3,000 sign words and 14 sign markers. Each sign word represents a separate entry in a standard English dictionary.

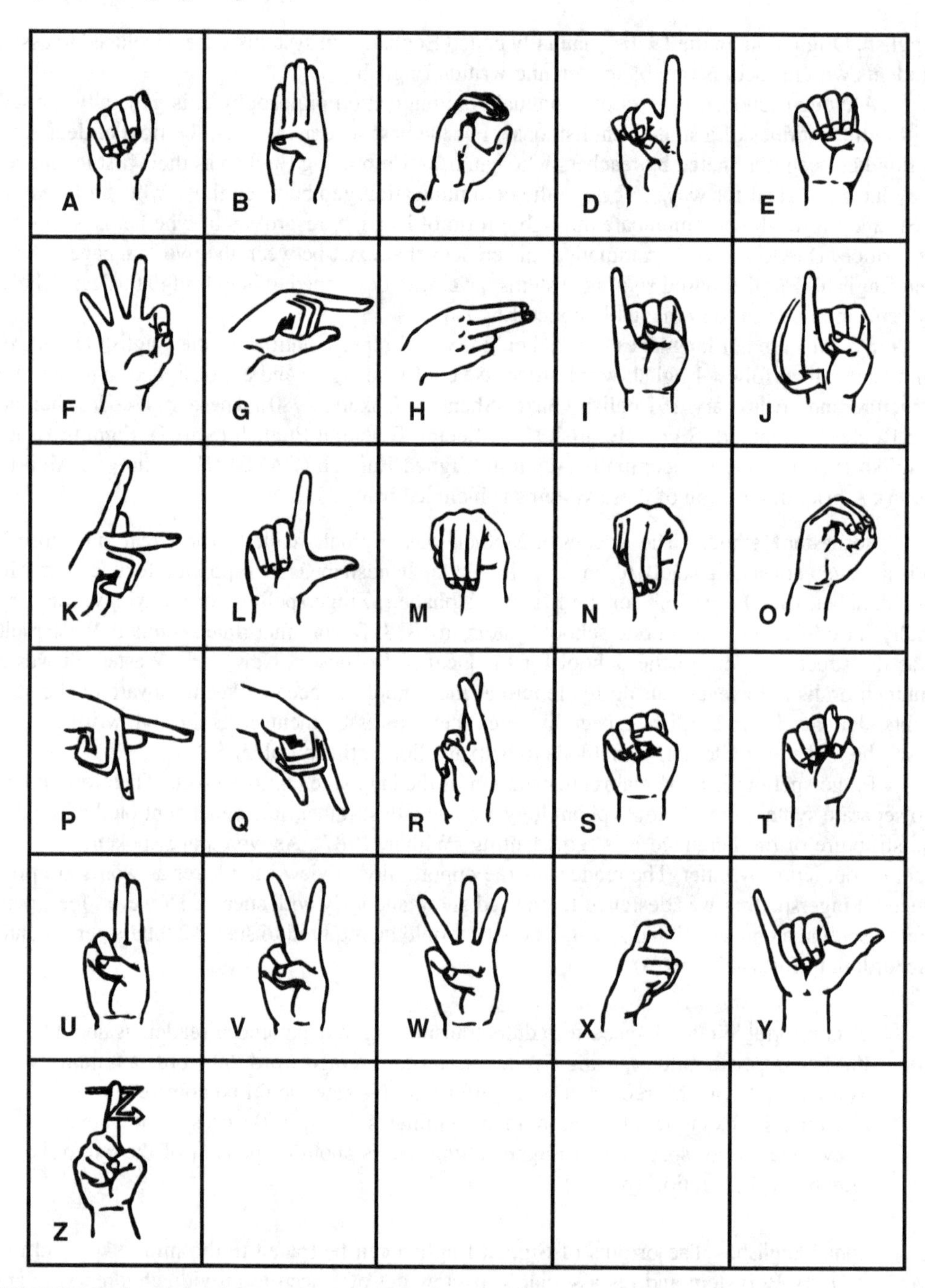

FIGURE 6.3 Letters of the American alphabet.

Source: Courtesy of Simon J. Carmel.

Sign markers are used to illustrate word form changes. Five of these markers were adopted from ASL; the remaining nine were contrived as part of the system. These markers are added to signs to indicate "regular and irregular plurals and past, third person singular, -ing verb form, participle, adverbial, adjectival, possessive, comparative, superlative, agent, and 'opposite of' prefix" (Bornstein, Saulnier, & Hamilton, 1983). ASL signs are used whenever possible, and only one sign marker per sign can be added to change the form of the signed word. However, in the event that a sign word together with a sign marker does not adequately represent the word, this system mandates that the entire word be fingerspelled. (See Figure 6.4 for illustrations of the sign markers.)

Seeing Essential English (SEE I). SEE I is the oldest of all the contrived sign systems. It was developed in the late 1960s by David Anthony, a Deaf instructor, and a group of his associates (all prelingually deaf individuals between the ages of 15 and 67 years). It is a concept, not a method, and is based on the linguistic structure of English. The philosophy of SEE I is "to provide a syntactical, visual sign system for English speaking parents and teachers who do not know the complexities of ASL for them to use with their children in order to develop within them a language structure that is more like their hearing peers" (Washington State School for the Deaf, 1972).

SEE I originated because of concern that ASL is a concept-oriented language that is unrelated to English. Anthony (1971) examined the signs that the average person who was prelingually deaf used. By doing so, they discovered that when signs were produced, they indicated a general rather than a specific word. For example, if one wanted to convey the concept of "ability," the individual might sign the word SKILL but probably would not know the meaning of the word *ability* as defined in the dictionary. As a result, the teacher would discover that the child's vocabulary was limited and his or her use of English syntax was nonexistent.

Based on these concerns, Anthony (1971) began examining the words contained in basic English and soon discovered there were no signs for half of them. Words such as *fruit, bag,* and *the* had no signs, whereas other words, such as *beauty, beautiful, beautifully, lovely, pretty,* and *attractive,* were expressed through the same sign. They also discovered that although some English sentences could be expressed completely through ASL, others could be only approximated.

In an attempt to present English as a viable, visual medium to complement speech rather than to communicate concepts, Anthony (1971) devised a sign system, and SEE I was developed. The system consists of approximately 5,000 signs, with each sign representing only one English word; each was designated as a "root" sign. Affixes, syllables, and free and bound morphemes are referred to as "part" signs. Persons communicating through SEE I can virtually express each word in English word order using correct, colloquial English signs.

Signing Exact English (See II). SEE II is an outgrowth of Anthony's original work on SEE I (1971). It was developed by Gustason, Pfetzing, and Zawolkow (1972) and is currently the most widely used sign system. It shares the philosophy of SEE I in that it is intended to be used simultaneously with speech, with every word signed in English word order.

SEE II attempts to parallel English morphology. English words are divided into basic, complex, and compound words. The system then defers to the "two out of three principle" to determine which sign will be used. That is, regardless of the meaning, if two English words are alike in any two of the three principles (pronunciation, spelling, and meaning), then the sign representing these words remains the same. For example, the English word *right* has three basic meanings: (a) You are right (correct). (b) Turn right (direction). (c) All right (affirmative). In ASL, three different signs represent these three distinct concepts. However, SEE II uses only one

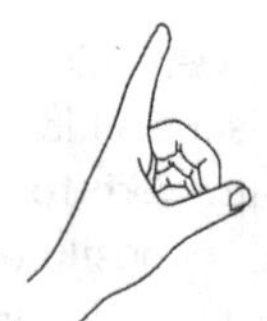

regular past verbs: -ed
walked

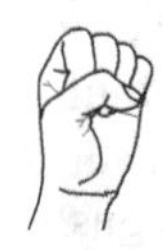

regular plural nouns:s books

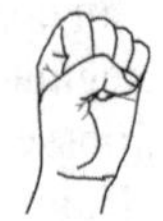

third person singular: -s
walks

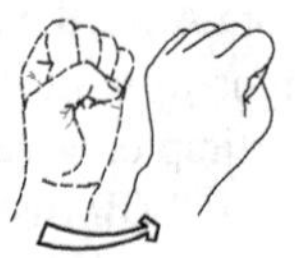

possessive: -'s
girl's

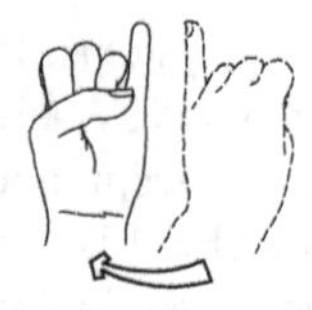

verb form: -ing
walking

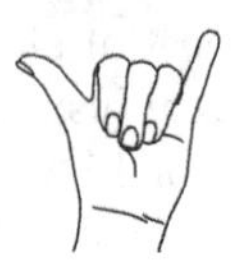

adjectives: -y
rainy

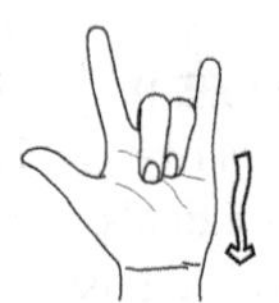

adverb: -ly
slowly

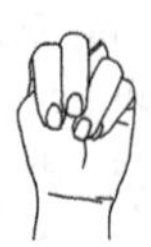

participle:
woken

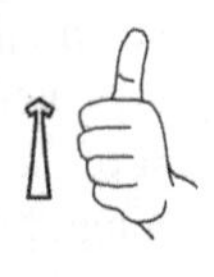

comparative: -er
bigger

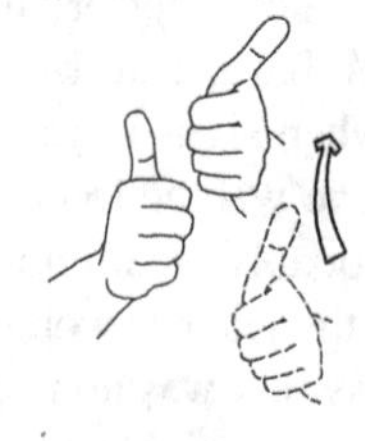

superlative: -est
biggest

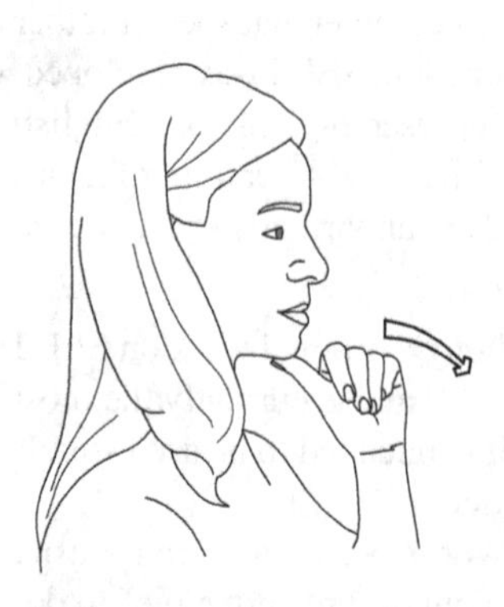

opposite of: un-, im-, in-, etc.
(sign prior to signing the word)
unchanging, impractical, etc.

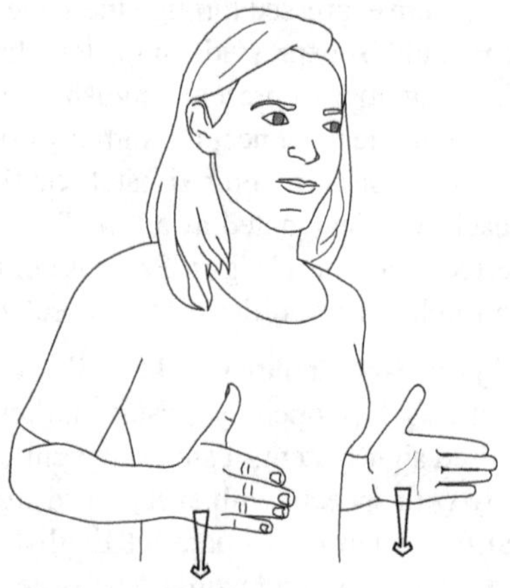

agent (person):
(sign made near the body)
baker, dancer, etc.

FIGURE 6.4 Signed English markers.
Source: Courtesy of Marie A. Scheetz.

sign for all three concepts; this is due to the fact that the spelling and the sound of the words are the same. If the parallel sign in ASL has more than one English translation, the supporters of SEE II have determined that a new sign may be invented.

Although SEE II has retained some of the ASL pronoun signs (ME, YOU, YOUR), initialized signs have been invented for the other pronouns. The E hand shape is incorporated for *he,* the M hand shape for *him,* and the S hand shape for *his.* This system indicates plural nouns by forming an S after the sign, and it forms possessives by moving the S hand sign in the shape of an apostrophe directly after signing the noun. Forms of the verb *to be* are indicated by signs for initials; complex forms are indicated by signs for affixes. The SEE II manual consists of 2,100 signs, 70 affixes, and 7 contractions (Gustason et al., 1972).

SEE II has been incorporated into several school systems. Its goal is to provide students who are deaf with a visually clear English model whereby they can master the English language and succeed academically.

Conceptually Accurate Signed English (CASE). CASE refers to the use of signs based on the meaning of the idea being conveyed rather than the English word that is being used (Humphrey & Alcorn, 1994). Those who use CASE for communication purposes rely on the meaning of the word rather than the spelling of the word when selecting the appropriate sign. When using this system, signs are produced following English sentence structure, frequently with simultaneously spoken or mouthed English. However, ASL features, including use of space and facial markers, are incorporated into this system. Unlike the examples used for RIGHT in SEE II, in CASE each of the concepts expressed by the word RIGHT would be conveyed using a different sign.

These sign systems have been used in various ways throughout the years. Originating for use in the schools, they have found their way into communities as students graduate and either enter the workforce or continue their education. Individuals who are well versed in a sign system frequently encounter Deaf individuals or professionals within in the field who are fluent in ASL. When this occurs, adjustments must be made in the way both English and ASL are presented for communication to take place.

Fluent ASL users wishing to engage in conversation with those who rely on one of the sign systems for communication oftentimes find they must rely on Pidgin Signed English, also referred to as contact signing or Total Communication, to facilitate the exchange of information.

Contact Signing or Pidgin Signed English. Because language provides a communication link with individuals residing in our environment, people must be able to adapt to the mode being used to express their ideas. As in other foreign languages, when two variant groups seek to interact with each other, a method for exchanging information must be developed. The system in foreign languages is referred to as a *pidgin;* when referring to sign language, it is identified as pidgin-signed English or contact signing (CS). It typically combines certain vocabulary items and grammatical structures from the native languages of each group.

Contact signing becomes the middle ground for communication between Deaf individuals whose native language is ASL and hearing or deaf individuals who are familiar with ASL but not fluent in it. By placing ASL and English in tandem with each other, one is able to see how CS interfaces with the two distinct language bases (ASL and English) and the English sign systems. (See Figure 6.5 for a continuum showing contact signing interfacing with English.)

Although home signs may be devised to foster communication between family members who are hearing and deaf, and variations of signed English systems may be developed to represent spoken English. One must not lose sight of the fact that only two distinct languages are

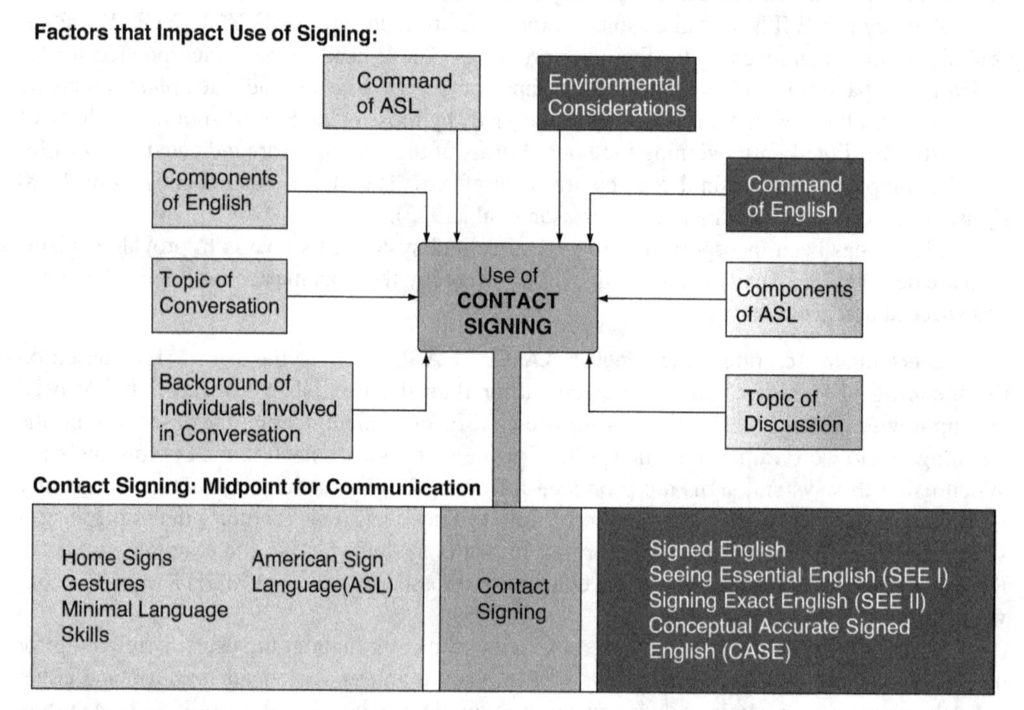

FIGURE 6.5 Continuum showing Contact Signing interfacing with English and ASL.

Source: Courtesy of Marie A. Scheetz.

being presented; the other communication modes overlap each system and are describable in terms of current variation theory in linguistics.

The hearing person's command of ASL, and the situation in which communication occurs, may determine to what extent ASL is used when conversing with individuals who are deaf. Professionals in the educational arena often prefer to use a more English-based signing system, similar to CS. Those who work within social service agencies and religious settings (depending on their sign backgrounds and how they acquired the language) may gravitate toward a more formal ASL format. One's command of the language and the environment in which the conversation takes place will influence the style of communication that is used. Figure 6.5 illustrates the factors that influence the use of CS. See Table 6.2 for a summary and comparison of the visual modes of communication.

Multimodal Communication Approaches

A number of other approaches combine spoken language while incorporating one of the forms of visual communication. In some instances equal emphasis is placed on speech and sign, whereas at other times signs are only utilized occasionally to support speech as the individual bridges to a totally oral approach. Each approach has distinct features and has found a niche in the field of deaf education. Five of these merit particular attention: cued speech,

TABLE 6.2 Visual Modes of Communication

ASL	Signed English	SEE I	SEE II	CASE	CS or PSE
• A visual rule-governed language. • Developed by and for use in the Deaf community. • Consists of its own grammar and syntax. • 3-D space, nonmanual markers, and conventional symbols are used to convey information.	• Origins traced to Harry Bornstein. • English-based sign system. • Consists of 14 sign markers. • Designed to present a visual model of the English language.	• Oldest of all of the sign systems. • Origins traced to David Anthony. • Designed to present a syntactical, visual sign system. • Root and part signs are used to convey English.	• Outgrowth of SEE I. • Origins traced to Gustason and colleagues. • Attempts to parallel English morphology. • Utilizes the 2 out of 3 rule.	• Based on the concept that signs should be used to reflect the concept rather than the English word. • ASL features such as use of space and facial markers are incorporated into this system.	• Designed as a communication mode to be used between ASL and English users. • May use CASE, or one of the other manual systems to communicate. • Based on the signers' command of the language and the topic being discussed. • Viewed on a continuum it, may incorporate more ASL structure or adhere more closely to manual sign systems.

sign-supported speech (SSS), simultaneous communication, Total Communication, and bilingual communication.

CUED SPEECH. Cued speech is basically a communication approach that is used to assist in the development of a spoken language (Paul, 2009). It is critical to note that it is not a language. Termed a multisensory approach, cued speech differs from the unisensory approaches in that it places equal stress on audition and vision. Similar in nature to the unisensory approaches, it promotes the need for early identification, amplification, and adequate auditory management (Paul).

Developed by R. Orin Cornett, cued speech is based on the hypothesis that several of the speech sounds in our spoken language look similar when produced on the lips. For example, when pronouncing the letters *g, z, e,* and *c,* all the letters look similar when produced on the lips and are, therefore, represented by a different hand shape. By providing the person who is deaf or hard of hearing with a different visual indicator for similar sounds, the person would receive a cue as to what sound is being produced. As a result, optimum comprehension can be achieved. Cued speech is designed to overcome the limitations of pure oral/aural methods without deviating from or compromising any of the objectives that are inherent in the oral philosophy. Concerned that many students who are deaf and hard of hearing do not have access to a completely spoken message (including the phonological or building blocks of the language), Cornett designed

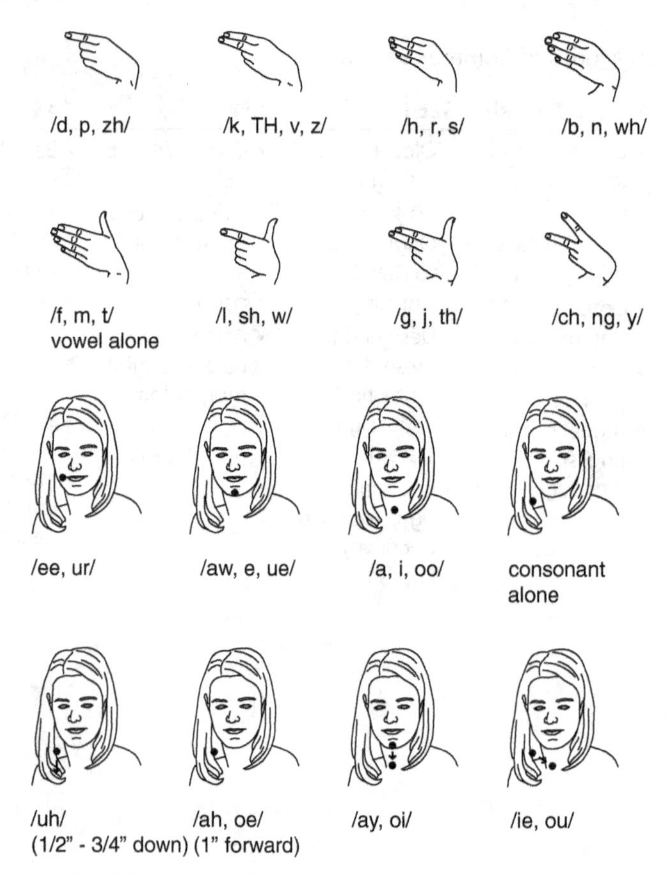

FIGURE 6.6 American English cued speech.

Source: Courtesy of Marie A. Scheetz.

Cued Speech so they could more effectively make a distinction between the various, discrete speech sounds (Paul, 2009, p. 132).

Cued speech is a communication method whereby one hand is used to supplement information on the lips. Within Cornett's system are 36 cues for the 44 phonemes of English. The vowel cues are represented by four hand configurations near or on the face. The eight handshapes represent various groups of consonants. To achieve various vowel-consonant pairs, consonant hand configurations can be combined at the location where the vowel is placed. (Figure 6.6 illustrates the hand shape and the position for the various vowel and consonant sounds.) It should be noted that the T Group cue is also used for an isolated vowel (those that occur without a preceding consonant).

SIGN-SUPPORTED SPEECH. The term *sign-supported speech (SSS)* began appearing in the literature in the late 1980s; coined by Johnson, Liddell, and Erting (1989), it was initially used to denote anytime individuals used signs to support what they were saying. Currently, when the term appears in the literature it refers to signs used in conjunction with an auditory method. In these instances the family's primary concern is for their child to develop speech. Therefore, signs are used to develop speech and language only until they are no longer needed. In this respect they basically become a bridge to enhance words that are not easily seen or heard. However, once the child can utilize the auditory information and produce the words correctly, the use of sign is eliminated (Stredler-Brown, 2010).

SIMULTANEOUS COMMUNICATION. Simultaneous communication involves speaking and signing at the same time. When individuals elect to use this form of communication, they sign while they are speaking, using one of the manually coded English sign systems (SE, CASE, etc.). In essence, their goal is to visually produce everything that is being said. Simultaneous communication cannot be used in conjunction with ASL due to the fact that one cannot communicate in two different languages at the same time (Stredler-Brown, 2010). Although simultaneous communication is used today, it bears mentioning that when speakers attempt to maintain conversational speeds and deliver an extensive amount of information, especially content that is technical in nature, the tendency may be to drop some of the signs, thus skewing the overall intent of the message.

TOTAL COMMUNICATION. The term *Total Communication* refers to a philosophy of education as well as a mode of communication. It was developed in the late 1960s when several studies revealed that children who were deaf of Deaf parents exposed to manual communication had English skills that were superior to those of children who were deaf whose parents could hear and relied primarily on speech to communicate (Moores, 1996, p. 14).

During the late 1960s and early 1970s, schools for the deaf were experimenting with a variety of instructional methods and sign systems. Whereas some incorporated SEE I into their classrooms, others introduced SEE II, Signed English, or CASE. These systems were used simultaneously with speech for instructional and conversational purposes. The goal was to provide students with a total form of communication, thus enhancing their English reading and writing skills. Total Communication quickly became a catchword in the professional community, with credit being given to Roy Holcomb for initiating its use. Holcomb later became known as the "father" of Total Communication.

This philosophy was initially embraced by the Maryland School for the Deaf. By 1976, the members of the Conference of American Schools for the Deaf provided this term with the following official definition: "Total Communication is a philosophy requiring the incorporation of appropriate aural, manual, and oral modes of communication in order to insure effective communication with and among hearing impaired persons" (Gannon, 1981, p. 369).

BILINGUAL COMMUNICATION: ASL AND ENGLISH. Bilingual communication refers to mastering fluency in two natural languages. When describing individuals who are deaf, it refers to those who are fluent in one oral language, in both the spoken and written forms, and one natural sign language, such as ASL (Wilbur, 2008). Artificial signing systems (SE, SEE I, SEE II, etc.) and simultaneous communication are not considered under the umbrella of bilingual communication.

The goal of bilingual communication is to provide individuals who are deaf with a solid foundation in ASL as well as English so they can become successful competitors in the academic arena. Karchmer and Mitchell (2003), Mayer and Akamatsu (2003), Wilbur (2000) and several others have indicated that when children who are deaf are fluent in ASL they become better readers. Drawing from a fully established language base they can use this foundation, much like children who can hear, to master the fundamentals required to become successful readers. (For further discussion of this topic, see Chapter 9. See Table 6.3 for a summary and comparison of the multimodal communication approaches.)

TABLE 6.3 Multimodal Communication

Cued Speech	Sign-Supported Speech	Bilingual ASL & English	Total Communication	Simultaneous Communication
• Originated with Orin Cornett. • Consists of 36 cues for the 44 phonemes of English. • A visual indicator for sounds that look similar on the lips. • Designed to be used in conjunction with speech.	• Coined by Johnson, Liddell, & Erting. • Utilized in conjunction with auditory approaches. • A few signs are added to speech when necessary to support speech and language development (Stredler-Brown, 2010). • Signs are used as a bridge to totally oral communication.	• The philosophy behind bilingual modes of communication is to foster fluency in both ASL and English. • English may either be acquired through print or through organizing signs in the same order as spoken English. • ASL fluency is gained by receiving content information through ASL.	• Roy Holcomb is designated as being the Father of Total Communication. • Developed in the late 1960s. • A philosophy rather than an approach. • Uses differentiated communication strategies to match the needs of the individual.	• Defined by Johnson, Liddell, & Erting (1989). • Signs (one of the manually coded English systems) are used in conjunction with speech. • Note: This can be produced only using one of the English sign systems; it cannot be done using ASL as these are two completely different languages.

IMPACT OF PRELINGUAL HEARING LOSS ON LANGUAGE DEVELOPMENT

Of all the topics discussed within the professional literature, the subject of language development in children who are deaf and hard of hearing has undoubtedly received the most attention. Professionals continue to identify and evaluate interventions, methods, and strategies that will enhance the linguistic abilities of this population. Conducting research studies that examine social, emotional, and academic development, the goal is to uncover new and existing inroads that will promote and enhance cognitive and linguistic growth.

Historically speaking, the controversy of whether to use sign language or speech to promote normal language acquisition has created and elicited heated debates among professionals, parents, and Deaf adults. With the implementation of universal newborn hearing screening programs, and advances in the technology available to improve the hearing experience, research continues to examine the most effective ways to promote language development in this population.

It is well documented in the literature that hearing loss in children invariably contributes to delays in speech and language development. A plethora of research indicates that even very young children with a relatively mild degree of hearing loss struggle as they attempt to acquire speech and language through the auditory channel (Bess, Dodd-Murphy, & Parker, 1998; Dodd, McIntosh, & Woodhouse, 1998; Meadow-Orlans, Mertens, & Sass-Lehrer, 2003; Moeller, 2000; P. Spencer, 2004). Consequently, several young children who are deaf do not have full access to language in any modality (Snodden, 2008).

With the advent of cochlear implants, there has been a proliferation of articles in the literature describing how these devices improve access to sound, thus impacting speech perception and production (Blamey, 2003; Blamey et al., 2001; Preisler, Tvingstedt, & Ahlstrom, 2002). Although the majority of these articles stress the positive outcomes of using an auditory-verbal approach in conjunction with cochlear implants, others document the benefits of using ASL as the foundation for developing spoken English word perception and production skills (Yoshinaga-Itano, 2006). In recent years the field has produced several texts, such as *Advances in the Spoken Language Development of Deaf and Hard-of-Hearing Children* (Spencer & Marschark, 2006), *Advances in the Sign Language Development of Deaf Children* (Schick, Marschark, & Spencer, 2006), and *Language and Deafness* (Paul, 2009), all of which provide a rich cadre of articles reflecting current sign, speech, and language research that has been conducted in the field.

Regardless of which approach is used, the consensus within the field is that early identification of hearing loss is critical, and input of language must occur before the age of 2 if normal language development is to occur. Without this early intervention, language delays inevitably occur and the gap between where the child needs to be and where he or she actually is continues to widen as the child enters school. Language delays experienced early in infancy can continue to plague the child throughout the academic years, leaving him or her to struggle with language exchanges the typical hearing child automatically takes for granted. What does the research say about using ASL to communicate with children who are deaf? What does it reveal about promoting oral language training and spoken language development? Can both be combined to enhance language development, thus providing the foundation for successful literacy outcomes? Is there one solution for all children who are deaf or hard of hearing?

Enhancing Language Development Through the Use of American Sign Language

Studies that examine the similarities of signed and spoken languages demonstrate that natural signed languages, such as ASL, exhibit the same linguistic properties as those found in spoken languages including phonetic, phonemic, syllabic, morphologic, syntactic, discourse, and pragmatic levels of organization (Newport & Meier, 1985; Petitto, 1994). Furthermore, D/deaf children who are exposed to ASL from birth acquire this language on a maturational time line that mirrors and parallels that of hearing children who acquire English (Petitto, 2000; Volterra, Iverson, & Castrataro, 2006). Research conducted by Morford and Mayberry (2000), Newport and Meier (1985), Schick (2003), and Spencer (2004) indicates that children exposed to sign language from birth to age 3 onward demonstrate identical stages of language acquisition, including syllabic babbling between 7 and 11 months, first-word attainment between 11 and 14 months, and two-word achievement between 16 and 22 months (Petitto, 2000).

These findings further support earlier research conducted by Kourbetis (1987) and Weisel (1988) that indicates deaf children of Deaf parents exposed to sign language perform significantly better than children who are deaf who have hearing parents when completing tests of academic achievement that include reading, writing, and social development. Previous research conducted by Israelite and Ewoldt (1992) reveals that native ASL users have higher English literacy abilities than children who are deaf and learn ASL later in life. Moreover, recent studies continue to substantiate these findings. Furthermore, Singleton, Supalla, Litchfield, and Schley (1998), and Strong and Prinz (1997, 2000) posit that highly ASL-fluent children who are deaf are able to achieve higher levels of English literacy regardless of the hearing status of their parents.

International studies are providing additional insights into early acquisition of ASL and spoken language. Research conducted in Sweden by Preisler et al. (2002) revealed that preschool children who had received cochlear implants between the ages of 2 and 5 had significantly more developed spoken language skills if they possessed well-developed sign language skills. Even though sign language skill level could not be solely attributed to spoken language development, those children with limited sign language skills also had limited or no spoken language abilities. Preisler's observations also indicated that as children improved their sign language skills, their spoken language also improved.

Parallel to the increased number of children receiving cochlear implants are the number of articles that have been written regarding vocabulary development and spoken language skills. Case studies cited by Yoshinaga-Itano (2006) describe three infants who acquired ASL and simultaneously received cochlear implants and auditory-oral stimulation. She notes that the broad ASL vocabularies exhibited in these children were instrumental in providing them with a foundation for developing spoken English word perception and production skills.

Enhancing Language Development Through an Auditory Verbal Approach

It has been well documented that with the advent of universal newborn hearing-screening programs combined with advances in technology that individuals who are deaf and hard of hearing are being provided with a new era of communication possibilities. With digital hearing aids readily available and the number of cochlear implants increasing annually, professionals are continuing to scrutinize the varying approaches being implemented to promote language development. An influx of articles during the past decade describe the outcomes of children with cochlear implants who are enrolled in speech and language programs.

Among professionals supporting the use of cochlear implants, the overall consensus is that the earlier in life children are implanted the better their chances are of developing spoken language. Studies conducted by Nicholas and Geers (2007), Dettman, Briggs, Dowell, and Leigh (2007), and Nikolopoulos, O'Donoghue, and Archbold (1999), reveal that those implanted early, before substantial delays in spoken language develop (between the ages of 12 and 16 months), generally achieve better outcomes in speech perception and speech intelligibility. Furthermore, these children experience language growth that matches growth rates achieved by their peers who can hear. Even though these growth rates are well documented in younger children, research also reveals that this does not typically hold true for children who receive an implant after 24 months of age. These children generally do not achieve the same levels of language proficiency as their hearing peers (Nicholas & Geers).

Although numerous articles have been published pertaining to language development in children who are deaf or hard of hearing that have received cochlear implants, representative findings of these studies are varied. Several researchers have investigated the factors that may relate to why some children experience tremendous benefits from their implants and others do not. Part of the variation has been attributed to the age of the child when the study was conducted. Recognizing that cognitive development and language development do not proceed linearly with age, it is well established that the rates of progress for each individual child may be affected by the child's developmental level at the time the study was conducted (Nicholas & Geers, 2007, p. 1050).

Keeping this in mind, Moreno-Torres and Torres (2008) have reviewed several studies and summarized pertinent factors that might explain the variability of spoken language development in children who receive cochlear implants. Although their list is noninclusive, it does provide insights into some of the more influential components. Significant factors include age at implantation (e.g., Kirk et al., 2002; Nicholas & Geers, 2006; Osberger, Zimmerman-Phillips, & Koch, 2002), preimplant experience with audition (e.g., Nicholas & Geers, 2006; Spencer, 2004), communication mode (e.g., Geers et al., 2002; Kirk et al., 2002), and family characteristics (Spencer, 2004).

Without a doubt, as the technology continues to improve and children are implanted at an earlier age, the development of their auditory skills after implantation continues to be enhanced (Allum, Greisiger, Straubhaar, & Carpenter, 2000). Studies such as those conducted by Geers, Breener, and Davidson (2003) indicate that children who receive their implants by 5 years of age exhibit speech and language skills that go far beyond those previously reported for children who are profoundly deaf. By collecting a nationwide sample, Geers et al. have reported that the majority studied scored 50% or better on open-set speech perception tests and had speech that was at least 75% intelligible to listeners who were not familiar with the speech produced by individuals who are deaf (Tobey, Geers, Brenner, Altuna, & Gabbert, 2003, as cited in Spencer & Marschark, 2006).

As the technology continues to evolve and this young population enters and progresses through the educational system, additional research studies will need to be conducted to monitor their progress. A substantial body of research reflects the characteristics of infants and young children prior to implantation. Throughout the next decade additional studies will need to examine the support services, educational programming, and types of auditory stimulation that will be needed to enhance spoken language development.

Summary

Infants enter the world biologically equipped to learn language. Early in infancy they are attending to and imitating facial expressions. Attuned to sound, they begin to develop both a receptive and expressive vocabulary. Starting slowly at first, within the first 2 years children develop a vocabulary that consists of approximately 200 to 300 words. Throughout the next year of life their vocabularies increase rapidly, and by the time they are 3 years old they may have heard several million words, acquired several thousand words, figured out how to build and understand complex sentences, and mastered the sound or phonological system of their language (O'Grady, 2005). Furthermore, their vocabularies continue to increase as they enter school and begin their educational journey.

Language becomes the master key unlocking the doors to socialization, education, and communication. It spans one's lifetime providing the lifeline for forming connections, accessing the curriculum, and allowing for the transmission of and sharing of ideas. Evolving from infancy, it provides the scaffolding allowing teens and young adults to begin exploring the world of abstractions while transforming word knowledge into world knowledge.

Children who are deaf born to hearing parents begin life in a linguistically altered environment. Unlike infants who can hear, who share a mutual language base with their caregivers, babies who are deaf are not privy to the benefits afforded by the auditory channel, a mechanism taken for granted by those who can hear. From the onset they are faced with the challenge of developing language and acquiring background knowledge through their visual domain.

Some parents, when discovering their child is deaf, will opt for surgery and select a cochlear implant. Others, due to choice, philosophical beliefs, or financial reasons will look for alternative solutions. Some parents will elect to use ASL or a form of manual communication with their child, recognizing the value of a visual language; others will search for strategies and techniques to enhance speech reading and speech production. All parents, regardless of the mode they select, share a common goal: to provide their child with a language that they can use to communicate with those around them, along with a mechanism to grow and develop into healthy, happy, well-adjusted individuals.

Language and communication will always lie at the heart of human existence. Helping children who are deaf and hard of hearing develop to their fullest potential first requires that they possess a rich and robust language. Recognizing that the mode of communication is secondary to the development of a strong language foundation, it is critical that children who are deaf and hard of hearing are provided with multiple pathways to form communication links with others. As Gannon (1981) so poignantly stated, "The ear no more than the eye is the unique window of the soul, and no less. Each one . . . [can] give insight about a living human person and his world."

7

Hearing Assessment, Hearing Aids, Cochlear Implants, and Modern Technology

Identification, Remediation, and Communication

Hearing loss and auditory processing disorders can and do occur at all ages, impacting the lives of infants, children, and adults. When one's ability to hear is affected, or one's ability to process information is altered, it has a direct bearing on how, when, and where communication takes place. The ramifications of hearing loss are complex and related to a multiplicity of factors, including age of onset, type and severity of loss, background knowledge of hearing loss, and familiarity with deafness. Once a diagnosis is made, recommendations for amplification and rehabilitation generally ensue.

Throughout the United States an estimated 36 million Americans have some type of hearing loss. According to the National Institute on Deafness and Other Communication Disorders (2010) more than 30% of people over age 65 have some type of hearing loss, and 18% of those between the ages of 45 and 64 have varying degrees of hearing loss. Furthermore, close to 8 million people between the ages of 18 and 44 have a hearing loss (American Speech-Language-Hearing Association [ASHA], 2009). Statistics also indicate that daily, throughout the United States, 33 children are born with congenital hearing loss (Leonard, Shen, Howe, & Egler, 1999; Stierman, 1994; White, 1997). Although experiencing a loss at any age can have an adverse affect on spoken language communication, for those who are born deaf or lose their hearing before the age of 2, the ramifications are far reaching, frequently creating delays in language development thus impacting academic achievement and later job satisfaction.

How is hearing loss identified? At what age are infants tested? What are the routine ages at which school-age children are evaluated? What is involved in a comprehensive hearing evaluation? What types of hearing aids, and assistive listening devices, are available to treat hearing loss? What types of amplification systems are available in schools and public meeting places that can be requested by those who experience difficulty hearing?

IDENTIFYING HEARING LOSS: THE HEARING EVALUATION

The primary purpose for any hearing evaluation, regardless of the person's age, is to measure the individual's ability to respond to a set of acoustic signals. When conducting an audiologic examination, trained personnel may conduct an initial hearing screening test or a more comprehensive assessment to determine if the individual has a hearing loss that merits amplification or surgical implantation. Although hearing screenings are useful to determine if any problems might exist audiologic evaluations provide audiologists with comprehensive information regarding the type of loss, the severity of loss, and the impact the loss can have on the individual's ability to receive information through the auditory channel.

The two major types of peripheral hearing loss are those that are conductive and those determined to be sensorineural (see Chapter 4). When an individual has a loss reflective of both types it is referred to as a mixed loss. Although the categories are broad and inclusive, the effects on individuals may vary considerably. Therefore, it is imperative that the audiologist ascertain the existence of a hearing impairment and make judgments regarding the severity and influence of the loss on the individual, identify the location and configuration of the lesion responsible for the pathology, and recommend possible solutions for remediation of the problem. To accomplish this, an extensive battery of tests must be administered.

Due to recent medical advances, the knowledge base surrounding hearing impairments has broadened, and techniques involving test procedures have become more exact and complex. Audiologists no longer rely on tuning forks or the sole results of an audiogram to make their diagnosis. Today most clinicians feel that the minimum audiologic examination must consist of pure-tone testing, both by air and bone conduction, accompanied by appropriate masking, speech reception threshold tests, auditory discrimination tests at suprathreshold levels, and immittance (tympanometry) and acoustic reflexes.

Furthermore, within the educational setting, evaluations are included that consider communication function, listening skill development, hearing loss adjustment, and environmental factors that can and do impact hearing, such as classroom acoustics and classroom communication patterns (Johnson, 2009). By administering a complete test battery, audiologists are able to obtain information that helps them identify the problem area and describe how it impacts the individual. Once this information is obtained, they can make appropriate recommendations for remediation.

PURE-TONE TESTING

Pure-tone audiometers, designed to test hearing sensitivity by air conduction and bone conduction, have been used professionally for approximately a hundred years. Results provide the examiner with a broad perspective on the type and pattern of hearing loss experienced by the individual. Pure-tone audiometers can be portable and allow the examiner to select a series of pure tones at a variety of frequencies. Hearing is usually tested at 5 dB increments with testable frequencies for air conduction usually including 125, 250, 500, 750, 1,000, 1,500, 2,000, 3,000, 4,000, 6,000, and 8,000 Hz (Schlauch & Nelson, 2009). The machine is calibrated such that a 0 dB hearing level is established at each frequency representing the lowest intensity at which the normal ear can detect the presence of the test tone 50% of the time (Schlauch & Nelson). Therefore, an individual's hearing loss can be determined by the number of decibels in excess of this zero point that the tone must be intensified for a person to recognize that sounds are being transmitted. In the audiometric test situation, tones are administered through earphones for air conduction tests. A matched pair of earphones is provided for the individual being tested, and an output switch directs the tone to either earphone. When conducting the bone-conduction test, a bone-conduction vibrator is used to evaluate inner ear function.

When audiologists evaluate a person's hearing, they assess their ability to hear sounds at varying frequencies. Frequencies that comprise the test battery generally begin in the range of 250 Hz through 8,000 or 12,000 Hz. The sound-pressure level required to make a sound audible for the average normal-hearing person is referred to as zero hearing level. Therefore, one can identify a hearing loss by the number of decibels required to make the sound audible. The hearing level required to reach that threshold is the amount of the audiometer's calibration that equates to the amount of hearing loss. The maximum hearing level (HL) in most pure-tone audiometers is 100 dB HL.

As with any other test instrument, the audiometer is only a tool; results will only be as accurate as the skill level of the individual conducting this evaluation. The audiogram does not present a complete picture of an individual's hearing loss but, rather, an estimate based on the audiologist's observation of the person's behavior throughout the test situation.

In essence, the audiogram provides information in five specific areas where it:

1. illustrates patterns of hearing sensitivity for tones at various frequencies;
2. provides a comparison of air and bone-conduction sensitivity;
3. reflects the individual's hearing in relation to the normative standard;
4. projects interaural symmetry or asymmetry; and
5. can be used to reflect the results of other pure-tone tests. (Schlauch & Nelson, 2009)

Pure-tone testing is administered to the better ear first, beginning with the frequency of 1,000 Hz or cycles per second (cps). After a threshold level has been established, testing continues at even octaves above and below 1,000 cps, with 12,000 cps being the highest frequency tested. When a complete measurement is obtained on the first ear, the second ear is tested. If the thresholds of the second ear differ from the first ear by 40 dB, masking should be applied to ensure that hearing in one ear is not being assisted by hearing in the better ear.

BONE-CONDUCTION TESTING

When a hearing loss is indicated through air-conduction tests, it is standard procedure to administer bone-conduction tests. The purpose is to determine whether the hearing loss is caused by conductive or sensorineural factors, or a combination of the two. Utilizing a headband with a bone-conduction vibrator, the audiologist places a small vibrator on the mastoid process of the temporal bone behind the pinna of the ear to be tested, or occasionally on the forehead. By conducting this procedure, the examiner is able to ascertain if an external or middle ear lesion exists, and the extent of the conductive hearing impairment can be further determined. It is assumed that the threshold for bone-conducted signals is a measure of the sensorineural system. When test results indicate that sounds are heard normally through bone conduction, it is inferred that the sense organ and the auditory nerve are normal and working properly. When air-conduction thresholds are obtained, they represent the functioning level of the entire auditory system. Therefore, when a discrepancy occurs in the threshold levels between air and bone conduction (air-bone gap), it is assumed that the difficulty must lie in that part of the mechanism that is responsible for the conduction of airborne sounds. However, when evidence indicates that the loss is purely conductive, the bone-conduction thresholds will be normal (Vento & Durrant, 2009).

In essence, when both types of tests are completed, it can be determined if the loss is conductive or sensorineural. However, if bone-conductive measurements reflect losses that are equal to those obtained by air-conduction testing, the loss is sensorineural. If there is some loss by bone but not as much as by air, the loss is termed a mixed loss (Vento & Durrant, 2009).

Hearing test results are plotted on a graph referred to as an audiogram. The two dimensions of an audiogram are frequency and intensity. The results of each ear are plotted separately by both air and bone conduction. The symbol *O* and the color red are used to plot the threshold points for each frequency tested for the right ear. An *X* and the color blue or black are used to identify frequencies and threshold levels for the left ear. (A sample audiogram reflecting an individual with normal hearing is included in Figure 7.1.)

Losses reflecting conductive, sensorineural, and mixed patterns are characterized by different configurations on the audiogram. Generally, conductive losses are evidenced by fairly equal losses at all frequencies, with perhaps slightly greater losses appearing in the lower frequencies. (An audiogram depicting a conductive loss is reflected in Figure 7.2.)

Sensorineural impairments are characterized usually, but not always, by close to normal hearing activity at the lower frequencies with rapid decreases at the higher frequencies. Bone- and air-conduction thresholds are approximately the same. (Figure 7.3 illustrates a sensorineural loss.)

Individuals exhibiting characteristics of conductive and sensorineural losses are identified as having a mixed impairment. In the event a conductive loss is present and with some secondary nerve involvement, the audiogram may depict a loss in both the high and low frequencies.

A typical mixed impairment will produce an audiogram that shows some loss by bone conduction but a more severe loss by air conduction. However, depending on the etiology of the mixed loss, it may manifest itself by demonstrating a conductive loss in the lower frequencies and a sensorineural loss in the higher frequencies. (See Figure 7.4.)

CLASSIFICATION OF HEARING LOSS

The degree of hearing impairment can be grouped according to five separate classifications, ranging from mild through profound. The classification can be made on the basis of sensitivity at a single frequency or on the basis of the average sensitivity of several frequencies, the pure-tone average (PTA).

Individuals experiencing mild, moderate, and moderately severe hearing losses are identified as hard of hearing. Through the use of amplification, auditory training, and speech and language therapy, they are able to engage in a verbal exchange of communication and receive information auditorily. The term *deaf,* from an audiologic perspective, refers to those individuals with severe to profound hearing loss who cannot hear speech through their ears, with or without amplification. Although they may hear some loud sounds, they do not rely on their auditory mechanism as the primary channel of communication. (Table 7.1 is an expansion of Table 4.2. Columns have been added to reflect the impact hearing loss can have with respect to psychosocial development and the educational needs of the learner. Table 7.2 reflects the degree and prevalence of hearing loss found within the school-age population.)

Although these classifications have been established to aid the consumer and professional in understanding the severity of the varying degrees of loss, one must be careful not to pigeonhole or label someone based on this information. Labels and classification systems provide professionals with an avenue whereby they can discuss the various types of hearing losses and determine which services will contribute the greatest amount of benefit to the consumer. In this respect, labels serve a very useful function to the extent that they provide professionals with identifying terminology used that can be used to make recommendations, and to secure services. However, labeling of any group can have detrimental effects. Individuals may be misclassified, labels may be misunderstood, and stereotypes can occur. In addition, parents and consumers who are not well versed in the vernacular of medical terminology may misconstrue what is said and fail to understand the significance of services deemed necessary to enhance educational and personal development.

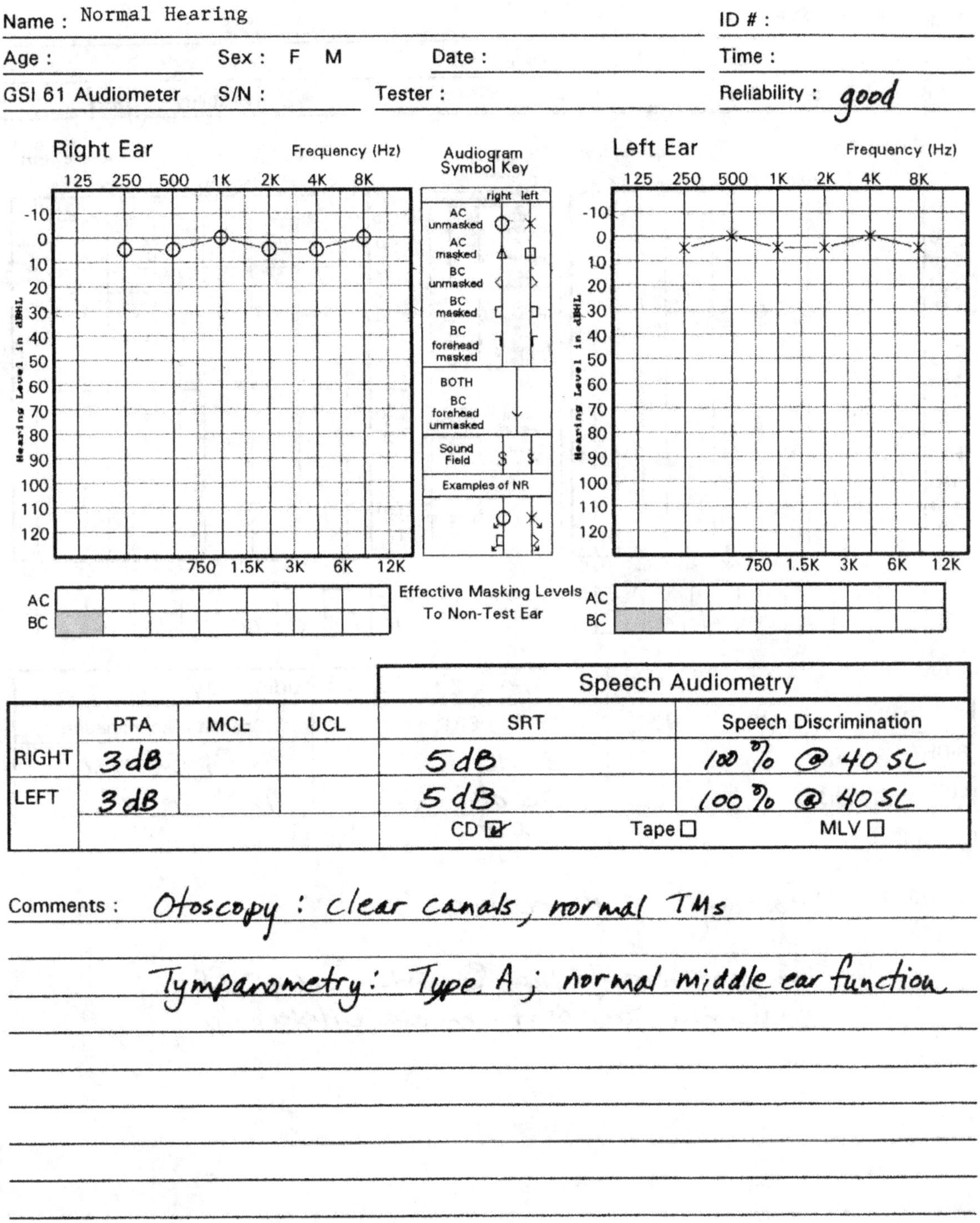

Name : Normal Hearing ID # :

Age : Sex : F M Date : Time :

GSI 61 Audiometer S/N : Tester : Reliability : good

Right Ear Frequency (Hz)

125 250 500 1K 2K 4K 8K

Hearing Level in dBHL: -10 0 10 20 30 40 50 60 70 80 90 100 110 120

750 1.5K 3K 6K 12K

Audiogram Symbol Key

	right	left
AC unmasked	O	X
AC masked	△	□
BC unmasked	<	>
BC masked	[	]
BC forehead masked	┐	┌
BOTH BC forehead unmasked	∨	
Sound Field	S	S
Examples of NR		

Left Ear Frequency (Hz)

125 250 500 1K 2K 4K 8K

Hearing Level in dBHL: -10 0 10 20 30 40 50 60 70 80 90 100 110 120

750 1.5K 3K 6K 12K

Effective Masking Levels To Non-Test Ear

AC
BC

AC
BC

Speech Audiometry

	PTA	MCL	UCL	SRT	Speech Discrimination
RIGHT	3dB			5dB	100% @ 40 SL
LEFT	3dB			5dB	100% @ 40 SL
				CD ☑ Tape ☐	MLV ☐

Comments : Otoscopy : clear canals, normal TMs

Tympanometry: Type A; normal middle ear function

FIGURE 7.1 Audiogram of an individual with normal hearing.

Source: Courtesy of Tish Consolini.

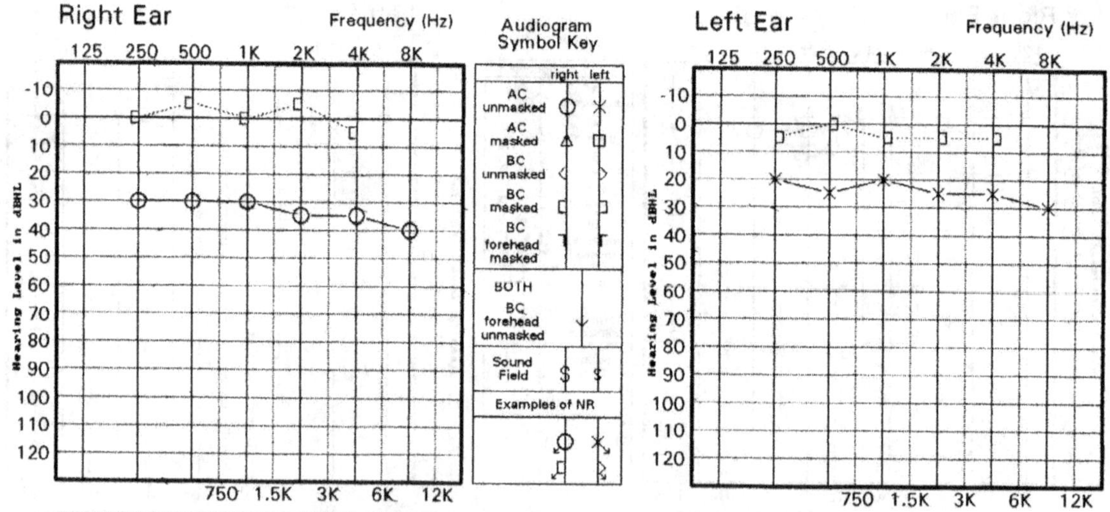

Name : Conductive Loss

ID # :

Age : Sex : F M Date : Time :

GSI 61 Audiometer S/N : Tester : Reliability : good

Effective Masking Levels To Non-Test Ear

Right Ear							
AC							
BC		40	45	40	45	45	

Left Ear							
AC							
BC		50	50	50	55	55	

Speech Audiometry

	PTA	MCL	UCL	SRT	Speech Discrimination
RIGHT	32 dB			30 dB	96 % @ 40 SL
LEFT	23 dB			25 dB	96 % @ 40 SL
				CD ☑ Tape ☐	MLV ☐

Comments : Otoscopy : TM redness

Tympanometry : Type B (flat, normal ECV); indicative of otitis media bilaterally

FIGURE 7.2 Audiogram depicting a conductive loss.

Source: Courtesy of Tish Consolini.

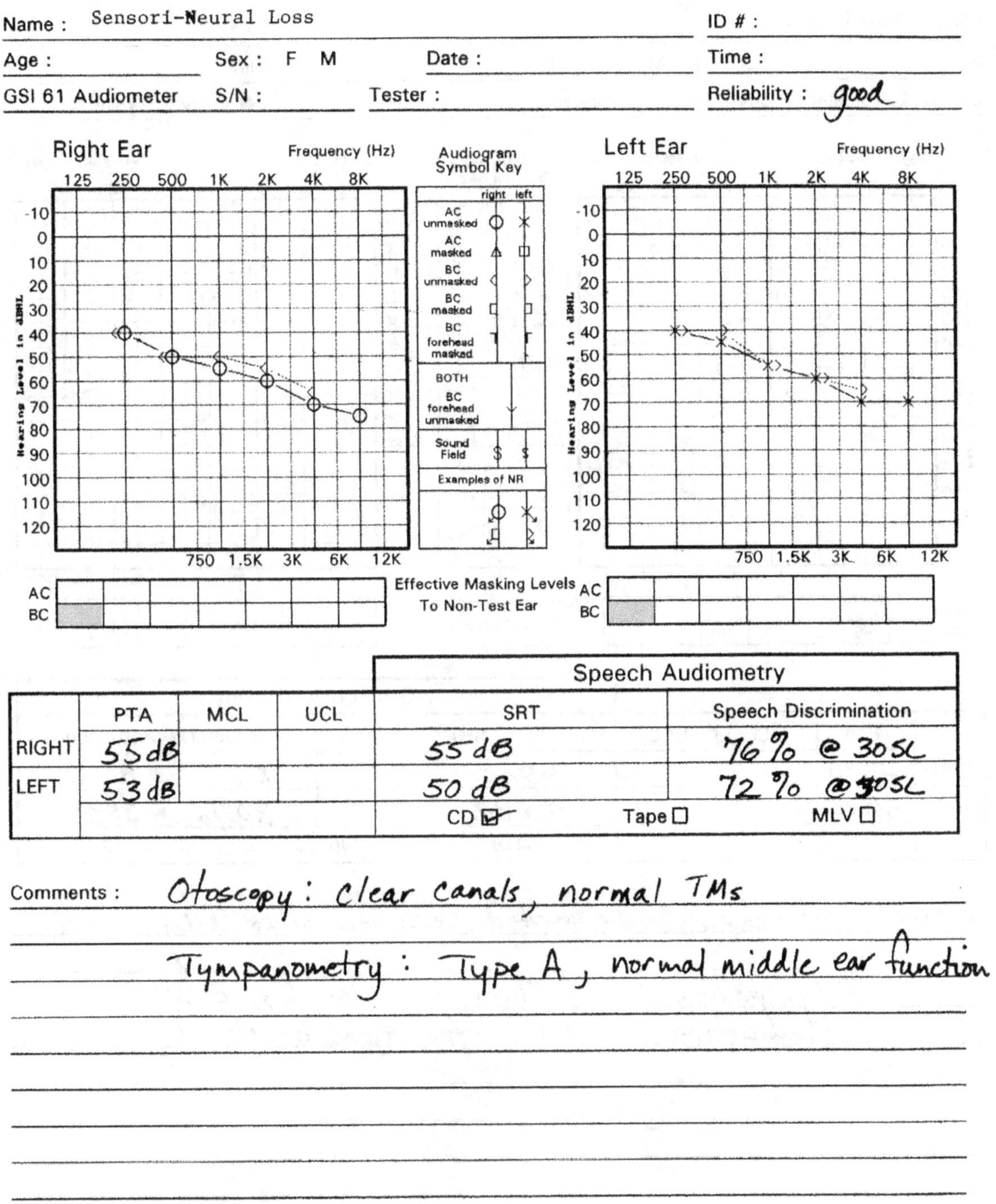

Name : Sensori-Neural Loss ID # :

Age : Sex : F M Date : Time :

GSI 61 Audiometer S/N : Tester : Reliability : good

Right Ear Frequency (Hz) 125 250 500 1K 2K 4K 8K

Audiogram Symbol Key: right left; AC unmasked; AC masked; BC unmasked; BC masked; BC forehead masked; BOTH BC forehead unmasked; Sound Field; Examples of NR

Left Ear Frequency (Hz) 125 250 500 1K 2K 4K 8K

Hearing Level in dBHL: -10 0 10 20 30 40 50 60 70 80 90 100 110 120

750 1.5K 3K 6K 12K

AC BC Effective Masking Levels To Non-Test Ear AC BC

Speech Audiometry

	PTA	MCL	UCL	SRT	Speech Discrimination
RIGHT	55dB			55dB	76% @ 30SL
LEFT	53dB			50 dB	72% @ 30SL
				CD ☑ Tape ☐	MLV ☐

Comments : Otoscopy : clear canals, normal TMs

Tympanometry : Type A, normal middle ear function

FIGURE 7.3 Audiogram depicting a sensorineural loss.

Source: Courtesy of Tish Consolini.

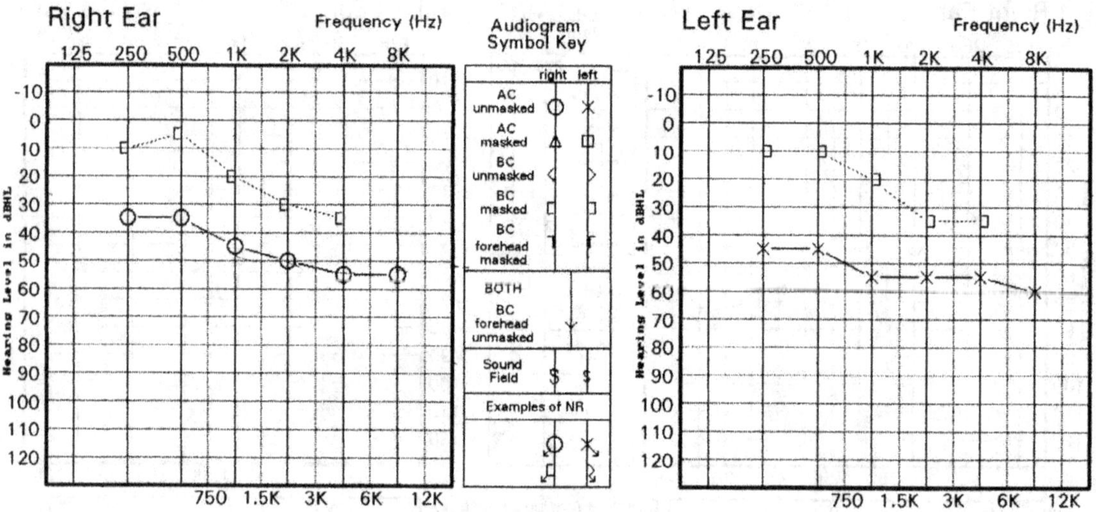

Name : Mixed Loss ID # :

Age : Sex : F M Date : Time :

GSI 61 Audiometer S/N : Tester : Reliability : good

Right Ear Frequency (Hz)

Audiogram Symbol Key

Left Ear Frequency (Hz)

Effective Masking Levels To Non-Test Ear

Right ear:

AC							
BC		65	65	75	70	75	

Left ear:

AC							
BC		55	55	65	70	75	

Speech Audiometry

	PTA	MCL	UCL	SRT	Speech Discrimination
RIGHT	43dB			45dB	84% @ 35SL
LEFT	52dB			50 dB	80% @ 35SL
				CD ☑ Tape ☐	MLV ☐

Comments : Otoscopy: Impacted cerumen bilaterally

Tympanometry: Type B (flat, high ECV) indicative of TM perforations bilaterally

FIGURE 7.4 Audiogram depicting a mixed loss.

Source: Courtesy of Tish Consolini.

TABLE 7.1 Categories of Hearing Loss with Implications for Communication, Psychosocial Development, and Educational Needs of the Learner

Degree of Hearing Loss	Classification of Hearing Loss	Impact on Understanding Spoken Communication	Impact of Hearing Loss on Psychosocial Development	Potential Educational Needs with Respect to Hearing Loss
−10 to 15 dB	Normal	No impact on communication		
16 to 25	Slight	If the environment is quiet there is usually no difficulty recognizing and understanding speech; however, in noisy environments speech can be difficult to understand.	Subtle conversational cues may be missed, as can fast-paced interactions with peers; this can have a potential impact on socialization and self-concept. Child may become fatigued due to the listening effort required when interacting with peers.	The learner may benefit from a personal frequency modulation (FM) system, or sound field amplification if instruction takes place in a noisy classroom. Student may benefit from favorable seating. General education teachers may need in-service training with respect to the impact of hearing loss on language development.
26 to 40 dB	Mild	When surrounded with a quiet environment and familiarity with the topic and limited vocabulary, communication can be established. However, speech produced faintly or at a distance can become difficult to hear. Typically placed in regular education program; preferential seating is important; may benefit from a speech reading program.	The child may struggle with suppressing background noise while trying to attend to the teacher and classmates. This can cause additional stress for the child. The student might be accused of daydreaming or not paying attention. Both can have a detrimental effect on self-esteem.	Students with a mild loss often benefit from a hearing aid and the use of a personal FM or a sound field system. Many also benefit from auditory skill building. Favorable seating and lighting are requirements. Attention might also need to be given to vocabulary development, articulation, speech reading, and academic support.

(continued)

TABLE 7.1 Categories of Hearing Loss with Implications for Communication, Psychosocial Development, and Educational Needs of the Learner (*continued*)

Degree of Hearing Loss	Classification of Hearing Loss	Impact on Understanding Spoken Communication	Impact of Hearing Loss on Psychosocial Development	Potential Educational Needs with Respect to Hearing Loss
41 to 55	Moderate	Has the ability to understand conversational speech at a distance of 3 to 5 feet. Can benefit from a hearing aid, auditory training, and speech therapy; preferential seating is beneficial. Group activities can be challenging.	When a student experiences a moderate loss, communication is generally significantly affected. It may become very difficult for the student to socialize with his/her hearing peers. If socialization becomes a problem, it can negatively impact self-esteem.	Students with moderate losses are usually referred to special education for language evaluations and follow-up services. It is critical to provide amplification. Emphasis is also placed on oral language development, literacy, and speech reading. Speech therapy might also be requested.
56 to 70	Moderate to Severe	Conversation will not be heard unless it is loud. The person will benefit from all of the above and should also receive enhanced language instruction. An individual who experiences this degree of loss may produce speech that is not completely intelligible.	The student may experience considerable difficulty with oral communication and struggle with one-to-one and group situations. As a result, the individual may isolate him- or herself from the mainstream. Lack of incidental social interactive opportunities may result in a poorer self-concept, social immaturity, and a sense of rejection.	Full-time amplification is essential. A teacher of the deaf and other support personnel are required to ensure student success. May require supplemental instruction in all areas of literacy development including vocabulary, grammar, syntax, pragmatics, and reading.
71 to 90	Severe	May identify environmental noises and loud sounds. May be able to distinguish vowels but not consonants; special education classes	If the student has contacts with other students who have a hearing loss, an opportunity is provided for the student to develop a positive self-concept	Students experiencing a severe loss may benefit from a sign language interpreter, teacher of the deaf who is fluent in sign language, or a full-time aural/oral

TABLE 7.1 *(continued)*

Degree of Hearing Loss	Classification of Hearing Loss	Impact on Understanding Spoken Communication	Impact of Hearing Loss on Psychosocial Development	Potential Educational Needs with Respect to Hearing Loss
		designed for deaf children may be beneficial. Speech is not always intelligible.	and a sense of cultural identity.	program for deaf students. It is critical that amplification in the form of hearing aids, cochlear implants, and personal FM systems are made available for the student.
91+dB	Profound	Does not rely on hearing for primary means of communication; may hear some loud sounds. Education services are beneficial. Speech may be difficult to understand, or may not be developed.	Depending on the student's mode of communication, parental attitudes, and educational environment, the student may or may not prefer to socialize with other deaf students and may begin to identify with Deaf culture.	Comprehensive support services must be available to encourage academic success. While some students will attend residential settings, many others will receive their instruction in included settings with a team of support personnel.

Source: Based on Keith (1996); Turbull, Turnbull, Shank, Smith, & Leal (2002).

In addition to the classification system, several other factors determine how well individuals with any given degree of loss will function within their surroundings. The following list contains several pertinent factors; however, it is certainly not exhaustive:

- The auditory environment in which listening occurs
- The individuals' ability to utilize speech reading, speech, and residual hearing
- Any secondary handicapping conditions such as physical impairments and/or mental handicaps
- The individual's vocational occupation

TABLE 7.2 Degree and Prevalence of Hearing Loss Within the School-Age Population

Mild	(from 27–40 db, ANSI)	13.3%
Moderate	(from 41–55 dB, ANSI)	14.2%
Moderate severe	(from 56–70 dB, ANSI)	12.3%
Severe	(from 71–90 dB, ANSI)	13.8%
Profound	(from 91 dB and above, ANSI)	27.5%

Source: Gallaudet Research Institute (2008).

- Personal lifestyle preference
- Educational background
- Etiological factors
- Psychological adjustment to degree of hearing loss

These factors are evaluated through a complementary battery of tests prescribed by the clinician.

SPEECH RECEPTION THRESHOLD TESTS

Audiometric testing would not be complete without an assessment of the individual's ability to hear and understand speech sounds. The focus of this testing revolves around the individuals' abilities to understand speech to the degree that they can repeat simple words or understand phrases or connected speech. The softest intensity level at which the individual can repeat words or understand phrases is referred to as the speech reception threshold (SRT). A common test administered to establish SRT consists of two-syllable words, which are referred to as spondees. One's SRT is defined as the hearing level at which the examinee can repeat 50% of the words accurately.

The ability to discriminate speech or words is also critical. Although some individuals have the ability to hear (i.e., detect) speech at increased amplitude levels, they may suffer an impairment in understanding what is heard. As similar sounds are produced, individuals may have difficulty discriminating one sound from another and, therefore, cannot understand the spoken words.

To test word discrimination skills, phonetically balanced (PB) word lists are administered at a minimum of 40 dB greater than the individual's SRT. Each list contains 50 monosyllabic words, equally representing samples of speech sounds that are found in typical spoken English phrases and sentences. Scoring of this test is based on the percentage of words the individual hears correctly.

SOCIAL ADEQUACY INDEX

Speech discrimination tests provide information pertaining to the individual's ability to perceive speech sounds. However, the test scores by themselves are of minimal use to the clinician. It is essential to relate these findings to the individual's ability to function socially in everyday settings. At the present time a specific formula has not been developed for equating speech discrimination scores with particular levels of social functioning. Rather, one must examine these scores as they relate to a multitude of variables. Those variables that have particular significance and contribute to communication performance include intelligence, motivation, experience, communication set, situational cues, expectation, redundance, and linguistic sophistication (Paul & Whitelaw, 2011).

Although valuable data are gained by administering speech discrimination tests, it is critical that the findings be integrated with additional data previously obtained during the audiologic testing process. It is of paramount importance that observations made by the clinician be coupled with the formal test results so that an accurate picture of the person's ability to communicate within his or her environment is established.

The purpose of an audiologic evaluation is to identify the cause and type of hearing loss the individual has and to determine what form of amplification, if any, will be beneficial. Frequently, a medical doctor (an otolaryngologist or an otologist) will do the initial evaluation to determine if the loss results from a medical problem. A hearing evaluation, performed by an audiologist or medical doctor, assists in determining the location of a hearing impairment along the auditory peripheral or central pathway. If no obvious problem is identified, the person may be scheduled for further evaluation with an audiologist.

Throughout the United States, the current trend is to conduct hearing screenings on newborns before they are discharged from the hospital. This relatively new practice was implemented in March 1993 when the National Institutes of Health (NIH) recommended that all newborns be screened for hearing loss (White et al., 2005). Prior to that time less than 3% of newborns in the United States were being screened. However, as recently as 2005, based on the endorsement of NIH, 93% of newborns nationwide were receiving the universal newborn hearing screening, data collected by the National Center for Hearing Assessment and Management (NCHAM, 2005). Currently, all states now have data collected by the National Center for Hearing Assessment and Management (NCHAM, 2005); they have also established that an early detection and intervention program ensures that all infants are screened before they reach 1 month of age. Infants who fail the screening receive additional evaluations prior to 3 months of age and are enrolled in an appropriate intervention program prior to 6 months of age (White, 2003).

What is involved in this screening procedure? What types of tests are administered to infants prior to their discharge from the hospital? What kind of information is usually gleaned from these early evaluations?

NEONATAL SCREENING

Two screening procedures are typically administered to newborns and infants. Both can detect permanent or fluctuating, bilateral or unilateral, and sensory or conductive hearing loss that averages 30 to 40 dB or greater in the frequency range critical for speech recognition (approximately 500–4,000 Hz) (ASHA, 2009). The two procedures include the otoacoustic emissions (OAEs) and/or automated auditory brain stem response (AABR). Both procedures can be administered without causing any pain to the infant while the child is resting quietly.

Otoacoustic Emissions

The use of otoacoustic emissions (OAEs) as a neonatal screening procedure has emerged rapidly in recent years. Designed to screen infants during their first few days of life while they lie quietly in their bassinets, it is being found to be an excellent screening mechanism to identify infants who have a hearing loss greater than 25 to 30 dB. The procedure involves the use of noninvasive technology.

To conduct the screening, a probe that contains a miniature loudspeaker is placed in the external auditory canal. The loudspeaker presents the stimulus while a tiny microphone picks up the emission and converts it from sound into an electrical signal. The stimulus causes the outer hair cells of the cochlea to vibrate; in turn, the vibration produces an inaudible sound that echoes back into the middle and outer ear. This sound is identified by the probe, indicating that the infant can hear. Those infants with normal hearing will produce emissions that can be measured by the probe. Those with a hearing loss greater than 25 to 30 dB will not produce the emissions (Martin & Clark, 2009; ASHA, 2009).

Frequently infants are screened first using a transient evoked otoacoustic emissions (OAEs) measurement to determine any cause to suspect hearing loss. In the event the newborn fails the initial evaluation, an automated auditory brain stem response (AABR) is usually requested.

Two screenings are typically conducted to confirm findings before a follow-up audiologic or medical evaluation is recommended.

Auditory Brain Stem Response

The purpose of an auditory brain stem response (ABR) is to measure responses from the brain. This screening requires that the infant be resting quietly. During administration of this test, electrodes are placed on the scalp behind the outer ear and on the vertex (top) of the skull, with a ground electrode placed on the opposite mastoid, the forehead, or the neck (Martin & Clark, 2009). These sensors measure electrical activity as the infant responds to auditory stimuli. Auditory brain stem responses (ABRs) can detect damage to the cochlea, the auditory nerve, and the auditory pathways located in the stem of the brain (Martin & Clark, 2009; ASHA, 2009).

Trained technicians can perform ABRs. Additional in-depth diagnostic ABR procedures are conducted by audiologists. Initially, due to the highly qualified personnel and the time required to conduct this screening, ABRs were not typically administered in well-baby nurseries. Rather, they were only used to screen infants placed in the neonatal intensive-care nurseries (NICS), due to the relatively high incidence of handicapping hearing loss found in babies placed in these nurseries (Herrmann, Thornton, & Joseph, 1995). However, a frequent strategy that is being used in various locations involves a two-stage screening protocol prior to babies being discharged from the hospital. Using this protocol, newborns are screened first with either "distortion product or transient evoked otoacoustic emissions (OAEs), and those who fail are screened with automated auditory brain stem responses (A-ABR)" (White et al., 2005). A major reason for the two-step process is to reduce the number of infants being referred for additional testing upon discharge from the hospital.

Even with universal newborn hearing screenings being conducted throughout the United States, the Centers for Disease Control and Prevention (CDC) estimate that 44% of the infants referred from these screening programs are "lost to the system" before completing a diagnostic evaluation (CDC, 2005). What happens when infants are not identified at an early age? What happens to those who are not scheduled for follow-up appointments? How is their hearing loss identified? What if an infant passes the screening tests but later shows signs of having difficulty hearing? What types of tests are used with infants, preschoolers and, later, school-age children?

INFANTS AND TODDLERS

If an infant does not pass the initial screening tests, they are generally referred for a follow-up medical and audiologic examination to take place within the first 3 months. The purpose of these evaluations is to confirm the presence of a hearing loss, determine the cause and type of loss, and identify options for treatment. Parents, whose infants show indicators for a progressive or delayed-onset hearing loss, are encouraged to receive audiologic monitoring every 6 months until their child is 3 years of age (ASHA, 2009). Two areas of pediatric audiologic evaluations can be conducted: behavioral, which requires responses from the child, and those involving electrophysiology tests. The electrophysiology evaluation tests in the pediatric battery often include ABR, OAE, and tympanometry. With very young children (6 to 8 months of age), behavioral observation audiometry (BOA) is often implemented. Two clinicians work together in BOA to present a variety of sounds. Although this type of screening can be used to indicate a hearing loss, it provides little or no information about the configuration of the loss (Martin & Clark, 2009).

However, as children continue to grow and reach 18 months of age, two screening techniques are typically used to indicate a loss. These include visual reinforcement audiometry (VRA) and operant conditioning audiometry (OCA). In VRA, children as young as 6 months receive auditory stimulation, either through earphones or a sound field consisting of varied tones and speech sounds. As the child responds, his or her response is reinforced by using anything that interests the child (i.e., a picture, animated toy, light, and so forth). In OCA, food, play (putting objects in a box or placing pegs in holes), and other tangible reinforcements can be used to encourage children (age 2½ to 5 years) to respond to sounds as they are introduced. In the event that these screening techniques are not successful, alternative procedures such as OAEs or ABRs can be used to obtain information.

SCHOOL-AGE CHILDREN

School-age children between 5 and 18 years of age should be screened for hearing loss as needed, when requested, or when conditions place them at risk for developing a hearing loss. The ASHA (2009) recommends that children should be screened on first entry into school, and, every year from kindergarten through 3rd grade, in 7th grade, in 11th grade, or if a student begins receiving special education services, repeats a grade, or enters a new school system. School-age children with no evidence of additional disabilities other than anticipated hearing loss can be evaluated by a clinician using the following test battery: pure-tone testing, both by air and bone conduction, with appropriate masking; SRT tests; auditory discrimination tests at suprathreshold levels; and tympanometry.

In conjunction with these tests the audiologist is also evaluating the student's communication function, listening skill development, hearing loss adjustment, and environmental factors that impact the child's ability to receive classroom information. By administering a comprehensive test battery, audiologists are able to obtain information that helps them identify the problem area and describe how it impacts the child (Johnson, 2009).

In the event a child's hearing tests within the normal range—but with evidence of poor listening skills, short attention span, or a communication or academic problem or problems—the child might be evaluated to determine if he or she has a central auditory processing disorder (C)APD. In 2005 ASHA discussed removing the word "central" from the title of this disorder to reflect the broad nature of the developmental or acquired communication problems it encompasses. However, rather than changing the designation, the ASHA reported that both terms—auditory processing disorder (APD) and (C)APD—were acceptable with the word *central* remaining in parentheses. (C)APD now appears in the literature. Encompassing a broader perspective, the current term allows for difficulties to be identified by the anatomical location (Tillery, 2009). With (C)APD affecting an estimated 2 to 3% of children, and with twice as many males thusly diagnosed (Chermak & Musiek, 1997), it has been recognized as a diagnostic category that merits treatment. Identification is based on a comprehensive assessment with input from audiologists, speech-language pathologists, educators, and psychologists.

Children who experience a (C)APD may exhibit poor listening skills, have short attention spans, and may experience difficulty mastering reading comprehension. Unlike children with a hearing loss that can be treated through amplification and support services, children who have (C)APD are provided with strategies to improve their listening skills, classroom listening devices, and spoken language comprehension. Those experiencing a loss other than (C)APD are frequently provided with amplification options that may include hearing aids, assistive listening devices, cochlear implants, or other implantable devices.

THE FUNCTION AND COMPONENTS OF HEARING AIDS

The basic function of a hearing aid is to amplify sounds, making them more intense or loud for the individual with a hearing loss. It operates like many other amplifying devices incorporating a microphone, amplifier, and receiver into its system.

Microphones

The purpose of the microphone is to pick up sounds in the environment. The two general types of microphones are directional and omnidirectional (Tye-Murray, 2009). Directional microphones were first used in hearing aids in 1972. Designed to pick up sounds from in front of the head, these microphones are less sensitive to other sounds occurring in the environment, thereby enabling listeners to hear the individual speaker in front of them. However, in rooms where a great deal of reverberant noise is present, the effectiveness of the microphone can be compromised (Paul & Whitelaw, 2011; Smaldino, Crandell, Kreisman, John, & Kreisman, 2009).

Omnidirectional microphones pick up sounds from all directions. In essence, they do more than just enable the listener to focus on an individual speaker; they also help listeners connect with their environment and the sounds that surround them. When dual microphones, incorporating the use of two omnidirectional microphones, are used by the listener, he or she has the advantage of equally picking up sounds that are being transmitted from a wide array of locations (Smaldino et al., 2009).

Amplifier

The amplifier serves two basic purposes. First, it amplifies the original environmental sound, which is received as a pulsating electrical signal from the microphone. This amplification is an optimal volume for assistance with hearing. Second, to avoid exceeding the user's level of comfort, it limits the amount of sound pressure that the aid can deliver.

The amplifier consists of a series of integrated circuits (ICs). These circuits are comprised of transistors, diodes, and resistors on a silicon chip to provide the individual with the desired electronic output (Bentler & Mueller, 2009).

Receiver

The function of the receiver is to convert the electrical signal back to an acoustical signal that is louder than the original environmental signal that was received by the microphone. The amplified acoustical signal is channeled through a receiver sending sound impulses into a plastic tube that directs the sound into the ear canal. When behind-the-ear hearing aids are utilized, the tube is guided into the ear canal by a supporting structure called an earmold.

Earmolds

Some earmolds are made from a hard material, such as Lucite, and others are soft and made out of materials such as silicone. The type of mold and material is based on the degree of hearing loss and related acoustic parameters as well as the person's desire for a particular color, pattern, or material. Regardless of the material used, all earmolds are designed to fit the ear so that sound can be transmitted into the car canal and onto the eardrum (Paul & Whitelaw, 2011). An earmold prevents sound from leaking out of the ear and has a strong effect on the overall performance of the aid. It is essential that the earmold be designed to enhance the sound as it courses down the ear canal, to fit comfortably, to appear cosmetically attractive, and to be easily cleaned.

The following are the three main types of earmolds (Bentler & Mueller, 2009):

The regular or receiver. In this type the earmold fills a considerable part of the concha and extends into the ear canal.

The skeleton or one of a similar type. With this mold, only the amount of material necessary for sealing, retention, and comfort is utilized. It is designed with a tip that extends into the ear canal and seals against its walls.

Open or nonoccluding. This type of mold is designed to keep the ear canal as unoccluded as possible. An open or unoccluded type of mold is used with tubing or a small diameter tip that projects into the ear canal.

If an earmold does not fit properly, the overall functioning of the aid will be affected. In addition, a loose-fitting mold may permit leakage of sound transmitted by the aid, thus producing a whistling sound commonly referred to as feedback.

Additional Components

Hearing aids have additional highly sophisticated circuitry to enhance their performance. Although not all the controls are available on all aids, most share the more common ones: volume control, telecoil circuitry, and batteries.

VOLUME CONTROL. Volume controls (sometimes referred to as gain controls) enable the hearing-aid wearer to adjust the level of sound to a comfortable listening level as it is delivered to the ear. If the control is set too loud, headaches and dizziness may occur.

PITCH OR TONE CONTROL. A pitch or tone control is used to alter the frequency response or the pitch emphasis of the amplified sound. Unlike the volume control, this control is set by the audiologist or hearing-aid dispenser and should not be altered. This circuitry is especially beneficial for people who have a loss in one primary frequency range. Individuals who experience normal hearing in only the low-frequency range can benefit from a hearing aid with the tone control set to emphasize high-frequency sounds.

TELECOIL CIRCUITRY. Many hearing aids have circuitry built into the aid to make it easier to hear what is being said over a telephone. In 1988 the Hearing Aid Compatibilities Act was passed by the U.S. House of Representatives (House Bill H-22213) and Senate (S-314), mandating that all public telephones be compatible for use with telecoils. Hearing aids incorporating this circuitry utilize a telephone switch, usually labeled T on the hearing-aid case. The T switch when turned on activates the telecoil.

Telecoils function by responding to a magnetic field generated by the receiver within the telephone handset. Due to the variability in how handsets are constructed, some units are not designed to generate an adequate magnetic field. Adaptors can be purchased and attached to the earphone portion of the handset to correct this problem; they will change the acoustic energy of the earphone into a useful magnetic field. Other modifications installed directly within the handset can also produce the desired magnetic field. In addition to providing the wearer with increased opportunity for telephone use, telecoils increase one's options for accessing various assistive listening devices, such as closed-circuit "loop" systems found in large meeting rooms, theaters, churches, and synagogues. The telecoil receives the magnetic energy produced by these other devices. Subsequently, the hearing aid amplifies and then converts the energy into an audible sound.

BATTERIES. Batteries supply the electrical power to the aid and consist of two main types: zinc and mercury. Currently, zinc air batteries are the most widely used They have a significantly longer shelf life than mercury batteries and will last approximately twice as long while in use in the hearing aid (J. Shelfer, personal communication, 1990).

TYPES OF HEARING AIDS

The earliest form of amplification utilized was probably man's hand cupped behind his ear. Acoustic amplifiers such as horns and speaking tubes followed the concept of cupping one's hand. These were followed by carbon hearing aids that were based on the principle of the telephone. Around 1938, vacuum tube hearing aids appeared and offered much greater amplification possibilities, wider frequency response, and lower harmonic distortion (Katz, 2009).

Today's hearing aids come in a variety of types and styles (see Figures 7.5, 7.6, 7.7, and 7.8) and are based on the invention of the transistor by Bell Telephone Laboratories. This discovery enabled manufacturers to design hearing aids that are much smaller and more powerful and to transition from analog to digital programmable aids. Individuals experiencing a hearing loss have a variety of aids from which to select.

Over the Ear or Behind the Ear

The Over the Ear, or as it has also been described as the Behind the Ear (BTE) was the principal type of aid used for several years. The aid fits behind the pinna with the tubing going over the ear and carrying sound to the earmold. This type of aid provides enough room for several fitting adjustments. They are durable and are easily serviceable. Because they are able to produce a significant amount of power, OTEs/BTEs are now being commonly used by individuals with mild and moderate, as well as severe to profound, losses. The basic design of this aid provides enough distance between the microphone and the earmold tip to facilitate increased power usage without encountering problems with feedback. In addition, many assistive devices are designed for use with OTE/BTE aids either through the use of the T-coil or a boot that can plug into the aid. The boot is a connection that is attached at the bottom of the hearing aid and allows a cord to be plugged into it. The cord is then connected to the signal-receiving device of the assistive listening device, enabling the hearing aid user to hear the sound being generated by the assistive listening device through the personal hearing aid (see "Assistive Listening Devices"). (See Figure 7.5 for an example of a BTE hearing aid.)

All In the Ear or In the Ear

All in the ear (AIE) hearing aids that fit entirely in the ear have become increasingly popular in the United States. In 1983 they accounted for 49.4% of hearing-aid sales (Hearing Industries Association, 1984). Recent technology has facilitated the miniaturization of electret microphones, correspondingly small receivers, and batteries. These advances have allowed the aid to be designed to fit within the concha and the ear canal.

In the ear (ITE) aids are primarily custom designed; however, modular units are also available. Custom aids are built into a shell made from an impression of the user's ear. Modular ITE aids are built into a case of fixed shape that fits into a matching depression in a custom earmold.

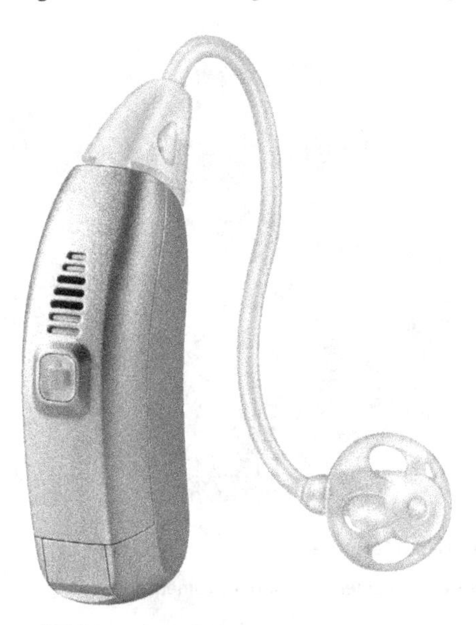

FIGURE 7.5 A behind-the-ear (BTE) hearing aid.

Source: Courtesy of Rexton, A division of Siemens Hearing Instruments, Inc.

There are three main styles of custom in-the-ear aids: in the ear (ITE), in the canal (ITC), and completely in the canal (CIC).

IN THE EAR (ITE). This is the most commonly utilized custom aid. It occupies the entire concha area of the ear and extends into the canal. It permits the greatest flexibility in circuit design and fitting flexibility. (See Figure 7.6 for an example of an ITE).

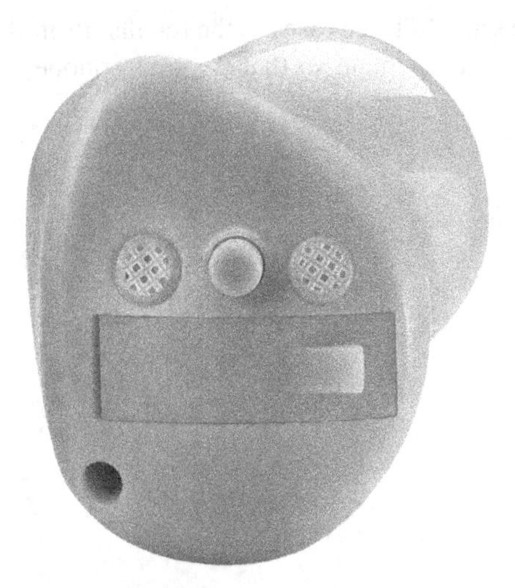

FIGURE 7.6 An in-the-ear (ITE) custom hearing aid.

Source: Courtesy of Rexton, A division of Siemens Hearing Instruments, Inc.

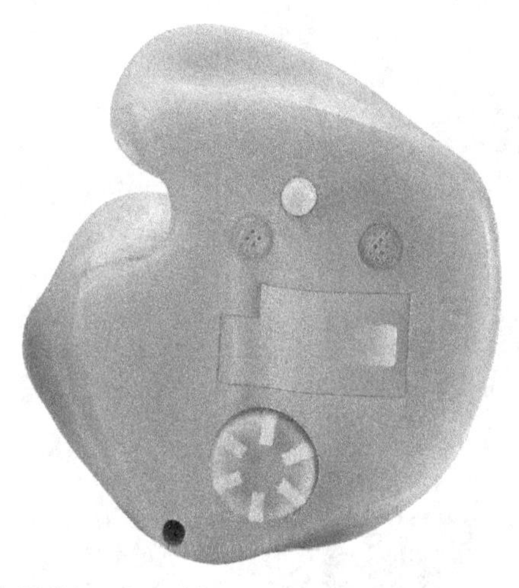

FIGURE 7.7 An in-the-canal (ITC) hearing aid.

Source: Courtesy of Rexton, A division of Siemens Hearing Instruments, Inc.

IN THE CANAL (ITC). This aid occupies the concha, cavum, and canal. Because it is smaller, less room is available for the circuits and components, limiting its potential for gain and output. (See Figure 7.7 for an example of an ITC.)

COMPLETELY IN THE CANAL. This style of aid is the least visible of all. It fits in a small space at the beginning of the ear canal. The sound quality of these aids can be quite good as the bowl of the ear is open and can help collect sounds. In addition, the tip of the aid is closer to the eardrum for better high-frequency hearing. (See Figure 7.8 for an example of a CIC).

Low-Profile Aids

This type of aid utilizes the same full size cases as the regular all-in-the-ear aids. However, it has an additional feature: an inset faceplate so that the microphone, battery cover, and volume

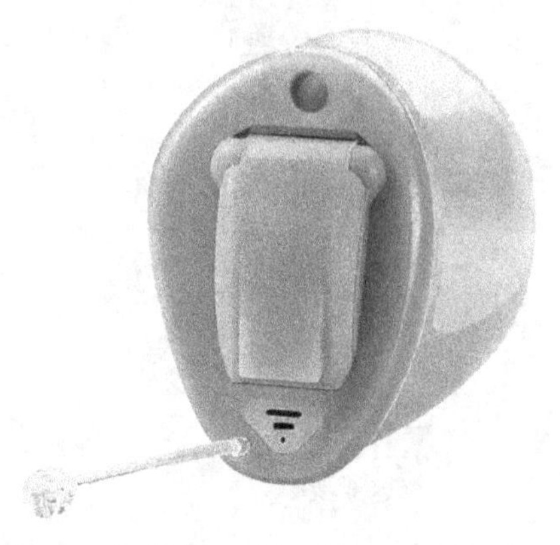

FIGURE 7.8 A completely-in-the-canal (CIC) hearing aid.

Source: Courtesy of Rexton, A division of Siemens Hearing Instruments, Inc.

control are recessed. Because those parts are less apparent, wind and noise are reduced and the ear bowl helps gather sounds.

CROS Hearing Aids

Contralateral routing of signals (CROS) hearing aids are designed for individuals who have an essentially nonfunctional or unaidable ear and a good ear. Encased in a hearing aid worn on the nonfunctioning ear, a microphone picks up sound from the nonfunctioning ear and routes it to the good ear. A hearing-aid device is also utilized on the good ear, receives sound from the poor ear, and directs it into the good ear. Both hearing-aid devices are connected by a cord that extends around the back of the head, or by a small, wireless FM radio transmitter, allowing the signal to be transferred from one ear to the other.

BiCROS Hearing Aids

Bi-contralateral routing of signals (Bi-CROS) hearing aids are particularly beneficial for the individual experiencing deafness in one ear and a high-frequency loss in the other. By utilizing a nonoccluding, open earmold design on the good ear, the tubing permits good amplification in the high-frequency range while reducing the low-frequency response. Sound from the poor ear's side of the head is transmitted to the good ear, which also receives added amplification needed by the good ear to assist in hearing sounds in the high-frequency range where the hearing loss exists (J. Shelfer, personal communication, 1990).

The transcranial CROS differs from the conventional CROS in the way that sound is transferred from the impaired ear into the good ear. When employing this technique, a high gain–high output ITE or BTE aid is placed in the impaired ear. The sound is then transmitted through the cranial structures of the temporal bone into the cochlea of the better ear. Thus, sound travels by way of bone conduction (Valente, Meister, McCauley, & Cass, 1994). Recipients of the transcranial cross have reported "that amplified sound presented through their transcranial CROS was more 'natural' than the sound processed through their conventional CROS" (Freyman, Nerbonne, & Cole, 1991, p. 420).

IROS Hearing Aids

Ipsilateral routing of signals (IROS) hearing aids have an open earmold. They came into use after the open tubing effect of the CROS aid proved beneficial for sharply falling sensorineural hearing losses. This design can be utilized with BTE/OTE aids. When incorporated, the tubing itself projects into the ear canal with a nonoccluding earmold. Those individuals exhibiting mild to moderate sensorineural losses are able to benefit from this type of configuration and enjoy the comfort of not having an earmold that is occluding the ear. This allows the ear's natural resonance to be utilized, enhancing the amplification of the high frequencies where the hearing loss is being experienced.

Bone-Conduction Hearing Aids

Bone-conduction aids operate by applying sound vibrations to the bones behind the ears. Although some sounds can be heard this way, the performance of this aid is poor when compared to aids that utilize earmolds (such as air-conduction hearing aids). Very frequently bone-conduction aids are used only where there is no ear canal or where there is chronic ear canal drainage.

Traditionally, bone-conduction aids were used in individuals who experienced a large discrepancy in their ability to hear sounds as they were received through the auditory canal and temporal bone vibrations. When the air–bone gap exceeded 35 dB, conductive aids were employed. However, because of the success of stapes surgery in reducing the air–bone gap, the need for bone-conduction aids has diminished.

Currently, two major types of conventional bone-conduction aids are being used. One incorporates a body aid, and the other utilizes the eyeglass aid. When a bone-conduction aid is used in conjunction with a body aid, a bone receiver is substituted for the air receiver and is held against the mastoid processes of the user by a headband. When eyeglasses or an OTE aid is used, the bone receiver is incorporated into one end of the eyeglasses or a headband is utilized.

Implantable Bone-Anchored Hearing Aid

For individuals who cannot utilize either the conventional bone- or air-conduction hearing aid but would benefit from a bone-conduction type of hearing aid, an implantable temporal bone stimulator has been developed. People who have chronically draining ears or an ear deformity, such as atresia of the ear canal or absent pinna, may be candidates for this type of device. The bone-anchored hearing aid (BAHA) is a medically implanted device that requires medical and audiologic management. Basically, this unit is an electromagnetic device that directly stimulates the cochlea via a magnet implanted in the temporal bone. Individuals whose bone-conduction thresholds are no worse than 40 dB HL in the speech frequencies appear to benefit most. Furthermore, research conducted by Snik, Mylanus, and Cremers (1994) indicated that implantable bone-conduction devices were found to be more effective than previously worn traditional bone-conduction hearing aids. Patients indicated that the quality of sound they received was good; the amount of acoustic feedback found in traditional hearing aids was less and, therefore, they preferred the implantable aid over the traditional hearing aid. The audiologist utilizes patient feedback together with test results to determine which device will provide maximum use of the auditory response of the cochlea.

Implantable Middle Ear Hearing Aid

Individuals who experience a conductive or mixed loss, due to middle ear transmission problems, may benefit from an implantable aid. These aids are designed to directly drive the ossicles, thus providing more "comfortable" speech reception for the listener.

Two designs are currently being explored: the partially implantable hearing device (PIHD) and the totally implantable hearing device (TIHD). Although they differ in which components are housed externally, both provide direct magnetic stimulation to the tympanic membrane or the ossicular chain (Goode, 1995; Maniglia, 1989).

Digital Technology

The term *digital hearing aid* can be used to encompass anything from an aid that incorporates touch volume controls to those instruments that have been computer programmed to meet the individual needs of the consumer. According to Kirkwood (2006) almost 90% of the hearing aids sold in the United States in 2006 were digital hearing aids. Designed to separate electrical signals into basic units of information representing the characteristics of sound input that include frequency, intensity, and timing aspects, individuals are able to move from one social environment into another. Digital hearing aids provide them with a mechanism whereby they can adjust the performance program by pressing the hearing aid's up or down digital control buttons. In certain situations the program tells the system to reject "noise" and amplify only "speech." In a noisy environment the hearing aid analyzes incoming noise and speech, compares both to coded data in its memory, and then processes the speech differently—all within 10 microseconds. Furthermore, digital aids allow the individual to connect with devices such as telephones or computers through wireless Bluetooth transmission (Levitt, 2007; Ricketts, 2009). This technology can be especially beneficial for individuals who have poor speech discrimination/understanding, even under ideal listening conditions.

Cochlear Implants

Cochlear implants (CI) have changed tremendously since they were first introduced in the 1980s. Improvements have been made to both the internal and external components. Now recognized as a safe and effective treatment for both children and adults who exhibit moderate to profound losses, CIs provide most users with the ability to detect speech sounds within the range of 100 to 6,000 Hz at approximately 20 to 40 dB. This provides individuals who are deaf and hard of hearing with access to high-frequency information that is not typically available through the use of hearing aids (Zwolan, 2009).

Children as well as adults are often strong candidates for CIs. Viable candidates are those who have profound bilateral losses and, ideally, have no additional disabilities. Children must meet the following guidelines to be considered as a CI candidate: have a severe to profound bilateral sensory-neural hearing loss, be at least 12 months of age or older, receive little or no benefit from hearing aids, have no medical or radiologic contraindications to surgery, be placed in an educational setting that is committed to providing auditory skill development, and be surrounded by a motivated family. Guidelines for adults include at least a moderate hearing loss in the low frequencies and a profound loss in the mid to high speech frequencies bilaterally, receive little or no benefit from hearing aids, have no medical or radiologic contraindications to surgery, and be motivated with realistic expectations (Zwolan, 2009).

CIs involve a surgical procedure that can last between 2 and 5 hours. During that time an array of electrodes is implanted into the ear within the cochlea. The implanted electrodes stimulate different hearing fibers that send messages on to the brain. Information is initially received from an external microphone and is then transmitted to a speech processor by a thin cable that connects them. Subsequently, the speech processor codes the sound signal and returns it to the transmitter. These electric codes are sent to the receiver/stimulator and then on to the electrode array implanted in the cochlea (DeBonis & Donohue, 2004).

Both children and adults have been successful implant recipients. These individuals have found traditional hearing aids to be of no significant benefit. For children to derive benefit from CIs, the implants must provide rudimentary hearing to profoundly deaf persons and improve their speechreading ability. Additional factors that contribute to the success of the implant include the person's motivation to optimize hearing and the determination to undergo the expense and discomfort of the surgical procedure.

Cochlear implants rely on several components; they include internal devices as well as external components. The internal device consists of a receiving coil/internal processor and the array of electrodes that deliver the signal to the inner ear. Placed surgically in the mastoid bone, the processor consists of a magnet so the external headset can be attached; it also has an antenna that receives the transmitted signal. The external components work together to collect, analyze, process, and deliver auditory signals to the internal components. The external part of a CI

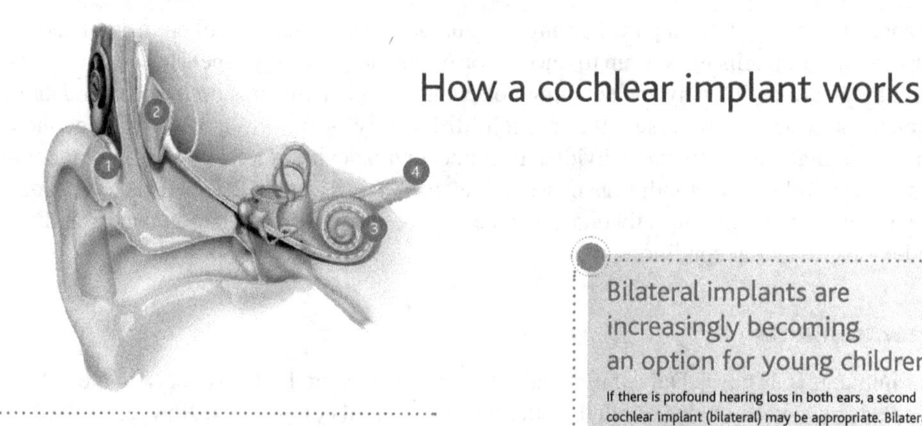

How a cochlear implant works

1. The external sound processor captures sounds, then filters and processes the sounds.
2. The sound processor translates the filtered sounds into digital information, which is then transmitted to the internal implant.
3. The internal implant converts the digital information into electrical signals, and sends them to a tiny, delicate curl of electrodes that sits gently inside the cochlea.
4. The electrical signals from the electrodes stimulate the hearing nerve, bypassing the damaged cells that cause hearing loss and allowing the brain to perceive sound.

FIGURE 7.9 How a cochlear implant works.

Source: Courtesy of Cochlears America.

consists of a microphone, speech processor, connecting cables, and a transmitter coil (Zwolan, 2009). (See Figure 7.9 for an illustration of a cochlear implant.)

BINAURAL AND MONAURAL HEARING AID FITTINGS

Research has been conducted over the past several years to determine if binaural aids (two aids) are more beneficial for the consumer than monaural aids (one aid).

Studies show that those wearing binaural rather than only monaural aids can discern sounds in ambient noise better. They also provide the individual with greater versatility in social situations (Ross, 2006).

People hear better with two ears than with one. Sounds are clearer and stronger with binaural aids, and they provide the listener with a stereo effect similar to that of normal hearing. In addition, two aids assist the individual as he or she attempts to determine the directionality of sound and locate the individual who is speaking. Today bilateral cochlear implants as well as binaural aids are also becoming increasingly popular.

HEARING-AID ORIENTATION

Following the hearing evaluation an appropriate aid is selected and an earmold is designed. Instruction is then necessary to familiarize the user with the device. The purpose of hearing-aid orientation is to help the consumers adjust to the use of their aid. At this time individuals learn how to use the aid and what benefits to expect. In addition to acquiring information regarding the physical characteristics of the aid, individuals may need to receive counseling addressing the psychological and emotional ramifications of hearing loss. Keep in mind that this is a diverse population with varying needs.

Physical Aspects of Hearing-aid Use

During the orientation period the person who is deaf or hard of hearing must be provided information pertaining to the following topics:

- How to insert, remove, and clean the earmold
- How to utilize the various switches:
  - On-off switch
  - Gain control
  - Telephone switch
  - Tone control
- What type of batteries the aid uses, where to purchase them, and how to change them
- What the device can and cannot do to improve communication
- What may be the user's communication abilities and limitations with the hearing aid

Psychological and Emotional Ramifications of Hearing Loss

Throughout the orientation session, it is imperative that the audiologist foster acceptance and objectivity regarding the hearing loss in a way that helps the consumer feel comfortable in utilizing an aid. (See Table 7.3 for tips on how to communicate with individuals who are deaf and hard of hearing.) The following topics may need to be discussed with the person who is deaf or hard of hearing:

- Understanding the nature of the hearing loss
- Understanding the nature, advantages, and limitations of hearing aids and cochlear implants
- Learning acceptance of the loss and making a commitment to use amplification
- Learning how to inform other people of the loss and providing them with communication tips that will benefit individuals who are deaf and hard of hearing

In addition, the person who is going to wear an aid needs to know when to wear it. This will be determined by the magnitude of the loss, the demands on the individual's hearing, and the environment in which listening occurs. Individuals with slight or mild hearing losses may benefit from wearing aids part time, utilizing them in quiet surroundings where people speak softly. Individuals experiencing a moderate loss may find wearing an aid most of the time beneficial, with removal in "cocktail party" listening situations helpful. Listeners with severe or profound losses who use amplification generally wear their aids on a full-time basis; although aids do not afford them the opportunity to understand speech, they do keep them in contact with the environment.

When individuals begin wearing an aid, they may become aware of environmental sounds that they had forgotten existed. Some new hearing-aid users make an easy adjustment and wear their aid from the moment they receive it. Other individuals, especially those with very mild or quite severe losses, may require a long time to adjust. Throughout the orientation period, the person who is deaf or hard of hearing is provided with suggestions, thus providing the necessary tools to effectively utilize their specific type of amplification.

TABLE 7.3 Tips for Communicating with Persons Who Are Deaf or Hard of Hearing

Physical /Environmental Considerations

- Face the person directly when communicating.
- Avoid talking with your back to a light source.
- Avoid talking with anything in your mouth (pens, pencils, etc.).
- Avoid covering your mouth while speaking.
- Refrain from turning your head during the course of the conversation.
- Maintain eye contact.
- Remain within 3 to 5 feet.
- Select a quite environment for communication exchanges.
- When possible, let the person with a hearing loss select the location for the dialogue to take place.
- When using visual aids, give the person time to look at the aid before attempting to speech read.

Spoken Communication Considerations

- Make sure the person is looking at you before you begin speaking.
- If more than one person is engaged in the conversation, identify/reference who is about to speak before he or she begins.
- When multiple people are engaged in a discussion (classroom settings, social gatherings, etc.), make sure that only one person at a time talks.
- Speak clearly and at a normal pace.
- If a person does not understand what you have said or asked, ask the person to tell you what part he or she missed.
- Rephrase rather than repeat messages that are not understood; oftentimes it is the word order or the word choices that are confusing.
- Avoid shouting—this will distort your message.
- Use open-ended questions to check for clarification.
- Don't be afraid of incorporating gestures and employing natural facial expressions.
- State the topic before you begin and let the person know if you change topics.
- Ask the person what will be of help in the communication process.
- Keep in mind that a person might be able to hear a voice and know that someone is speaking but might not be able to not understand the words that are spoken.

Communicating Through Signs or Through the Use of an Interpreter

- If you know some basic signs, don't be afraid to use them.
- When signing to a deaf person, if a hearing person comes up, continue to sign; don't leave the deaf person out of the conversation.
- When using an interpreter speak directly to the deaf person; the interpreter will respond in the first person.
- Rely on writing if you reach a communication impasse.
- Use open-ended questions to check for clarification.

GROUP LISTENING SYSTEMS

In addition to individual aids, group listening systems are available for people with severe losses. Such a system can also prove helpful for someone experiencing a mild loss, provided the individual accepts the loss and is willing to seek help. The four major types of group systems are audio loops, FM systems, AM systems, and those incorporating infrared light waves.

Audio Loops

Audio loops consist of a microphone, an amplifier, and a length of wire that loops the seating area. Within an audio loop sounds are convened to magnetic forces that emanate from wires under floors and around the walls. Hearing aids with telephone switches (T-coils) pick up these forces and change them back into sounds.

FM Systems

The frequency modulation (FM) system is very easy to install. Within this unit, transmitters broadcast sound using the same methods as radio stations. The listener uses a personal receiver for making sounds available to the ear. This system is easy to install, and the signals can be transmitted over a 300-foot range.

AM Systems

The amplitude modulation (AM) system works on the same principle as the FM system: however, it is more prone to static. Because it uses amplitude modulations instead of frequency modulations, it is comparable to an FM radio, which provides better sound fidelity than the same radio tuned to an AM station.

Infrared Systems

Infrared systems are one of the newer types of group listening devices. These systems are designed to convert sounds into infrared light waves that are converted back to sounds by the listener's infrared receivers. This system is easy to install and is virtually free of static. However, the range is limited to line-of-sight propagation, and the infrared light waves will not pass through obstructions such as walls or around corners. The devices are also subject to interference from some light sources.

INDIVIDUAL AMPLIFICATION SYSTEMS

Assistive Listening Devices

Assistive listening devices (ALDs) are designed to be used alone or in conjunction with a hearing aid. They send the desired signal directly from the sound force into the listener's ear. The signal is not affected by room noise or room acoustics. This allows listeners the opportunity to perceive the sound as if they are listening under ideal conditions. They require both the speaker and the listener to wear a unit about the size of a cigarette pack. The signal is usually transmitted by an infrared or FM signal. These systems are equipped with a microphone (for the speaker), amplifier, and receiver (for the person who is hard of hearing) and can be utilized one-on-one by those individuals attempting to participate in lecture or one-on-one communication situations. For individuals whose hearing loss involves (central) auditory processing problems, conventional hearing aids often provide little benefit. Personal ALDs tend to be much more effective due to the superior signal-to-noise ratio they achieve, which significantly reduces, if not entirely eliminates, unwanted background noise.

Telephone Amplifiers

Some individuals who are hard of hearing can better communicate on the phone if their telephone is equipped with an amplified handset. The amplifier, which is built into the phone handle, can be adjusted to an appropriate sound level.

Portable amplifiers are also available and are small enough to be carried in one's pocket or purse. These slip over most telephone receivers and virtually serve the same purpose. Not all phones are designed to work with portable amplifiers. However, telephone adaptors can be purchased to facilitate usage.

ADDITIONAL DEVICES FOR INDIVIDUALS WHO EXPERIENCE DIFFICULTY HEARING

Hearing aids, cochlear implants, assistive listening devices, and portable amplifiers are only some of the aids available to assist individuals with hearing losses. Other products have been devised to alert the persons who are deaf or hard of hearing to sounds within their environment.

Visual signals have been developed to alert persons with varying degrees of hearing loss to doorbells, telephones, alarm clocks, smoke alarms, and security systems. Additional devices have been designed to alert parents when their infant is crying. Light sources, increased amplification, and vibrotactile methods are employed when designing such assistive devices.

Summary

A variety of aids and assistive listening devices are available today. Modern technology has made great strides in providing individuals who are deaf or hard of hearing with stronger and more powerful forms of amplification. These new devices, coupled with orientation and consumer usage training programs, provide the wearer with opportunities not previously available.

In the next decade one can expect to see additional research into the development of implantable hearing aids designed for the middle ear as well as the auditory brain stem. Continued attention will be paid to cosmetics as aids that fit entirely in the ear canal are modified and perfected. Furthermore, research will continue in the area of digital technology to enhance these aids.

Although hearing frequently cannot be restored to within the normal functioning range, these devices can enhance users' ability to become aware of sounds within the environment, thereby assisting them in communication.

8

Educational Settings
From Tradition to Current Practice

Across the United States educational reform has undergone a tremendous metamorphosis since the 1960s. Producing a heightened sense of awareness within the public sector, this transformation has drawn attention to the quality of the curriculum, the teachers' mastery of their subject matter, and their knowledge of related pedagogy. Consequently, today's public school teachers are no longer considered effective based solely on their classroom management strategies and grade-level report cards; rather, their efficacy is ultimately measured by the scores their students earn on standardized tests.

Milestones, such as the Civil Rights Act of 1964, the inception of the Elementary and Secondary Education Act (ESEA) of 1964, and the No Child Left Behind (NCLB) Act of 2001, have all been instrumental in altering the landscape of American education. Throughout the past 40 years, the passage of these mandates in conjunction with other key pieces of legislation created a salient force influencing the reengineering of America's public education system. A brief historical overview of this legislation provides a foundation to examine pertinent topics relevant to the field of deaf education today. Embedded in this legislation are specific mandates that have influenced the way students with special needs are educated, particularly students who are deaf and hard of hearing, thus impacting their overall academic development and success.

What are the key pieces of legislation that have influenced the educational arena today? How has this legislation impacted the education of students who are deaf and hard of hearing? Where and how are these students being educated? How successful are education programs for students who are deaf and hard of hearing? What modes of communication are being used to deliver instruction? What are the evolving roles and responsibilities of school personnel serving these students? How can we characterize teachers of the D/deaf student population today? What role does the educational interpreter play in settings from pre–K through 12th grade? These are only some of the questions that are vital to the field. By examining these topics we can gain a deeper understanding of the issues, concerns, and future goals for today's students who are deaf.

HISTORICAL OVERVIEW: SCHOOL REFORM SINCE THE 1960S

Elementary and Secondary Education Act (1965)

The Elementary and Secondary Education Act (ESEA; Public Law 89-10) was enacted as part of the broad sweeping Civil Rights Act of 1964. The political tone of this era reflected presidential views that believed education was the key to social mobility and that a vast number of American schools lacked the necessary resources to provide fundamental skills to students from disadvantaged backgrounds. Designed to improve educational opportunities for students attending the poorest schools in the United States, Title I of the ESEA became the vehicle for providing financial assistance to meet the needs of educationally deprived children. The intent of this legislation was to assist disadvantaged children living in low-income areas by hiring additional educational staff members and purchasing additional classroom equipment. (See Table 3.1 for a synopsis of legislation that has made an impact on the education of students who are deaf or hard of hearing.)

Vocational Rehabilitation Act (1973)

Less than ten years after the ESEA was enacted, legislation was passed that would specifically define the term *handicapped person* and would further delineate the meaning of an "appropriate education" for individuals identified as having a handicapping condition. The landmark Vocational Rehabilitation Act (VRA; Public Law 93-112, Section 504) prohibits discrimination against students with disabilities in federally funded programs and entitles those with disabilities to a free and appropriate education.

Educational Amendments Act (1974)

Within the next year the Educational Amendments Act (Public Law 93-380) was passed, granting federal funds to states to establish or continue funding programming for learners who were exceptional. By providing the first federal funding for students who were gifted and talented, families were granted the right of due process in special education placement.

Education for All Handicapped Children Act (1975)

In 1975 the Education for All Handicapped Children Act (EAHCA; Public Law 94-142, Part B) was passed, frequently referred to as 94-142. Also known as the Mainstreaming Law, this particular legislation has had a dramatic effect on the education of students who are deaf and hard of hearing. Public Law 94-142 defines the term *least restrictive environment* as those classroom settings where chronological peers who are disabled and nondisabled receive their education alongside each other. It further requires states to provide a free and appropriate public education for children with disabilities between the ages of 5 and 18. Schools are obligated to develop individualized education programs (IEPs) for students with disabilities and provide educational opportunities for them in the least restrictive environment. Further discussion of how this legislation has impacted students who are deaf and hard of hearing is discussed later in this chapter.

Education of the Handicapped Act Amendments (1986)

Approximately 10 years after the EAHCA was passed, it was amended (Public Law 99-457) to include children with disabilities between birth and age 5 years. Requiring that states extend a free and appropriate education to children with disabilities between the ages of 3 and 5, this landmark legislation provided the impetus for the establishment of early intervention programs for infants and toddlers with disabilities from birth to age 2 years. Specific intervention programs designed to identify and serve infants with hearing loss have emerged as the result of this legislation and are discussed later in this chapter.

First Wave of Educational Reform

Although the 1980s are known for legislation pertaining to students with disabilities, the early 1980s are also noted within the public education sector as that period of time when the first wave of educational reform spread throughout the United States. With the release of "A Nation at Risk: The Imperative for Educational Reform," produced by the National Commission on Excellence in Education, the initiative for educational reform began. This report cited declining test scores, highlighted the number of functionally illiterate adults, acknowledged the large socioeconomic and racial achievement gaps among students, and compared the performance of U.S. students with students in other industrialized nations, indicating that students in the United States have considerably weaker test scores. As a result of this report, states were challenged to raise educational quality by requiring more courses and implementing more testing of student and teacher performance. Furthermore, states were to assume the leadership in improving existing practices.

Second Wave of Educational Reform

The second wave of educational reform began in 1986. The first wave of reform was initiated by politicians and business leaders; the second wave was spearheaded by educators such as Theodore Sizer, John Goodlad, and Ernest Boyer. This initiative stressed the need for basic reform of school practices. Recommendations emphasized that students should study fewer subjects but study them in depth and that teachers who were more highly trained in their content areas should be hired (Sadker & Zittleman, 2009).

Third Wave of Educational Reform

By 1988 a third wave of educational reform was initiated, calling for a reformulation of schools throughout the nation. The first two waves of reform had focused on raising the standards and restructuring the schools; the third called for schools to become comprehensive, full-service centers by providing students with a network of support services including nutrition, health care, transportation, counseling, and parent education, thus ensuring that the child could be transformed into a successful adult.

The following year education was further featured in the political spotlight when President George W. Bush convened a National Educational Summit. "Education 2000," a by-product of the summit, was later modified as "Goals 2000" under President William "Bill" Clinton's administration. Embracing a list of worthy but perhaps unrealistic goals, the objectives outlined in the document served to guide the nation on a course of self-examination as states developed standards of learning that would dominate the field of educational literature throughout the 1990s (Sadker & Zittleman, 2009).

Americans with Disabilities Act (1990)

By 1990 additional legislation focusing on people with disabilities had come to the forefront. The Americans with Disabilities Act (ADA; Public Law 101-336) was designed to protect those with disabilities against discrimination in the private sector. Furthermore, it was written to ensure that this group of individuals would be provided with equal opportunities for employment, public services, accommodations, transportation, and telecommunications.

Individuals with Disabilities Education Act (1990)

Other noteworthy legislation that transpired in 1990 was the passage of Public Law 101-476, the Individuals with Disabilities Education Act (IDEA). Intended to rename and replace Public Law 94-142 (EAHCA), it established "people first language" and extended special education services to include social work, assistive technology, and rehabilitation services. It also extended provisions for due process and confidentiality for students and added two new categories of disabilities: autism and traumatic brain injury. In addition, it required states to provide bilingual education programs for students with disabilities and to educate students with disabilities for transition to employment. By requiring the development of individualized transition programs for students with disabilities by the time they reach the age of 16, and providing them with transition services, students would be more fully served as they prepared to enter the world of work.

Individuals with Disabilities Education Act (1997)

As part of the authorization of Public Law 105-17, the Individuals with Disabilities Education Act (IDEA), schools were required to continue providing services to students with disabilities, including students who were expelled from school. In addition, states were allowed to extend their use of the developmental delay category for students through age 9. By 1997 the emphasis began to shift to requiring schools to assume greater responsibility for ensuring that students with disabilities have access to the general curriculum. Furthermore, it allowed for special education staff members, working in mainstream settings, to assist general education students when needed. Public Law 105-17 also requires that a general education teacher be part of the IEP team and that students with disabilities must participate in statewide as well as districtwide assessments. Other requirements under this mandate include that states offer medication as a voluntary option to parents and educators, and that a proactive behavior management plan be included in the student's IEP if a student with disabilities is experiencing behavior problems.

No Child Left Behind (2002)

In 2002, new federal legislation entitled No Child Left Behind (NCLB; Public Law 107-10) entered the forefront of American education. Described by both Democrats and Republicans as "the most significant change in federal legislation of public schools in three decades" (Sadker & Zittlman, 2009), it has dramatically changed and expanded the federal role in elementary and secondary education policy. According to McGuinn (2006), this new law represents the consolidation of a reform movement that began in the wake of 1983.

No Child Left Behind contains four major provisions. The first provision pertains to annual testing. States are now required to administer math assessments in Grades 3 through 8 and once in high school; each state determines which test is to be used. In 2007–2008 students also began taking standardized science tests at least once each in elementary, middle, and high school.

The second major provision applies to academic improvement. States must define academic proficiency for all students, and all students must be proficient in reading and math by

2013–2014. States are required to report Adequate Yearly Progress (AYP); if a school does not meet its AYP for 2 consecutive years, it is labeled as underperforming.

The third provision relates to report cards. States and school districts must provide the public with report cards of district and school progress.

The fourth and last provision relates to faculty qualifications. All teachers must be highly qualified (certified or licensed) with an academic major in the field in which they are teaching.

Without a doubt, the legislation contained within the NCLB mandate has caused a great deal of concern and consternation on the part of school administrators and personnel. The ramifications of it are far reaching, impacting students, teachers, administrators, and related service providers. Further discussion of how this legislation has impacted the education of students who are deaf and hard of hearing appears in various sections throughout the remainder of this chapter.

Reauthorization of IDEA (2004)

The Reauthorization of IDEA (Public Law 108-446) of 2004 is closely aligned to NCLB and focuses on academic results, early intervention, parental choice, and assessment. Note that short-term objectives and benchmarks in IEPs will be replaced with the NCLB system (except for the 1% of students taking alternative assessments), which measures academic progress toward state standards and accountability for academic achievement. As such, children with disabilities must conform to the state systems established under NCLB (Moores, 2005). Doubtless, schools are being held accountable to provide an educational foundation that prepares the majority of students to meet the rigors set forth by the state's curriculum as demonstrated by achieving adequate yearly progress.

In Summary

All of this legislation has made an indelible mark on the education of students who are deaf and hard of hearing. It has influenced where they are educated, how they are educated, and what they are expected to accomplish. A closer look at the education of students who are deaf and hard of hearing reveals the impact that previous and current legislation, as well as political and professional philosophies, have had on shaping the educational growth and development of this population.

At the heart of deaf education lies the fundamental question of how to deliver instruction to this unique population. The mode of communication selected reflects philosophical and cultural beliefs and remains very dear to members of the Deaf community as well as those outside of the community who believe strongly regarding whether individuals who are deaf should sign or be encouraged to speak.

Since the inception of the field, heated debates have remained in the forefront regarding the best mode of communication for delivering classroom instruction: sign or speech. Woven throughout the history of deaf education, this topic is still relevant and merits further discussion as it forms an integral thread in the fabric of who Deaf people are and how they view their heritage. A brief historical review of the educational arena indicates that the setting where these students obtained their education in tandem with the mode of communication used to deliver classroom instruction have been instrumental in shaping the Deaf community.

Where did deaf education establish its roots in America? Where did the majority of students who were deaf receive their instruction? How do contemporary educational programs serving students who are deaf and hard of hearing compare with early educational endeavors in the United States?

ESTABLISHING SCHOOLS FOR THE DEAF IN AMERICA

We know little about the community comprised of individuals who were deaf and resided in the United States before 1817. However, research indicates that between 2,000 and 6,000 people who were deaf lived in the eastern United States as early as the mid 1700s, and these individuals relied on some form of sign for communication (Baker-Shenk & Cokely, 1980; Vernon & Andrews, 1990).

One community that merits special consideration lived on Martha's Vineyard, an island off the coast of Massachusetts. Studies by Groce (1985) reveal that a large population of people who were deaf lived on the island from the late 1600s to the 1900s. These individuals migrated from the Kentish region of England and communicated through Old Kentish sign language (Moore & Levitan, 1993). During this time, generations of individuals married within their families. Those involved carried a pool of recessive genes for deafness, thus contributing to a marked increase in the population in the population comprised of individuals who were deaf. The community was bilingual; all the residents, both hearing and deaf, used sign language to actively and fully participate in the social and political events of the day. Although no formal description exists of the form of sign communication used on Martha's Vineyard, it is presumed to have influenced the early development of ASL, the preferred mode of communication adopted by the first school for the deaf in America (Moores, 2001).

Before the 1800s no educational facilities had been established in America for children who were deaf. Parents living in the colonies had the following three choices: teach their children themselves, hire a tutor, or send their children overseas to the Braidwood Academy in Edinburgh, Scotland (later London and Manchester, England) (Moore & Levitan, 1993, p. 32). Those who were poor could either keep their children at home or place them in an asylum. Unfortunately, no formal training was available to them.

However, the educational opportunities and the formalized use of sign language began to change during the early 1800s. This was largely due to the efforts of Thomas Hopkins Gallaudet and Laurent Clerc. Thomas Gallaudet was a graduate of Yale University and was enrolled in a ministerial program. While at home recuperating from an illness, he became acquainted with his neighbor, Dr. Mason Cogswell, whose daughter Alice was deaf. Alice was 9 years old at the time and was virtually without language. Gallaudet had a natural affinity for children and wanted to communicate with her. He became intrigued with the idea of teaching her and became determined to discover methods that would enable her to incorporate reading and writing skills into her communication system.

Cogswell became so impressed with Gallaudet's efforts to teach Alice that he initiated a fund-raising campaign in New England. His goal was to send Gallaudet to Europe where he would master the "oral method" and acquire teaching techniques deemed appropriate for use with children who were deaf. After working with the masters in Europe, he would return to Connecticut where he would establish a school for the deaf. Funds were secured, and Gallaudet sailed to Great Britain to visit the Braidwood School, an institution with an excellent reputation for working with persons who were deaf.

When he arrived in England, he soon discovered that he would need to remain at the Braidwood School for 4 years to become trained sufficiently in the oral method. Reluctant to do so, he left the school without receiving the training (Moores, 2010). However, while in London, he attended one of the public demonstrations conducted by Abbe Sicard, one of the French educators of the deaf. At the conclusion of the presentation Gallaudet sought out Sicard and found him to be open and willing to share his teaching methods. Sicard invited Gallaudet to visit the French National Institute and study its teaching techniques.

Upon his arrival, Gallaudet had the opportunity to work with Jean Massieu and Laurent Clerc (an instructor who was deaf). He was able to learn the sign system invented by Abbe Charles Michel de L'Eppe while becoming familiar with some of the teaching techniques used to educate pupils who were deaf. When the time arrived for Gallaudet to return to Connecticut, he had convinced Clerc to accompany him to the United States. There, the two of them were instrumental in establishing the first school for the deaf in America.

On April 15, 1817, with funding secured from the State of Connecticut and other groups who supported this unique population, Gallaudet and Clerc established the Institute for Deaf Mutes. It was later renamed the American Asylum at Hartford for the Education and Instruction of Deaf and Dumb (now named the American School for the Deaf). The school was established to meet the needs of 89 individuals who were then residing in Connecticut.

Throughout the 19th century the impetus for providing formal educational opportunities for students who were deaf continued, with numerous states establishing schools for the deaf. A number of these schools were created under the direction of Deaf professionals. Some of the professionals became superintendents; several others became part of the first group of Deaf instructors to teach within residential school settings. By 1850 more than 15 residential schools had been founded, and approximately 4 of every 10 instructors employed by these schools were deaf individuals (Marschark & Spencer, 2003).

The establishment of these schools marked a turning point for children who were deaf residing throughout the United States. During this era, residential settings frequently provided students who were deaf with a haven in which to congregate, a mecca for language and culture to flourish, and an opportunity to receive a quality education for the first time in their lives. Prior to the establishment of these schools, people who were deaf throughout the United States were scattered, and the majority lived in relative isolation from one another (Jankowski, 1997, as cited in DeLuca, Leigh, Lindgren, & Napoli, 2008). Once this isolation was broken, individuals who were deaf found themselves in situations where they could share stories based on experiences that were unique to them as a collective whole, while developing a strong camaraderie with others like them. Often misunderstood by hearing people, these dialogues provided children with a way to validate their identities while allowing them to behave as Deaf individuals.

Within these early school settings ASL was used in both educational and social settings, providing a mechanism for administrators, instructors, and students to share their personal opinions, beliefs, and life stories. This provided students with an open forum where communication flowed freely between peers and with professionals. Many students developed permanent bonds that would be maintained long after they finished school and left the classroom. These bonds provided Deaf graduates with a conduit for sharing their common cultural values of what it meant to be Deaf. The early network, characterized by the use of ASL to communicate, helped foster the initial organization and development of the Deaf communities throughout the nation. These early exchanges would eventually extend far beyond the classroom walls and become the cornerstones of Deaf communities. Under the auspices of these communities Deaf culture would thrive, be cherished, and shared with generations to follow.

These early schools provided more than an education for people who were deaf. They provided an opportunity to develop friendships, establish socialization patterns, meet future spouses, and acquire a visual language. Schools for the deaf afforded those in attendance with much more than an academic education so often associated with public school education.

Educating Deaf Students: The Oral/Manual Controversy

Although the majority of the original schools for the deaf in the United States embraced ASL and supported the use of manual communication for both instructional and extracurricular activities, this was not the philosophy endorsed by several professionals on the international scene. Throughout Europe the belief had always been very strong that individuals who were deaf should be educated orally. Known as the oralist philosophy, educators such as John Baptist Graser and Frederick Moritz Hill of Germany were staunch supporters of this philosophy and are credited for leading the German oralist movement that quickly spread throughout Europe during the 19th century (Lang, 2003). This movement would find its way to the United States under the direction of Horace Mann and Samuel Gridley Howe. Touting the benefits of using oralism in the educational arena, by the second half of the 19th century the proponents of this philosophy would find themselves in a bitter debate with those who supported manual communication (Lang, p. 15).

Until the 1880s, the Convention of American Instructors of the Deaf (CAID) had viewed all modes of communication as acceptable within educational settings. Throughout America at this time, approximately a dozen schools used the oral approach; others employed a combined approach (sign and speech), and still others supported the use of sign language (manualists) as the primary mode of communication. As the oralist movement spread across Europe it sparked a bitter debate within the United States regarding the best way to educate children who were deaf. Prominent leaders engaged in the debates were Alexander Graham Bell, a staunch oralist, and Edward Miner Gallaudet, referred to as "the champion of deaf people," who fought to have the combined system used for instruction and sought to preserve sign language (Lang, 2003, p. 15). The debates culminated at the 1880 Conference of Milan when hearing educators of the deaf voted to make the German oral method the official method used within schools serving deaf students. Speech was considered superior over sign language, and as a result many of the Deaf professionals employed by the schools for the deaf were terminated from their teaching positions.

Even though many of the residential schools were skeptical of Bell's views of teaching speech and relying on speech for instruction, Bell was instrumental in influencing the National Education Association to support him and the oralist movement by declaring that this approach should be used when educating students who were deaf. By 1920, 80% of these students were educated without using any signs (Van Cleve & Crouch, 1989). In enforcing the oralist teaching framework, children frequently were subjected to sitting on their hands or having their hands tied behind their backs (Cerney, 2007). Creating a definite division within the field, the century-long battle regarding how children who were deaf should be educated raged throughout the United States. It was not until the 1960s that sign language began to surface again within this educational arena (Cerney, p. 13).

From the underpinnings of this historical backdrop, the settings where students who were deaf began receiving their education were founded and developed. Today, these educational settings are as diverse as the students receiving the education. Where are the majority of students who are deaf and hard of hearing receiving their education today? What mode or modes of communication are they using? What types of support services are they receiving? How are they doing academically? How do the students perceive the quality of the education they are receiving today?

EDUCATIONAL ENVIRONMENTS

Students who are deaf or hard of hearing are receiving their education in a variety of settings. According to the National Center for Education Statistics (2009) 51.9% are receiving the majority of their education in regular education settings; 17.6% are receiving up to 50% of their education outside general education within regular education settings; 16.8% receive more than 60% of their education outside general education within regular education settings; 12.3% are being educated in residential facilities or special schools; 0.2% are being home schooled; and 0.1% are receiving their education in correctional facilities. Of these students, 50.7% rely on sign language (with or without speech) to communicate within instructional settings and 47.8% communicate through speech only. Keep in mind that many of these students are identified as being hard of hearing (GRI, 2008).

Statistics reported by GRI (2008) further indicate that although many of these students attend public schools, of those who attend, approximately 64% receive their education with hearing peers for at least part of the week, while 33.6% of them are not integrated at all with hearing peers. Those integrated in public school settings receive a variety of support services: 23% rely on sign language interpreters; 1.2% utilize the services of oral interpreters; 9% receive tutoring; and 60.3% receive speech training. Itinerant teacher/services are provided to 40.5% of the students, and audiologic services are provided to 41.6% of the students.

An overview of each of these settings provides insights into where students who are deaf and hard of hearing are being educated today. It further sheds light on the impact these educational settings are having on Deaf culture and Deaf communities, as well as on the modes of communication being used in the classroom. Throughout the history of deaf education, a tremendous amount of time and emphasis has been placed on the development of communication skills and the development of English proficiency (Woolsey, Harrison, & Gardner, 2004). How has this emphasis influenced the overall achievement levels of students who are deaf and hard of hearing? Before this question can be addressed, it is beneficial to glean a basic understanding of the characteristics of each of the settings.

Education programs for children who are deaf and hard of hearing are generally classified within two general categories: special schools and regular educational programs. Special schools may be designed as a residential facility or established as a separate day school. Regular education programs include early intervention programs, day classes, resource rooms, and itinerant services. In addition, day classes may foster a mainstreaming approach or be structured in the form of self-contained classrooms.

Residential School Programs

Formal education opportunities for students who are D/deaf began within the confines of residential school settings. Publicly or privately funded, they were constructed following a boarding school concept and offered students educational opportunities while affording them a place to live within dormitory environments. Conceived with a low-incidence population in mind, one of the primary goals of the residential setting was to serve the small and scattered population of students who were deaf residing outside of metropolitan areas.

Residential schools have traditionally employed Deaf and hearing teachers and a support staff specifically trained in the area of deaf education. Typically serving between 150 and 200 students, they provide an excellent range of support services, including audiologists, counselors, and psychologists. Students are provided with an array of academic and vocational courses as well as a wide range of athletic and social programs (Stinson & Kluwin, 2003). Class sizes are typically small, with some instructors teaching between three and eight students at a time, and all the classrooms are designed to provide students with visible access at all times to the teacher as well as the other students. Recognizing the importance of language acquisition and expression, residential facilities embrace a variety of communication methods including ASL, Total Communication, or a bilingual-bicultural (Bi-Bi) approach.

The ASL/English Bi-Bi approach to educating deaf students came to the forefront in the 1990s. For decades manually coded English systems were used extensively in residential and day school settings; however, even when requiring students to sign following the structure of English word order, reading levels remained low. Dissatisfaction with these low achievement levels prompted three professionals within the field—Johnson, Liddell, and Erting (1989)—to develop a position paper entitled "Unlocking the Curriculum: Principles for Achieving Access in Deaf Education." Disseminated across the nation, the authors advocated for a radical change in the language used to deliver classroom instruction. Stating that ASL and English should be kept separate, they encouraged the use of ASL as the first language (L1) when instructing children who are deaf, reserving written English for expressing oneself via written text (LaSasso & Lollis, 2003).

"Unlocking the Curriculum" was widely distributed among educators, and it has become the impetus for several schools to adopt a Bi-Bi approach. According to the *Directory of the American Annals of the Deaf,* 19 schools identify themselves as following a Bi-Bi approach; 16 of them are residential schools, and 3 are day schools. They are located in a number of states including California, Massachusetts, Texas, New Mexico, Maryland, Minnesota, Colorado, Utah, New York, Kansas, and Arizona (LaSasso & Lollis, 2003). Promoting the use of ASL, students are able to engage in classroom activities and receive instruction visually through their L1 language.

Within the residential school setting, students have the opportunity to interact with their peers who are deaf both inside and outside of the classroom. Socializing in the cafeteria, in the dormitories, and during athletic events, these interactions and encounters with Deaf adults have provided students with social, cultural, and linguistic models. Furthermore, these exchanges have played a vital role in shaping Deaf children's identities while contributing to the overall development of one's self-esteem.

From a Deaf perspective residential schools have always been viewed in a positive light as a locus for academic and cultural instruction; in these settings ASL is revered, cultural values have been transmitted, and long-lasting friendships have been formed. By affording those in attendance with a unique environment conducive to unimpeded and effortless communication, these schools have provided the historical cornerstone on which the Deaf community and culture have been founded (DeLuca et al., 2008).

Residential school enrollment peaked in the 1970s as a result of the earlier rubella epidemic. During that time one third of the students attended residential schools while another one third attended special school programs designed specifically for students who were deaf (Marschark, Lang, & Albertini, 2002). Many of these special school programs included day schools for the deaf that were also established to accommodate the increased population. However, due to legislative mandates, advances in technology, and parental attitudes, enrollments have declined in the 21st century. Based on a report provided by the National Center for Education Statistics (1999), 16.8% of students who are deaf receive their education in residential or day schools.

Day Schools

Day schools are public schools that have been established to accommodate students who are deaf who reside at home. Intended to offer an academic curriculum commensurate with those attending residential facilities, day schools also employ Deaf and hearing faculty and staff members who are specifically trained to work with students who are deaf and hard of hearing. The majority of these schools are located in metropolitan areas, and although their student populations may vary, they continue to provide an environment conducive to academic and social growth and development.

Regular Education Classes

EARLY INTERVENTION PROGRAMS. Although residential and day school programs have served this student population for decades, by comparison, early intervention programs are a relatively new addition to the field. These programs are broad in scope, vary in design, and have become integral to the field. Developed to encourage effective communication and enhance social interactions, early intervention programs have been established to work with families while providing them with counseling, strategies for language development, and activities to enhance cognitive development.

Furnishing parents with a support system and information on deafness and child development, these programs vary in their approach to promoting modes of communication and educational opportunities. Some of the early intervention programs stress a Bi-Bi approach by emphasizing spoken and sign language and the cultures of both hearing and Deaf populations, and others advocate for the use of one communication mode over another (Marschark, Lang, & Albertini, 2002). Early intervention programs are administered by a variety of agencies including public schools, residential schools, departments of human services, and departments of education.

It has been well documented in the literature that hearing children who have had access to preschool programs are oftentimes better prepared both socially and linguistically to enter kindergarten settings. Although the benefits of early intervention programs for children who are deaf have not been researched as extensively, one can only posit that by providing them with early language and social skills they will likewise benefit from these programs.

Programs such as the ones offered by the John Tracy Clinic located in California, the Colorado Home Intervention Program, the Parent-Infant Program at Boys Town National Medical Research Hospital in Omaha, Nebraska, the SKI*HI Institute located in Utah, and the Parent-Infant Program (PIP) sponsored by the Kendall Demonstration Elementary School located at Gallaudet University provide comprehensive early intervention services (Sass-Lehrer & Bodner-Johnson, 2003). Focused on a family-centered service delivery model, early intervention specialists strive to form effective relationships with family members while modeling developmentally appropriate practices. By collaborating with parents, they assist them in establishing goals for their child while identifying ways they can evaluate their child's progress. Recognizing that hearing loss directly impacts one's ability to communicate, all these programs place a tremendous emphasis on language acquisition as well as overall communication.

MAINSTREAMED PROGRAMS. Mainstreamed programs came to the forefront in the mid 1970s when President Gerald Ford signed into law the Education for All Handicapped Children Act of 1975 (Public Law 94-142). This act emphasized placing students in the least restrictive environment. The goal of mainstreaming has been to provide students with disabilities with educational opportunities that are equivalent to those of their peers who are nondisabled. Educational opportunities include academic content as well as social experiences (Kauffman, 1993).

Mainstreaming was based on the premise that students with disabilities, who were able to adapt to general education classes, could receive their education in the mainstream setting. This legislation opened the doors for students who were deaf and hard of hearing to attend regular education classes. It provided accommodations for them, including interpreters, tutors, and note takers so those with varying degrees of hearing loss could sit in the same classrooms and compete with their peers who could hear. The focus of mainstreaming changed in 1997 when Public Law 94-142 was reauthorized.

INCLUSION PROGRAMS. In June 1997 Public Law 94-142 was reauthorized and became identified as the Individuals with Disabilities Education Act (IDEA; Public Law 101-476). This new mandate stated that "all children with disabilities are entitled to a (1) free and appropriate education which must occur (2) to the maximum extent appropriate ... with children who are non-disabled (P.L. 101-476, subsection 1412(1), 1412(B)" (Wright, 1999, p. 11).

Inclusion has placed a greater emphasis on schools to adapt the general education classroom to the child. Many of the previously mainstreamed programs had placed students with disabilities in self-contained classrooms or had mainstreamed them in select classes, sometimes doing nothing more than seating them next to students who were nondisabled in classes such as physical education.

This changed with the impetus to move toward inclusion. Inclusion differs in philosophy from mainstreaming. Rather than focusing on the student, the inclusion movement has focused on general education classrooms to determine if appropriate adaptations have been made to meet the needs of students requiring special accommodations.

Students who are deaf and hard of hearing who are included in general education classes receive the same support services made available for mainstreamed students. Because the student population is diverse, the services provided vary from student to student. According to Antia, Stinson, and Gaustad (2002), inclusion, when engineered correctly, reflects more than the physical placement of the student in the classroom; it embodies the philosophy that all students are full members of the classroom and school community.

This segment of the population, who are receiving their education in included settings, represents a diverse group. Some are hard of hearing, others have severe to profound hearing losses, and although the majority of them have hearing parents, others have D/deaf members in their families. Even though many of the older students rely on traditional hearing aids for amplification, a substantial number of the elementary-school population are arriving at school with cochlear implants. Representing a variety of ethnic groups and communication modes, these students may still receive a portion of their education in resource rooms and/or separate classes for students who are deaf.

RESOURCE ROOMS AND SEPARATE CLASSES. According to Stinson and Kluwin (2003), the primary difference between resource rooms and separate classes is the amount of time students who are deaf spend in regular education classes. Students attending separate classes receive the majority or all of their education from a teacher trained specifically to work with this population; those attending resource rooms are outside of the general education classroom for only one or two subject areas. Oftentimes school districts will employ a teacher or teachers—specifically trained to work with students who are deaf—to remain at one school and instruct these students in separate classrooms. However, based on the needs of this student population, other school systems may rely on the services of itinerant teachers to provide educational support to these students. What are the responsibilities of resource room and itinerant teachers who work with students who are deaf?

Teachers working in resource rooms provide direct instruction to students, often providing remediation, pre-teaching or post-teaching content that is covered in the general education classroom. In addition, they may provide consultative services to general education teachers, assisting them in making modifications to their classroom instruction. Functioning as collaborative partners, they assist in the development of academic, social, or behavioral goals while providing general education teachers with strategies and materials specifically designed to promote academic success.

• Itinerant teachers provide these same services to students attending school in a variety of different locations. Typically, students served by itinerant teachers have a moderate hearing loss, have been educated orally, and do not have any additional handicapping conditions.

CO-TEACHING/CO-ENROLLMENT FOR STUDENTS WHO ARE DEAF AND HARD OF HEARING. Co-teaching, or team teaching, has been practiced in various settings by general education teachers for a number of years. Gleaning from the expertise of two professionals, students reap the benefits of having a team of teachers deliver academic content. Within the field of deaf education, co-teaching implies a team comprised of a teacher of students who are deaf and a general education classroom teacher instructing both hearing and deaf students within included classroom settings. As a team they focus on the academic, social, and communication needs of all students (Bowen, 2008).

In schools with co-enrollment programs, four or more students who are deaf are typically placed together in general education classes where they receive their instruction in concert with their peers who can hear. Designed to provide students with a challenging curriculum and an opportunity to socialize with others, this model differs significantly from many included settings. Typically found in public schools today, included settings are frequently characterized by classrooms that are predominantly comprised of students who can hear, with perhaps only one student who is deaf in attendance.

Many of the included settings provide a wide array of excellent academic offerings; however, invariably students who are deaf find they are placed in situations where they are the sole student in their class who cannot hear, and sometimes the only student who is deaf in their entire school. This can contribute to feelings of social isolation with limited opportunities to form friendships. Although the number of reported co-enrollment/co-teaching programs is sparse, initial research conducted by Kluwin (1999) and Bowen (2008) on some of the existing programs suggest that this model has the capability of providing a learning environment that promotes student achievement while fostering social acceptance.

• Students who are deaf and receive their education in included settings frequently rely on an array of support services so they can access the curriculum. These accommodations can include the services of an itinerant teacher, an oral or sign language interpreter, a note taker, a real-time captioner, a tutor, or perhaps a speech-language pathologist. Based on the students' needs, all or only some of these services may be requested. What role do these support personnel provide? What are their qualifications, and what credentials do they hold?

The Role of the Itinerant Teacher

• The primary role of the itinerant teacher is to provide direct instruction to students from 2 to 21 years of age who are deaf and hard of hearing. Daily, they travel between and among schools serving a number of students with varying degrees of hearing loss and academic abilities. Throughout the day they consult with other professionals and parents, providing recommendations for the students that they serve. Itinerant teachers provide their instruction in a variety of ways. "More than 75% of the students taught by itinerant teachers are served on a pull-out basis; about 15% of the time, teachers work with students while they are in the general education class, and only about 5% routinely team teach with the regular education teacher" (Stinson & Kluwin, 2003).

The Role of Interpreters in Inclusive Classrooms

When students who are deaf and hard of hearing are taught by general education teachers, they frequently rely on the services of a sign language interpreter to engage and participate in these learning experiences. According to Burch (2005) an estimated 60% of sign language interpreters work with approximately 60% of students who are receiving their education in included settings. Although many of the interpreters hired to serve in this capacity are graduates from reputable interpreter training programs, and they possess the needed skill set to provide this service, others hired to provide this same service may have acquired their signs through independent study or informal observations while watching working interpreters.

Educational interpreters work with a diverse population serving students enrolled in pre–K through postsecondary settings. The quality of their interpreting can have a profound impact on the child's language development, social acceptance, and academic achievement (Cerney, 2007). Since they function as a channel for communication, it is critical that working interpreters possess a complex skill set: They must understand the content being delivered, process the information into another language, and then accurately convey the intent and meaning of the message to the recipients. The interpreter's perception of what the speaker wants to communicate "speaker's intent" coupled with their ability to process this information affects the outcome of how the message is delivered. Although interpreters strive to provide an accurate interpretation, once the message is filtered through the interpreter, the message is affected to some degree (Winston, 1994).

Although interpreter training programs prepare these professionals to facilitate communication in a variety of settings, they cannot prepare them for the exact content they will encounter in every situation. Throughout the course of their careers, interpreters may find they are asked to interpret everything from algebra to sociology, as well as challenging courses such as trigonometry and chemistry. Their ability to provide an effective interpretation depends on their mastery of a complex skill set. To provide message equivalence, interpreters must cultivate their ability to navigate between two languages—English and ASL in a fraction of a second—while producing the vocabulary and syntax that are inherent in both languages.

Within the confines of education, interpreters are required to interpret for multiple speakers and to reflect shifts in register while engaging in different types of discourse. Throughout the course of the day, they typically are asked to interpret for both teachers and students. Oftentimes these communication exchanges require conveying information about the speaker's beliefs, expectations, and understanding that is frequently expressed through aspects of speaking such as tone of voice and prosody (Schick, Williams, & Kupermintz, 2005).

Educational interpreters provide one dimension as students attempt to gain full access to the intricacies and complexities found within the hearing classroom. In the pre–K setting educational interpreters function as language role models as well as interpreters; throughout the elementary and middle school settings they may also be asked to serve as tutors (Humphrey & Alcorn, 2001). Although their primary function is to interpret, they are frequently asked to assume other tasks.

With these support services available, how do students who are deaf perform academically? Are they performing on grade level commensurate with their hearing peers? Are they able to fully participate in included settings? Do they develop friendships with their hearing peers? Are they in fact reaping the benefits of a free and appropriate education?

Achievement: A Look at Deaf Students in the K–12 Setting

A tremendous amount of diversity is found within the field of deaf education. One does not have to look far within this student population to find students who are hard of hearing, or those who are characterized as having a moderate to severe degree of hearing loss, as well as those who exhibit severe to profound hearing loss. Regardless of the degree of loss, the mode of communication that is utilized, or the classroom setting where the students receive their education, the ultimate goal is the same: provide them with a rigorous academic program, challenge them to utilize their full intellectual potential, and prepare them to leave the K–12 setting functioning as independent and socially competent young adults.

Despite a long history of educating students who are deaf and hard of hearing, the field continues to grapple with the low achievement levels that are characteristic of the school-age population. In the area of academic achievement, the majority of hearing students continue to outperform students who are deaf. Furthermore, in the area of literacy, the reading levels achieved by students who are deaf remain consistently lower than their peers who can hear (Traxler, 2000). This has continuously plagued educators of students who are deaf who routinely question how they can effectively teach this population when the students they are charged with instructing arrive in their classrooms with "daunting language and experience gaps" (Woolsey et al., 2004).

Educational research conducted with hearing children demonstrates that academic achievement gains are correlated with time on task. However, literature describing the field of deaf education throughout the past 200 years reveals that the instruction of students who are deaf has primarily focused on the development of English language proficiency and communication skills (Woolsey et al., 2004). A plethora of articles germane to language development is evident in the literature. However, research findings which address specific variables that impact academic achievement of students who are deaf are virtually nonexistent (Mertens, 1990). Furthermore, Moores (2001) postulates that these low achievement levels can, in part, be exacerbated by professionals who lack sufficient skills to teach students who are deaf effectively, thus resulting in less than favorable academic outcomes.

Knowing what to teach and how to teach have significant implications for classroom instruction. The work of Bloom (1984) and Walberg (1984) within the field of general education has shed light on the variables that impact student learning. These variables include tutorial instruction, reinforcement, mastery learning, cues and explanations, student classroom participation, student time on task, improved reading/study skills, cooperative learning, graded homework, and classroom morale (Bloom). One can surmise that these same variables are applicable to and merit implementation within classrooms serving students who are deaf and hard of hearing, and if instilled they could be instrumental in further enhancing the delivery of instruction for these students.

According to Moores (2001), these variables can be directly applied to deaf education. By placing the variables into three domains—instructor, program, and those relating to the home environment—Moores delineates a list of activities that, if implemented, can assist in enhancing achievement levels found within this population. Noted among the instructor variables are the abilities to provide reinforcement and positive feedback, administer meaningful homework coupled with timely student feedback, and the investment of time on task while maintaining a goal-focused, cohesive classroom environment. Within the area of program variables, attention should be devoted to developing reading strategies for a variety of genres, placing high achievers in accelerated programs, and providing tutoring, either on an individual basis or through small group instruction. Home variables include working with parents to ensure leisure reading is encouraged, school progress and activities are discussed, and homework is monitored (pp. 333–334).

All these variables depend on fluent communication in order for them to be effective. The students must possess a foundation in language so they can receive instruction, positive feedback, and take advantage of strategies needed for decoding reading passages or discussing homework. Without this foundation, the variables listed above remain ideals that can never fully materialize into viable activities. Keeping in mind that learners who are deaf are visual language users, it is critical that individuals interacting with the students possess fluency in a variety of communication modalities. These include ASL, manually coded English sign systems, and strategies that promote and facilitate speech reading. Even though the field acknowledges vision as one of the primary avenues that people who are deaf rely on to access information, research continues to indicate that many teachers of students who are deaf do not possess the level of sign language, or sign system fluency, needed to convey information or engage in classroom discourse (Luckner, 1991). The ramifications of this are far reaching, not only by impacting the delivery of instruction, but also by imposing limits on the classroom discussions that follow.

What effect does this have on how students who are deaf and hard of hearing perceive the quality of education they are receiving and their participation in the classroom? What are their views on attending residential school programs as well as included settings? How do they perceive their identities in these settings? Do they have peers and a social network they can communicate with readily?

Within the past decade a number of published interviews have appeared on video as well as in print showcasing individuals who are D/deaf. Throughout these interviews school-age D/deaf children, as well as adults, have shared their sentiments regarding various educational environments, including residential and included settings, while expressing their perceptions with respect to academic offerings, socialization, communication, and support services. These poignant reflections embody the values, beliefs, and concerns of a complex and diverse population.

Janet Cerney's *Deaf Education in America: Voices of Children from Inclusion Settings* (2007) contains a number of interviews with children who are deaf between the ages of 10 and 18. Although these dialogues represent a small number of children, they capture the essence of the students' feelings that so often permeate the student population comprised of learners who are deaf residing in these environments. Cerney emphasizes that it is apparent while reading through the student responses that there is a "dividing line" between the students who utilize some residual hearing and speak and those who are profoundly deaf and communicate through the use of sign language. Some of the students received all of their education in one setting; others experienced both residential and included classroom experiences. Several of their comments merit discussion.

• Students were asked to describe what it is like being a student who is deaf and attending a school surrounded by a community of their peers who can hear. Overall, responses of the students reflected a social rather than an academic perspective. Those who relied on spoken communication had a more favorable outlook on included environments; those using sign communication indicated that they experienced a barrier to interacting with their hearing peers. One stated, "I'm not so lonely as those who can't talk. Learn to speak. If you can talk, it is much better." Another indicated, "Sometimes I feel lonely, like if people talk a million miles an hour. I just sit there and listen to them." And a third stated, "I can't understand them. They speak and I don't understand them. I can't talk... . I sign so they don't understand me. It's hard to communicate" (Cerney, 2007, pp. 64–65, 90). Even though some indicated they enjoyed going to a hearing school, the topic of learning about and being part of Deaf culture was a repeated theme.

• Communication is the key to navigating social encounters. For students to successfully network and become part of the social milieu, they must be able to speak the language as well as engage in appropriate conversational topics. Without these exchanges, quality relationships are not formed and feelings of social isolation can develop. Students addressed the issue of feeling lonely and isolated when asked questions pertaining to this topic. Two of the students linked feelings of loneliness to lack of motivation to learn. Others addressed the issues of feeling embarrassed, shy, or inferior. One student, when referring to hearing students in the classroom, stated, "I'd try to talk with them sometimes. . . . I felt lower than them, so I didn't even try." Another indicated, "Being deaf in a hearing school, I found that sometimes the other kids thought less of me" (Cerney, 2007, p. 70).

Rachel McKee, in *People of the Eye: Stories from the Deaf World* (2001), provides additional insights from D/deaf people's experiences in classroom situations. One of the stories, written by Sara Pivac, illustrates her frustration when she made the transition from the residential setting into an included classroom:

> "I remember the first day I was introduced to a hearing girl who was picked to be my buddy. Off we went to a hearing class, along with a person who was meant to interpret for me, but within a few minutes I ran out upset and crying. The interpreter came after me to find out what was wrong. It was hard for me to explain it to her, but I just felt so out of place, because I couldn't follow what was going on in the classroom. Before that, I'd been used to being with Deaf people who were signing, and I could easily talk with everyone and feel part of what was happening. But this class was a shock for me; I felt completely stranded. I'd always been in a small class, and now I was in a room of 30 kids, with a hearing teacher and an extra teacher of the Deaf to interpret for me. It was a bit traumatic." (McKee, 2001, p. 229)

School communities represent microcosms of society. They furnish the infrastructure for students to master academic subjects while providing an environment where social skills and psychological development can flourish. The school community for most students who are deaf and hard of hearing is within included classrooms. Although some integrate into the hearing mainstream with little if any difficulty, others experience feelings of inadequacy and social isolation.

Fitzgerald (2000) and Greenberg, Lengua, and Calderon (1997) note that children and adolescents who are deaf attending mainstreamed settings are at risk for developing feelings of alienation and delays in cognitive as well as social-cognitive processing. Further studies conducted by Hocutt (1996) reveal that students who are hard of hearing do not generally perform as well academically as students who can hear and that the difference can become exacerbated with age. Stinson and Antia (1999) have revealed that when students cannot easily participate with their peers due to communication difficulties, they tend to identify themselves as being helpless and may avoid participating in school activities.

Kluwin, Stinson, and Colarossi (2002) have summarized a series of studies that focus on the social processes and outcomes that occur when students who are deaf receive their education in included settings. Their review of the literature reveals additional insights into the challenges faced by these students. In essence the studies reveal that, within the public school setting, students who can hear are more socially mature than their counterparts who are deaf. Furthermore, students who are deaf interact more frequently with their peers who are deaf rather than with their classmates who can hear. Additional findings indicate that students who are deaf are somewhat accepted by their hearing classmates, and their level of self-esteem is not related to the amount of time they attended general education classes.

Summary

Students enter the educational arena at an early age and remain in their school communities until young adulthood. Throughout these formative years they experience a myriad of changes that impact them socially, psychologically, and academically. While being prepared to enter the realm of adulthood they are faced with opportunities to expand their horizons while developing their overall potential. For some, this journey is filled with positive learning experiences, leaving them with a sense of fulfillment and feelings of accomplishment. For others, the challenge of competing and rising to meet the demands imposed by the rigors set forth by the academic curriculum can be daunting if not altogether overwhelming.

Students who are deaf and hard of hearing enter the educational arena filled with the same hopes and aspirations as their hearing classmates. Faced with a complex constellation of challenges, they too explore ways to successfully navigate through the educational system. Enrolled in a variety of school settings, some are placed in environments that are conducive to their mode of communication and educational needs. When this occurs they are provided with the ultimate setting in which they can flourish. Others find themselves in environments that are not conducive to their communication style. In the event this happens they may succumb to frustration and eventual failure.

The face of deaf education is rapidly changing, and educators are being challenged to focus on academic subjects and remediate students to standards not previously attained by this population. The field is charged with providing students with the strategies and skills they need to succeed. Teachers must become fluent in the languages used by the students they are educating. They must become highly qualified in the content areas they are teaching and must master teaching techniques that focus on visual learners. Furthermore, they must learn how to form partnerships and become collaborators, consultants, and effective co-teachers. With these skills in place they can provide learning environments for students who are deaf and hard of hearing, thus enabling them access to the curriculum.

9

Literacy

Unlocking the Curriculum Through Reading and Writing

Language, whether signed or spoken, avails us with a socially shared code, whereby we express our ideas and exchange information with others. It is a powerful tool, one of several, that enables us to crack the code, and unlock the door to literacy. In its broadest sense, literacy can be categorized within three domains: personal, school, and community (Gallego & Hollingsworth, 2000). Extending far beyond the traditional classroom, it encompasses culture, technology, discourse styles, and individuals' critical awareness of themselves. Contemporary literacy can be viewed in terms of describing a person's "literacy profile," whereby the individual can exhibit an array of different literacies in a variety of social contexts (Unrau, 2008). In this respect one can be computer literate, possess math literacy, or have mastered musical literacy. However, of all the literacies within the realm of academia, the one that commands the most attention is the primary and traditional way the word *literacy* has been used to describe one's ability to read and write.

Numerous articles and texts have been devoted to the topic of literacy. Recognized as a complex process, academicians have invested countless hours probing, investigating, and identifying skills that, when applied, will enable children to become successful readers. Beginning with emergent readers and culminating with those who have gained fluency, teachers, reading specialists, and those engaged in research continually explore approaches, skills, interventions, and strategies that will ultimately assist readers in their quest to decode, decipher, and glean understanding from the printed word.

When students master these skills and become proficient readers, they are capable of accessing a variety of printed materials and, if motivated, can become highly successful students, embarking on a journey of lifelong learning. However, for those who struggle with the reading process, the task can become arduous, if not altogether seemingly impossible. When this occurs it can lead to academic failure, leaving students at risk for dropping out of school and becoming unemployed or at best underemployed.

Information provided by the The Nation's Report Card: Reading 2009 (National Center for Education Statistics, 2009b) reveals that 33% of fourth-graders across the nation perform at or above a Proficient level, with about 67% of fourth-graders performing at or above the Basic level. According to the NAEP, the Basic level denotes that students have partial mastery of prerequisite knowledge and skills that are fundamental for proficient work. Furthermore, statistics indicate that of the 10% to 15% of students who eventually drop out of school, over 75% of them have experienced difficulties learning to read (Carnine, Silbert, Kame'enui, Tarver, & Jungjohan, 2006).

Children, at a very young age, can begin to encounter difficulties while trying to learn how to read. If these difficulties are not resolved and the child continuously struggles, feelings of inadequacy can ensue. Over time, this can lead to a sense of failure and can negatively impact a child's self-esteem. Subsequent struggles with reading create ongoing frustration, prompting children to associate reading with their own sense of inadequacy. With each progressive grade level, they are presented with classroom material that continues to challenge their ability to decipher text. While trying to escape feelings of defeat, many of them avoid reading altogether, therefore placing them at higher risk for school failure.

By middle school, children who can read well read at least 10,000,000 words during the academic year; however, those who experience reading difficulties read less than 100,000 words during that same time period, thereby becoming part of the group referred to as at-risk readers. Those lagging behind their peers in vocabulary development and in the strategies needed to comprehend what they read frequently arrive at high school with a disdain for reading (Carnine et al., 2006, p. 4).

A myriad of questions must be considered in evaluating the role of literacy in human development. The following comprise a sample of questions germane to any discussion of literacy:

- What can be done to help the at-risk reader?
- What has the National Reading Panel found to be key elements for literacy programs designed to promote literacy on the part of all students?
- How does this research apply to students who are deaf and hard of hearing?
- What are the characteristics of this population of readers?
- Can these strategies be applied in classrooms where students who are deaf or hard of hearing are receiving instruction in the content areas?
- What other approaches are deemed applicable to this population?
- How can interventions designed to ensure that all students can read on grade level be adapted to meet the needs of these students?

The topic of literacy has been of interest to scholars for decades. The scope of the subject matter is broad and complex and obviously cannot be covered in detail in one chapter. However, by providing the reader with background information regarding the approaches, interventions, and strategies used to promote literacy within the context of deaf education, it is anticipated that further insights can be gained, and a basic understanding of effective reading practices with learners who are deaf and hard of hearing can be achieved, thus prompting new lines of research within the field.

READING: A PROCESS INVOLVING LANGUAGE AND COGNITION

A substantial body of literature describes the various theories and models that have emerged while attempting to explain the reading process. Although each of the theories differs in the strategies believed to assist students, they are all designed to support them as they strive to comprehend printed text. Three of the major approaches, sometimes referred to as theories or models for teaching reading, include Bottom-Up Theories, Top-Down Theories, and Interactive Theories.

Bottom-Up Theories

Bottom-up theories rely heavily on phonemics, word recognition, and the ability to use word-to-text information to construct word and sentence meanings (Carver, 1990; Gough, 1984; Perfetti,

1985). When this model is incorporated, identification of letters and words is stressed with comprehension receiving very little attention. Based on a hierarchical philosophy, the reader must first be able to master sounds before he or she can advance to the next level, which is comprehension. Therefore, meaning is extracted through the use of decoding skills.

Throughout the first three grades, emphasis is placed on phonetics with the assumption that once word recognition becomes automatic the child can focus on higher level comprehension tasks. According to this theory, children experience difficulty reading because they lack the ability to make the connection between English speech sounds and printed letters. Therefore, printed texts remain abstract until the mastery of phonemic patterns occurs.

Top-Down Theories

Top-down theories, also known as problem-solving models, focus on the cognitive task of deriving meaning from what lies in the reader's head. These theories are grounded in the premise that individuals form hypotheses and make assumptions about what they are reading based on their prior knowledge and experience. Based on this theory, the reader comprehends information "that is in the readers' heads, not what is on the printed page" (Paul, 2009, p. 272). In essence, the reader starts with meaning and then proceeds downward to the letters and words. This model is couched in the philosophy that children do not need to be taught how to read. Thus, the top-down theory deemphasizes the need to teach decoding skills and comprehension subskills. Instead, it directs its attention toward providing students with activities that will assist them in developing, activating, and applying prior knowledge to the text at hand, thus fostering comprehension (McAnally, Rose, & Quigley, 2007).

Interactive Theories

In recent years, interactive theories have been receiving more attention. Emphasizing the reader as an "active information processor whose goal is to construct a model of what the text means" (Paul, 2009, p. 272), the framework for the model lies in the premise that beginning readers are "text driven" whereas mature readers, for the most part, are "reader driven."

According to McAnally et al. (2007) interactive theories embrace two important premises: first, that prior knowledge plays an essential role in constructing meaning from the text and, second, that "readers develop and apply a large repertoire of processing strategies ranging from strategies for decoding print to complex metacognitive strategies" (p. 13). Using this type of model, both word identification and comprehension are stressed. Emphasis is placed on understanding the association between sounds and letters through the teaching of phonetics. By promoting this at an early age, it is postulated that these skills can then be incorporated into the top-down model, in which comprehension is stressed.

Furthermore, this approach stresses that instruction should capitalize on the prior experiences of the reader. Within the classroom setting, questions are asked and the use of semantic maps are incorporated. Semantic maps involve a series of questions through which one can demonstrate vocabulary and key points contained in a story. This enables the reader to organize information and store important points in his or her memory.

One particular group of interactive theories that merits discussion consists of the schema theories. This approach applies the concept of schemata as an organizing framework allowing for the storage and retrieval of information. As individuals process what they are reading they are able to rely on this organizational system to construct meaning from the printed word.

Schemata activation refers to the mechanism whereby readers can access what they know and match it to the information that they are reading. This allows them to build on and augment their previous knowledge. According to Vacca, Vacca, and Mraz (2011), when students can make a match between their prior knowledge and the text, they can use this schema to search for and select information that is aligned with their purpose for reading. In addition, they can use this information to make inferences and predictions by filling in gaps while they are engaged in reading. Furthermore, it helps them organize, remember, and elaborate on what they have read (p. 24).

Regardless of the approach that is applied, the ultimate goal is to equip the child, and later the adult, with the ability to construct meaning from printed text. Individuals must be able to extract information from their personal experiences and relate it to their linguistic and cognitive knowledge bases. When this interaction occurs, perceptions can be formed and comprehension can be facilitated.

REPORT: NATIONAL READING PANEL

All these approaches provide insights into the sophisticated skill set required to successfully engage in the reading process. These skills include a command of orthography and grammar, background experiences, cultural influences that embody readers, and the type of genre they are given to read. In essence, the reader must possess linguistic, cognitive, and social abilities to comprehend print or text.

Due to the complex nature of the reading process, and a desire to determine the most effective ways to teach children how to read, a national panel was convened in 1997 to review the scientific literature pertaining to reading research. Based on a review of approximately 100,000 reading research studies published since 1966, and an additional 15,000 that had been published prior to that time, the panel outlined five areas that it determined were essential for children to become accomplished readers (Carnine et al., 2007, p. 4): phonemic awareness, phonics, fluency, text comprehension, and vocabulary.

Phonemes are the smallest elements of speech and include vowels and consonants. As children develop phonemic awareness, they become cognizant of the fact that words are composed of letters and that these letters relate to phonemic segments found within the language. In essence they develop knowledge of the alphabetic principle. They recognize that words can be divided into a sequence of phonemes represented by letters of the alphabet (Paul, 2009; Wang, Trezek, Luckner, & Paul, 2008).

Phonics refers to how the sounds of speech (phonology) are represented by letters and spelling (orthography). Developing a phonological awareness implies that a child understands that each of the letters represents a sound, but the sounds in isolation have no meaning. Rather, when presented with a letter the child can produce the sound that it represents. When children develop phonological and orthographic awareness, they are developing the prerequisites required for mastering the alphabetic principle (Stanovich, 1986). Subsequently, this principle is what children use to map letters onto individual sounds. Without this, children struggle with decoding words, which is a skill they must develop to use independently while they are reading. When children master the alphabetic principle it becomes a very powerful mechanism that enables them to acquire a reading vocabulary by mapping new written word forms onto known spoken word forms (Hermans, Knoors, Ormel, & Verhoven, 2007).

Fluency refers to the individual's ability to read a text orally with speed, accuracy, and proper expression; it is one of several critical factors required for reading comprehension. Fluent readers express text in the same manner as if they were speaking. Becoming the bridge between word recognition and comprehension, fluency allows the reader to focus on the meaning rather than decoding the words (Carnine et al., 2006).

Text comprehension, or reading comprehension, is a complex cognitive activity comprised of a variety of skills and strategies. Initially, beginning readers focus on comprehension, sequencing, and the basic story line. Later the focus shifts to inferential comprehension, summarization, comprehension monitoring, and determining the main idea. Throughout the course of any formal reading program students are taught a series of strategies and skills intended to promote understanding, recollecting, and the art of communicating about what they have read.

The last of the skills emphasized by the National Reading Panel pertained to vocabulary. The majority of the words we acquire are learned indirectly, with students' vocabularies growing at a rate of about 3,000 words per year (Graves & Watts-Taffe, 2002). From the onset, children's vocabularies appear to be reflective of adult vocabularies; they include words that are representative of nouns, verbs, adjectives, and function words. Although initially common nouns account for approximately 40% of the child's first 50 words, by the time the child has amassed a vocabulary of over 600 words approximately 40% are nouns, 25% are verbs and adjectives, and about 25% are function words (Bates et al., 1994).

Readers enter school from a variety of cultural and socioeconomic backgrounds. When English is the primary language used in the home, students typically enter school with an English vocabulary of approximately 8,000 words. Once in school, they learn between 2,000 and 4,000 words a year and have acquired approximately 40,000 to 50,000 words by the time they are ready to graduate from high school (Anderson & Nagy, 1993; Graves, 2006). Even though vocabulary acquisition occurs the most rapidly between the ages of 6 and 18, semantic development continues throughout one's lifetime (Gleason & Ratner, 2009).

ADDITIONAL FACTORS CONTRIBUTING TO LITERACY

Literacy begins within the home during infancy and stems from an array of activities. Storytelling, shared reading, paper and pencil activities, exposure to print materials, and social interactions with family members all contribute to the foundation that will later support young readers when they enter school. Children who are raised in literate homes can have over 1,000 hours of informal reading and writing experiences before they arrive at school (Adams, 1990). While young children are engaged in these activities, the value and importance of literacy are being reinforced. These values are later reaffirmed for children when they experience success with reading and writing not only in the classroom but later as adults within the workforce.

Family values, culture, and attitudes all play a vital role in the development of literacy. This, coupled with the identities children develop, how they perceive themselves as competent students, and their degree of motivation to learn further impact this process as students progress through the educational system. The school community, peers, and development of one's sense of autonomy are only a few of the factors that contribute to the shaping of one's literacy profile.

For the hearing child, entering school possessing cognitive abilities, a well-established vocabulary, and linguistic competence are where the groundwork is laid for the child to begin working on developing decoding skills. However, if any of these components are weak or underdeveloped, the child arrives at school ill equipped to face the challenges imposed by formal education. Such is often the case for children entering the classroom who are deaf and hard of hearing.

IMPACT OF DEAFNESS ON READING DEVELOPMENT

Contemporary classrooms include students who are deaf and hard of hearing and who may exhibit a myriad of characteristics representing all levels of literacy skills. They come from all walks of life, portraying a variety of ethnic and socioeconomic backgrounds. Representing families in which all or the majority communicate through sign language, to those who rely on residual hearing and speech to communicate, they depict a diverse population. Some have received cochlear implants at an early age and are relying on aural/oral methods to decipher classroom materials; others access classroom information through ASL.

Historically speaking, regardless of the mode of communication used within the classroom, students who are deaf and hard of hearing have experienced a tremendous amount of difficulty learning to read. This has been well documented in the literature. Two points in particular merit discussion; first, upon graduation from high school the majority of students with a severe to profound hearing loss do not read above the fourth-grade level when compared to their hearing peers (Allen, 1986; Paul, 1998, 2009; Traxler, 2000). Second, throughout the course of the student's academic career in the K–12 setting, growth in reading level is less than a half a grade per academic year (Paul, 2009, p. 284). What are some of the factors that have contributed to these statistics? What types of interventions and strategies can be employed to foster English language literacy among learners who are deaf and hard of hearing?

Barriers to Reading Comprehension: Factors That Impact Students Who Are Deaf and Hard of Hearing

Paul (2001, 2003) argues that reading involves two broad entities: process and knowledge. Process refers to those skills associated with accessing print, such as word identification and letter-sound relations; knowledge refers to the skills related to metacognition, prior knowledge, and other cognitive skills related to the reading process. These components are interwoven and ultimately provide readers with the tools they need to comprehend printed materials. Although word identification skills imply that readers can decode words, one cannot assume that they comprehend what the words mean. Word knowledge, word mastery, or vocabulary acquisition suggests that the reader understands what the word means in isolation or can gain an understanding based on how the word is used in context. How do children who are deaf and hard of hearing identify words? What strategies do they use for decoding? What do they use to comprehend text? What does the research reveal regarding modes of communication, parental hearing loss, and school settings?

Phonemic Awareness in Children Who Are Deaf and Hard of Hearing

Schirmer and McGough (2005) conducted a review of the literature on the development and reading instruction of students who are deaf using the same topic areas presented by the National Reading Panel (NRP). Aligning their review within the same time period as the NRP, they examined articles from 1970 forward. The brief summary that follows highlights the research relating to phonemic awareness.

Phonological coding was first cited in the literature with early research conducted by Conrad (1979). Interested in determining if deaf readers used *internal speech,* the term he used for phonological codes, Conrad studied the way 15- and 16-year-old students who were deaf used phonological information with respect to word recognition. His findings suggested that individuals who were deaf could access and apply phonological information in word processing. Further research conducted by Hanson, Liberman, and Shankweiler (1984) suggested that deaf students used speech and fingerspelling to code letters when presented with individual letters. They further indicated that the child's ability to use speech coding was not related to the child's speech production skills.

Other research in this area has focused on the use of ASL and fingerspelling to facilitate the development of letter and word identification skills. Noteworthy studies conducted by

Hirsh-Pasek (1987) assert that fingerspelling can be used to separate words into parts, thus increasing word identification skills. Andrews and Mason (1986) advocate for matching internal ASL signs to printed words. Although it appears that readers who are deaf use these visual codes for word recognition, no empirical data to date suggest how these strategies can be taught.

Additional studies regarding phonological knowledge have produced conflicting results. Although Schaper and Reitsma (1993) found that students between the ages of 6 and 9 who are deaf and relied on the oral method for communication initially learned new words by coding the printed configurations, as they got older and were more experienced they tended to use speech-based coding. This is further supported by Waters and Doehring (1990) who concluded that the phonological forms of words are less useful for these young readers. Kelly (1993) determined that high school students who were deaf and were skilled readers showed a greater tendency to access phonological information; but this tendency did not correlate highly with accuracy of recall or increase of word processing time.

Schirmer and McGough (2005) surmise that although more skilled readers who are deaf are able to access phonological information, no evidence indicates the strength of their phonological knowledge. It is conjectured that students developed these skills through the use of residual hearing and amplification rather than through formal instruction.

Use of Phonics by Readers Who Are Deaf and Hard of Hearing

Research indicates that some children who are deaf or hard of hearing are more adept at acquiring phonological processing skills than others (Sterne & Goswami, 2003). While there are those who tend to use these skills when engaged in reading and benefit from instruction in traditional phonics, others struggle with mastering phonological coding skills and therefore rarely, if ever, use them. One body of research (Marschark & Harris, 1996; Padden & Hanson, 2000) indicates that young readers who are deaf do not develop their phonological coding skills as quickly as their peers who can hear. Although this skill is often mastered by hearing children by the time they are between 5 and 7 years of age, children who are deaf may not develop these skills until they are between the ages of 9 and 11 or while attending fourth or fifth grade. The literature does contain a few articles that describe the benefits of visual phonics; however, little empirical data support its use (Woolsey, Satterfield, & Roberson, 2006).

Fluency Among Readers Who Are Deaf and Hard of Hearing

A review of the literature indicates that approximately a dozen articles relate to reading fluency with respect to readers who are deaf and hard of hearing. Of those published, approximately half pertain to spoken reading fluency, and only a few meet the basic standards of research rigor (Easterbrooks & Houston, 2007). Reading fluency involves automaticity, which means the individual can engage in basic reading operations without expending an undue amount of mental energy. Those who can read fluently are said to be able to devote the majority of their working memory to prosody, rather than becoming bogged down in basic reading operations such as decoding vocabulary, deciphering grammar, and comprehending syntax (Kelly, 2003). According to Easterbrooks & Houston, reading fluency in signing deaf children requires their ability to go beyond the simple reading of words at an appropriate rate while forming a mental visualization of the printed English text. Once this is formed they must then render it expressively through ASL, spoken English, or one of the manually coded English systems (p. 40).

Comprehension of Text

One of the most pervasive difficulties experienced by numerous readers who are deaf and hard of hearing lies in the fact that they are attempting to learn and master the English language while they are concurrently being asked to read. Unlike their peers who can hear, who frequently bring an extensive bank of word knowledge to the reading process, the word knowledge possessed by readers readers who are deaf and hard of hearing can be scant by comparison. A study conducted by LaSasso and Davey (1987) indicates that vocabulary knowledge is an effective predictor of reading comprehension. Garrison, Long, and Dowaliby (1997) have also examined the relationship between background knowledge, vocabulary knowledge and comprehension. They likewise determined that vocabulary knowledge was a strong predictor of reading comprehension.

Although these studies have looked at vocabulary as a predictor of reading comprehension, by far the most extensive research within the field of deaf education has been within the area of syntax. Beginning with the seminal work of Quigley, Wilbur, Power, Montanelli, and Steinkamp (1976), numerous studies have been conducted that examine knowledge of syntactic structures with respect to reading comprehension. Quigley et al. focused on the performance of deaf students in their efforts to master sentences with respect to nine of the major English syntactic structures. These include negation, conjunction, question formation, pronomilization, verbs, complementation, relativization, disjunction, and alternation (Paul, 2009). They determined that students who were deaf had specific difficulties with sentences that used verb inflectional process and auxiliaries, relative clauses such as embedded phrases, and sentences that did not adhere to a typical subject-verb-object format. Furthermore, sentences containing figurative language were also found to be problematic.

Schirmer and McGough (2005) note that the research literature on reading comprehension can be viewed from two major perspectives: first, the prior knowledge the reader brings to the text and, second, the cognitive strategies the reader uses before, during, and after reading (p. 96). Prior knowledge includes knowledge of vocabulary, syntax, topic, and knowledge of the text structure. Cognitive strategies refer to the monitoring process readers use to consciously check their comprehension of the text and their abilities to use a variety of strategies to enhance understanding.

Beginning with one of the earliest studies on use of prior knowledge by Wilson (1979) and continuing today, Paul (2009) indicates that there is no comprehensive model for understanding the role of prior knowledge and how a student who is deaf reads. However, studies that have been conducted provide insights into the abilities and difficulties students encounter. Wilson hypothesized that one of the reasons many of these students hit the third/fourth grade plateau was due to their inability to make inferences. Recognizing that reading materials beyond the third grade require students to make use of prior knowledge to understand both implicit and explicit information, he designed a series of text-explicit and inferential questions for the students to answer. His findings indicated that those of a text-explicit nature were significantly easier for them to answer.

Additional research conducted by Andrews, Winograd, and DeVille (1996) demonstrate that when ASL is utilized to elicit and build prior knowledge preceding reading activities, improvement is evident in reading comprehension. A study conducted by Donin, Doehring, and Browns (1991) produced similar findings. Focusing on orally educated children who are deaf and hard of hearing, they determined that age and language experiences had a positive bearing on their understanding of textual content structures. Further research conducted by Jackson, Paul, and Smith (1997) determined that when students were questioned extensively before reading a selection, prior knowledge might assist them in recalling pertinent and relevant information.

Studies focusing on the metacognitive processes readers who are deaf and hard of hearing utilize to ensure they comprehend what they are reading have shed additional insights into how they know they understand what they are reading. The early work of Davey (1987) employed a "look back" condition where students were allowed to look back at the text before responding to questions. Although this strategy enhanced reading comprehension, these learners were not cognizant of the fact that their comprehension improved.

Additional research conducted by Ewoldt, Israelite, and Dodds (1992) examined rereading and retelling among 13-to 17-year-olds. Their results revealed that students used self-monitoring of comprehension to complete the task. Andrews and Mason (1991) examined the strategies used by students who are hearing and deaf to fill in incomplete sentences by supplying a word that had been deleted. Using a think-aloud strategy, it became apparent that readers who were deaf relied more frequently on rereading and background knowledge and readers who could hear made greater use of context cues. Further research by Strassman (1992) indicated that when students responded to a questionnaire pertaining to the characteristics of a good reader, they cited school-related tasks they had been taught rather than comprehension-monitoring strategies.

Vocabulary Development

It is well documented that word knowledge contributes significantly to reading comprehension (Anderson & Freebody, 1985; Snowling & Hulme, 2005; Stahl & Nagy, 2006). Having command of a sizeable vocabulary and the ability to comprehend figurative language, idiomatic phrases, multiple-meaning words, and nuances implied by specific word choices all assist the reader when faced with a variety of genres. Acquiring an extensive and meaningful vocabulary involves a complex process. Although a great deal of knowledge about words is not taught, skilled readers tend to develop their understanding of words through extensive reading, incidental learning experiences, and interpersonal interactions.

Within the field of deaf education a multitude of empirical studies document the low vocabulary levels of students who are deaf and hard of hearing when compared with their peers who can hear (Paul, 1996). These studies reveal that students who experience difficulty hearing generally comprehend fewer words when reading print and the words they understand are directly related to the words they use when they write (Paul, 2003). In essence, they tend to use more nouns and verbs than adjectives, adverbs, and conjunctions.

An additional body of research has demonstrated that vocabulary difficulty can be impacted by both knowledge and the processes involved in deciphering text. Because many students who are deaf struggle with critical English components, such as phonology, morphology, orthography, and syntax, they may experience tremendous difficulties as they attempt to decode and learn new words in context (Davey & King, 1990; deVilliers & Pomerantz, 1992). Many never develop the extensive vocabularies possessed by their hearing peers; this and their weak phonological skills hamper their abilities to utilize spoken forms of the language to decode words, especially those they are not familiar with when they encounter them in a written format. Further compounding the problem is the way numerous sentences are structured syntactically; syntactic structure can further prevent a student from decoding unfamiliar words.

Within the short confines of a chapter, one cannot begin to provide an in-depth look at reading development. Rather, the intent here is to acquaint the reader with some of the issues that merit further consideration. Authors such as Paul (2009) provide an excellent synopsis of the research that has been conducted on vocabulary development involving readers who are deaf and hard of hearing. For an in-depth review of this information, see Paul (2009), *Language and Deafness.*

PROGRAMS, INTERVENTIONS AND STRATEGIES DESIGNED TO PROMOTE LITERACY AMONG STUDENTS WHO ARE DEAF AND HARD OF HEARING

Bilingual Programs: Teaching Children Who Are Deaf to Read

Deaf children of Deaf parents consistently outscore their peers who are deaf and who have hearing parents when administered tests of English reading proficiency. This has been attributed to the fact that children who are deaf cannot rely on their spoken language skills when they are learning to read. Therefore, professionals have been prompted to examine the efficacy of employing a bilingual model. Across the United States there are 19 schools for the deaf, 16 residential schools, and 3 days schools that identify their programs as being bilingual. This implies that they are using ASL as a first language, with English introduced as the second language. These programs all build on the seminal work of Cummins's (1984) theoretical framework.

Cummins (1981) postulates that, regardless of the language, when one develops skills and proficiency in a first language the person can then use these skills to acquire, through transfer, a second language. Cummins refers to this as the Linguistic Interdependence Model. Theorizing that all languages are linked to a common conceptual core, he implies that as one gains experience and proficiency in one language it promotes proficiency in the second language. It is through this level of proficiency that the transfer of cognitive/academic or literacy-related skills can occur across both languages. These skills, critical to learning, include conceptual knowledge, subject-matter knowledge, the ability to use higher-order thinking skills, reading strategies, and writing composition (Evans, 2004).

Bilingual programs designed to work with students who are deaf differ from those traditionally designed for individuals who can hear. This is due to the unique characteristics of the deaf learner. Unlike hearing second-language learners who have acquired a mastery of their L1 language in both its spoken and written forms, those who use ASL (a visual, spatial, conceptual language) as their L1 language have gained a mastery in a language that does not possess a written form. Furthermore, individuals who are deaf are not privy to learning through the auditory channel; therefore, incidental language learning does not support the reader who is deaf when presented with materials in the L2 language. In addition, the lack of or inconsistent exposure of children who are deaf to the first language often leaves them with a less robust L1 language to draw from when they are presented with printed materials in the L2 language (Evans, 2004; Mayer & Akamatsu, 2003). Recognizing these fundamental differences, several strategies have been developed to promote literacy among deaf second-language learners. Three of these strategies merit discussion. For a more extensive review see Mayer and Akamatsu, in M. Marschark and P. E. Spencer (Eds.), 2003, *Deaf Studies, Language, and Education.*

The first of these strategies is referred to as chaining in the literature. Based on the work of Erting, Thumann-Prezioso, and Sonnenstrahl-Benedict (2000), Padden (1996), and Padden and Ramsey (2000), chaining refers to the use of fingerspelling to connect ASL to print. Describing a classroom strategy where the target word is signed, followed by fingerspelling, signed again, and then related to print, the "chaining structures" can be used to strengthen the relationship between the various language elements (Mayer & Akamatsu, 2003).

A second strategy has been described by Supalla, Wix, and McKee (2001). Using a four-step process students begin by signing narratives in ASL while being videotaped. They are then able to watch the narratives and translate them into a written code developed specifically for ASL. Following this, students translate their written form of ASL to English glosses and, finally, they transfer their glosses into standard English (Mayer & Akamatsu, 2003, p. 141). Working entirely in a print modality, the philosophy behind this strategy is that it will offer students who are deaf the same opportunity as other late learners of English: a way to enhance their academic performance. To date, no research supports this strategy; however, it does merit future study.

A third strategy has examined the value of using contact signing, originating with the work of Johnson (1994), who ascertained that the features used within this mode of communication could be used as a "natural and timely access" to the features contained in the structure, grammar, and lexical features of English. Stating that the mouth movements that are produced synchronously with English-based signing could facilitate the delivery of important phonological information, he suggested this model as a possible tool for the bilingual deaf learner. Used as a bridge to connect ASL and English literacy, Akamatsu, Stewart, and Becker (2000) found that when teachers used a concerted effort to use English-based signing as a bridge, students made relatively large gains in reading comprehension over a 3-year time span when measured by the Standard Achievement Test.

Based on Cummins's interdependence theory, it can be posited that L1 sign language can transfer positively to L2 literacy learning. However, additional longitudinal studies are needed to provide an increased understanding of which strategies do in fact enhance English literacy, thus unlocking the curriculum for learners who are deaf and hard of hearing. Research to date indicates that employing a bilingual approach provides one avenue for enhancing the reading and writing abilities of this student population. However, with the majority of students who are deaf and hard of hearing being educated in the mainstream today, and a significant percentage of them enrolled in programs where they are the sole recipient of services, they are frequently not privy to the benefits offered by a bilingual program. What other strategies, interventions, and materials are available to assist these readers?

SHARED READING PROGRAM. One of the early precursors to literacy development is the time invested by family members during infancy and early childhood. Providing parents with an opportunity to instill values in their young children, these parent–child interactions contribute to the child's knowledge of literacy and the role reading and writing play in everyday activities. From the beginning, while parents are teaching their children how to hold a book, turn the pages, read from front to back, top to bottom, and left to right, they are furnishing them with the fundamental skills they will later employ as young readers. Starting with the stories parents read to their children, and later supporting them as they begin to read independently, they are setting the stage for positive literacy experiences when their children enter school.

Shared reading is often an enjoyable experience shared by hearing parents and their hearing children; however, if their child is deaf, parents frequently struggle with how to read to their child. Recognizing that they cannot hear, some search for ways to read to them, and others resign themselves to the fact that it is a task for which they are ill equipped and unprepared to execute. When this occurs, it has a dramatic effect on their early literacy development, leaving them at risk to become struggling readers.

It is well established that all children benefit from shared reading at an early age. Cognizant of this fact, David Schleper (1996) developed a Shared Reading Project to assist parents and caregivers in reading books to their young children who are deaf. Modeled after Holdaway's (1979) shared book experience with preschool and primary school-age hearing children, the child's natural language is used to engage the child in stories read by adult reading models (McAnally et al., 2007). Through this interactive approach children are introduced to print through reading and rereading.

Based on this model Deaf adults become the model readers. They incorporate concepts of print, phonemic awareness, and language through shared reading experiences. Incorporating 15 principles deemed necessary for reading success, Schleper (1996) highlights some of the features of the shared reading program. These principles include using ASL by Deaf readers to translate the stories, and making both ASL and English visible to the child who is deaf as books are being read. This is done by expanding sentences found in stories, reading and rereading stories, letting children select the books, and taking implied meaning and making it explicit. The remaining principles include using spatial signs to convey meaning, while reading makeing adjustments in one's signing to bring the characters to life, connecting events in the stories to real-world experience, using attention maintenance strategies, relying on eye gaze to encourage participation, using role play to extend concepts, engaging in sign variations to represent repetitive English phrases, establishing a positive and reinforcing environment for reading to occur, and expecting deaf children to become literate.

Literacy materials provided through the Shared Reading Project include multiple sets of family book bags containing a storybook, a videotape of the story presented in ASL by a Deaf adult, an activity guide for parents, and a card with reading strategies. By providing families with tutor/readers who make weekly visits to the home to read, parents and family members are provided with support during the emergent literacy stage with the anticipation that serious literacy delays or frustrations can be prevented.

READING MILESTONES/READING BRIDGE. Children who are exposed to print at home generally fare better upon entering the traditional classroom; the same holds true for students who are deaf and hard of hearing. However, even with frequent exposure to print, when children who are deaf arrive at school they are often presented with text that is syntactically challenging for them. Research has repeatedly demonstrated that when most of these children are beginning to read they do not have a command of the vocabulary and syntactic structures contained in most grade level readers. Consequently, when faced with reading they are required to master vocabulary and orthographic and decoding skills while striving to gain comprehension. These gaps between their basic skills and the language level of the materials they are given to read can cause frustration and ultimately lead to reading failure.

Realizing these issues, Quigley and his colleagues designed a reading series, *Reading Milestones* and *Reading Bridge* (Quigley, McAnally, King, & Rose, 1991, 2001; Quigley, McAnally, Rose, & Payne, 1991, 2003) for children who are deaf and hard of hearing and those who are acquiring the English language. Determined to promote student success, texts from early reading to approximately the beginning of the fourth-grade level were developed that reflect specific structures and vocabulary already known to the child, so the emphasis can be placed solely on reading (McAnally et al., 2007, p. 215).

Based on the premise that when students experience success while reading they will be motivated to read more, the *Reading Milestones* reading series uses a balanced approach to reading while incorporating strategies to promote cognitive and metacognitive growth and development.

Reading Strategies: Literacy Practices Used with Students Who Are Deaf and Hard of Hearing

Understanding how children read and how deafness impacts reading acquisition has led professionals to explore the wide array of strategies that are being incorporated to promote literacy. By conducting research on a national scale, literacy practices used by teachers of the deaf have been delineated in the literature. Based on research conducted by Easterbrooks and Stephenson (2006), 10 currently cited practices have been identified in the literature. These practices include the use of level-appropriate reading materials for independent reading, technology, phonemic awareness, phonics, development of metacognitive skills, content area reading materials, activities that promote student collaboration, vocabulary meaning through semantic-based activities, teaching vocabulary through morphographemic-based activities, and incorporating specific strategies to promote either spoken reading fluency in oral students or signed reading fluency in signing students.

When selecting level-appropriate reading materials for beginning readers, attention should be given to concept books, predictable books, those that are well illustrated, ones that invite discussion, those that offer a framework for writing, and ones that support the curriculum. In addition, books should be linked to children's cultures and lend themselves to independent reading. Teachers of students who are deaf should explore CDs, captioned materials, and DVDs, such as those created by Newbridge and AlphaKids that connect text to sign to encourage young readers to attend to print. By exposing students who are deaf and hard of hearing to fluent-sign-models reading, students can read along, follow the story, and build vocabulary based on the models.

Phonemic awareness and phonics can be taught either through structured, auditory-based programs with appropriate modifications for oral students or through specialized materials and techniques designed to provide visual support. Programs such as those developed specifically for students who are deaf and hard of hearing, such as Visual Phonics, Cued Speech, and Lindamood Bell, should be explored as a resource to add visual support.

Metacognitive strategies can be incorporated and used as pre-reading and post-reading activities when students participate in guided reading as well as independent reading situations. Instructing them in how to use visual tools to predict and assist in text comprehension is as vital as providing them with cognitive strategies they can use later with more complex reading materials. Using graphic organizers, such as semantic webs or maps, Venn diagrams, and anticipation guides can be instrumental in promoting reading success. In addition, teaching students how to review titles, images, and captions prior to reading, as well as how to make predictions, will assist them in the reading process.

Content area reading provides its own set of challenges for readers who are deaf and hard of hearing. Unlike narratives, subject-based reading materials contain challenging vocabulary as well as new and unfamiliar concepts. May (1994) has estimated that students are expected to read approximately 33,000 pages of content-related material prior to the completion of the 12th grade. To accomplish this task, scaffolding and other content area techniques can be used to promote reading comprehension. Strategies such as previewing, skimming and scanning, using advanced organizers, self-questioning, developing study guides, outlining, underlining key words, and employing mnemonic devices are only a few of the tools students can use when faced with challenging material. By embedding literacy instruction in subjects such as social studies, science, and mathematics, students are provided with strategies that will assist them as they attempt to master subject matter knowledge.

Additional literacy practices include designing activities that require students to collaborate with each other through shared reading and writing projects and teaching vocabulary meaning through semantic-based activities. Semantic webbing or mapping is a strategy that builds on a student's prior knowledge (Heimlich & Pittelman, 1986). When forming this type of a map, students usually begin with brainstorming a topic. As ideas are formed a diagram is constructed to illustrate the connections among the various subcategories of the topic. Students draw on their previous experiences as they design maps. Through this process they begin to see words they know from a different perspective, formulate new meanings for words previously in their vocabularies, while simultaneously forming connections among and between the words they have chosen. Shared reading and writing activities as well as semantic mapping further promote literacy development.

The remaining two strategies discussed by Easterbrooks and Stephenson (2006) include teaching vocabulary meaning through morphographemic-based activities using structural analysis as well as incorporating specific activities and strategies to promote either spoken reading fluency in oral students or signed fluency in signing students. Structural analysis teaches students how to recognize prefixes and suffixes so they can decode words that are unfamiliar to them. By teaching students to initially focus on the root word they can then examine how the meaning changes when prefixes and suffixes are added.

Fluency can be described as one's ability to read material quickly and accurately with ease and expression (Carnine et al., 2004). Because fluent readers do not have to focus on decoding words, they can direct their energies to comprehending the text. There is widespread agreement among reading professionals that the best way to teach fluency is through direct instruction (Vacca, Vacca, & Mraz, 2011). Students who are deaf should be encouraged to practice with predictable texts and engage in retelling the story; those who are hard of hearing can benefit from these strategies as well as taking advantage of automated reading. Automated reading involves listening to a story in an audio format prior to reading it orally. Students repeatedly replay the story until they can read it fluently by themselves. Students who use ASL to communicate can repeatedly watch stories signed by an ASL model and follow the same procedures, watching it repeatedly until they can sign it fluently by themselves; in these instances students can read along with signed videos or DVDs.

Several of the strategies used with readers who are deaf and hard of hearing are the same strategies used with students who can hear. Reed (2003) examined the practices of itinerant teachers focusing on literacy development with students who have mild to profound losses. All the itinerant teachers within her study worked from a meaning-centered theoretical framework; however, their practices were eclectic, depending on the student's needs. Practices included using cloze procedures, chunking, corrections, drill, experiences, explanations, making connections, peer/teacher help, pre-reading and pre-teaching, questioning and discussion, reinforcement, sequencing, summarizing, and retelling. Recognizing that students must be actively engaged, many of these teachers have infused literacy in natural ways throughout the curriculum.

WRITING, SPELLING, AND STUDENTS WHO ARE DEAF. The goal of any literacy program is to prepare students to become functionally literate young adults prior to graduating from high school. Based on a set of standards established by the International Reading Association and the National Council of Teachers of English Standards for the English Language Arts, students are required to become proficient and literate users of language (Schley & Albertini 2005). Becoming a proficient and literate user is characterized by the individual's ability to read as well as his or her capacity to write.

An extensive body of research highlights the difficulties and challenges students who are deaf and hard of hearing experience when given writing assignments. Research indicates that students frequently struggle with verb agreement and correct use of tense, misuse function words such as articles and prepositions, and use fewer adverbs and conjunctions (Heider & Heider, 1940; Greenberg & Withers, 1965; Mykelbust, 1964; Stuckless & Marks, 1966; Yoshinaga-Itano & Snyder, 1985). Recent studies reveal that 18-year-old deaf students' writing samples, from a grammatical standpoint, are comparable on the average to those produced by hearing students who are 8 to 10 years old (Paul, 2003).

Although students who are deaf are frequently engaged in written communication at home when they write notes to their parents, send thank-you notes, exchange text messages, or become immersed in instant messaging (IM) to talk with their friends, these types of personal communication vary significantly from the writing that is required in the classroom. As determined by the teacher or the curriculum, students are asked to write reports, engage in writing drills that require appropriate use of vocabulary and grammar, and complete assignments that reflect their knowledge and perspectives on an array of topics.

Students who are deaf or hard of hearing can find writing to be as challenging as reading. Writing requires students to map the written form of a language onto a linguistic system they already know and understand. However, the majority of students who are deaf strive to complete this task while relying on a reduced set of understandings of the language. Struggling with a solid language base in either English or ASL, and a limited knowledge of the rules of conversation and discourse as well as vocabulary and syntax, their attempts to write are often lost in a panacea of confusion if not altogether stymied. Evidence of this can be seen in the writing samples included in Figures 9.1a–9.1d. Representing a variety of grade levels, these samples demonstrate a wide range of competencies.

Soon I don't need
My dog. I'll have brother
or sistter. Madye I haved s.
I wish I'll be trans formers
I buy trans formers.
Writing Sample #1
I Love My mommy.
I play foot ball.
I play Basket ball
My friend love me.
My mommy love me
Writing Sample #2

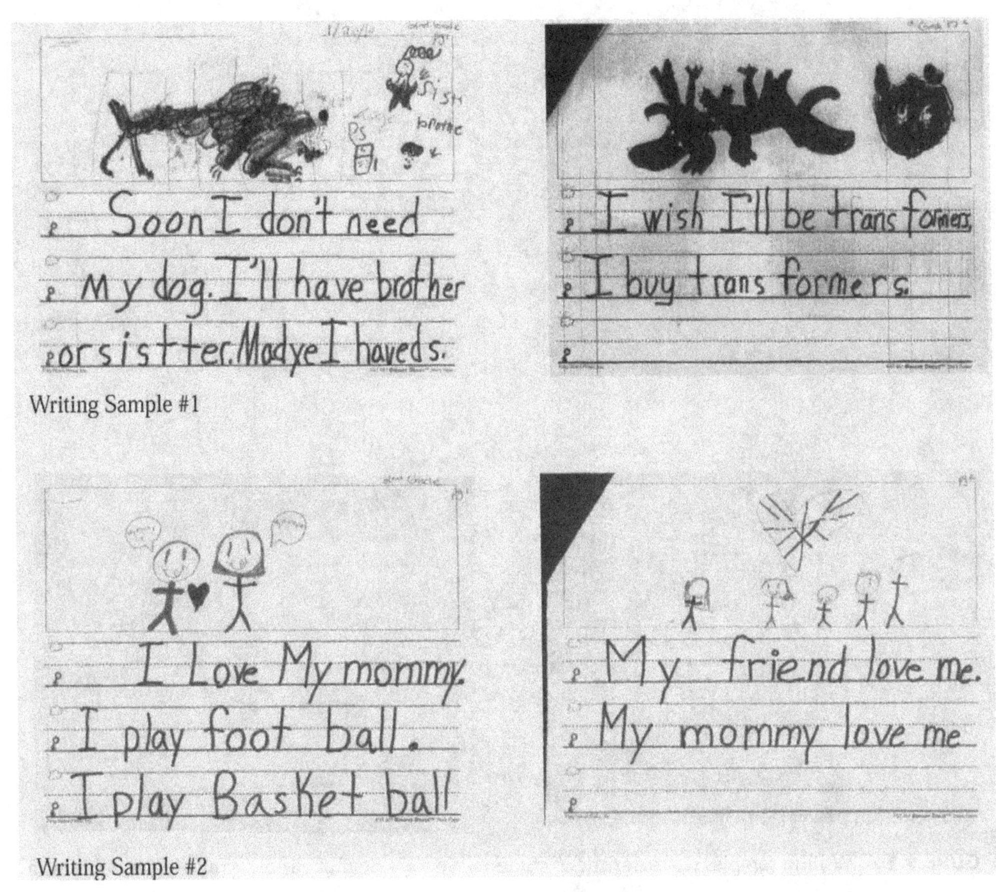

FIGURE 9.1a Writing samples characteristic of students who are deaf at various grade levels: 2nd grade.

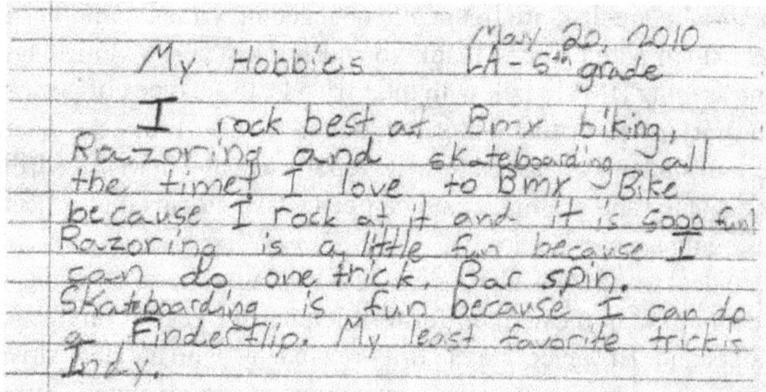

My Hobbies   May 20, 2010
LA - 5th grade

I rock best at Bmx biking, Razoring and skateboarding all the time! I love to Bmx Bike because I rock at it and it is sooo fun! Razoring is a little fun because I can do one trick, Bar spin. Skateboarding is fun because I can do a Finder Flip. My least favorite trick is Indy.

Writing Sample #1

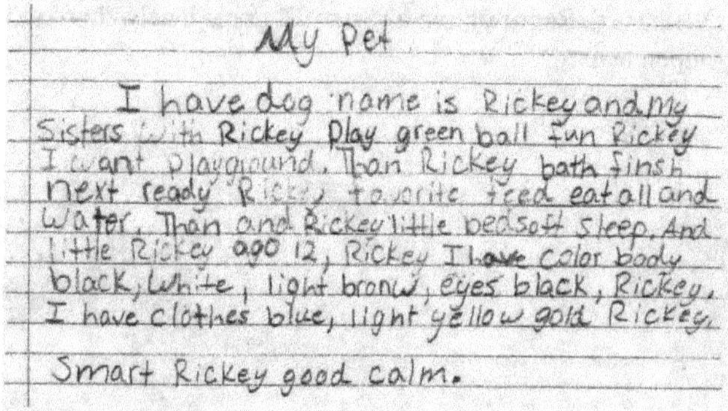

My Pet

I have dog name is Rickey and my Sisters with Rickey play green ball fun Rickey I want playground. Than Rickey bath finsh next ready Rickey favorite feed eat all and water. Than and Rickey little bed soft sleep. And little Rickey ago 12, Rickey I have color body black, White, light bronw, eyes black, Rickey. I have clothes blue, light yellow gold Rickey.

Smart Rickey good calm.

Writing Sample #2

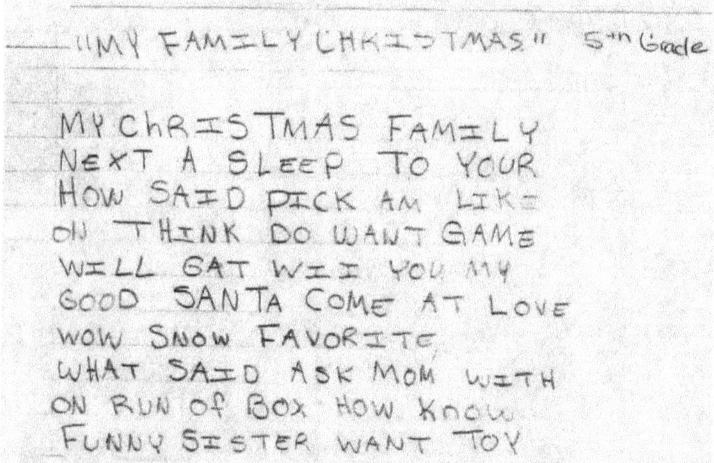

"MY FAMILY CHRISTMAS"   5th Grade

MY CHRISTMAS FAMILY
NEXT A SLEEP TO YOUR
HOW SAID PICK AM LIKE
ON THINK DO WANT GAME
WILL EAT WII YOU MY
GOOD SANTA COME AT LOVE
WOW SNOW FAVORITE
WHAT SAID ASK MOM WITH
ON RUN OF BOX HOW KNOW
FUNNY SISTER WANT TOY

Writing Sample #3

FIGURE 9.1b Writing samples characteristic of students who are deaf at various grade levels: 5th grade.

I felt good about summer. I really
little boring at my home. I said
want more fun meself.
This is summer on June. Where
I went? My dad, uncles, me
went to South Carolina for work
jobs. Fewing for 3 days. Where
they went to sleep live in South Carolina.
In the moring, my dad and me went to
work, let they went to arrive here.

Writing Sample #1

I love read books. Because I alway
read book. I am use computer for AR.
Because I maybe go to Six flag or anywhere.
my family watch me then I am use read books.
my family was happy for me.

my brother ask my family talk about buy
new kitten. My brother said "please buy
pet kitten" then my family said "fine".
my brother was happy. My family and brother
in car. They go to animal store. My brother
favorite black kitten. my brotler was buy
kitten. My brotler want name kitten is lucky.

Writing Sample #2

FIGURE 9.1c Writing samples characteristic of students who are deaf at various grade levels: 10th grade.

When I had the most fun ever

When I had the most fun ever
in Six flags.. I enjoyed Sixflags
rides with my parents on Oct.
30 2007. We waited in
long line to rides. The fun was
worth waiting like wait at line
to any rides. When we get on
a roller caster then the carts
start to move to high park of
roller coster rail.

Writing Sample #1

Anyway, life is not always perfect. I wish I can
rewind my whole life and do it the right way without break
somebody's heart. Not only that, it can be relate to
school, family, friend, and yourself. Like, while you
in school, you got one big fat F on your test.
That grade pull everything down, and you
want to re take it. Some teacher don't
approve it, but if you got it re take then
you're locky. If not, then it is hard
to keep up with a good work.

Writing Sample #2

FIGURE 9.1d Writing samples characteristic of students who are deaf at various grade levels: 11th grade.

Determining how to provide students with the tools they need to become successful writers has prompted professionals to examine the most effective approaches to teaching writing. Writers rely on grammar, spelling, and punctuation when putting their thoughts on paper. Furthermore, they draw from their experiences, language, and world knowledge to construct, organize, and share their information. Marschark, Lang, and Albertini (2002) note "writing is a process, but it need not be a lock-step sequence. How individuals write varies according to their goals and personalities, among other things. One way of looking at this process presents writing as a set of cognitive, linguistic, physical, and social activities" (p. 175). Therefore, as one engages in the process of writing, all these levels interact. Considering all these factors, various approaches to teaching writing have been examined. The approach that appears to hold the most promise for students who are deaf and hard of hearing is the process approach to writing.

PROCESS APPROACH TO WRITING. The process approach to writing is based on the premise that instruction should focus on writing tasks that are meaningful and purposeful for the student. Concentrating on process first and product second, students are encouraged to put their thoughts on paper, recognizing that their product will later be edited and corrected for grammar, word choice, and spelling. The writing process contains several components. These elements are not linear in nature; rather, students move back and forth among the elements based on where they are in the writing process. The components consist of prewriting, composing, revising, editing, publishing, skill instruction, and conferencing.

Prewriting includes anything that prepares the student for the writing assignment. Topics are selected, thoughts begin to be formulated, and ideas are frequently shared with peers or in a small group. This allows writers the opportunity to determine how and what they want to say. During the composing stage students begin to write their first draft. Teachers encourage students to concentrate on their ideas and place them on paper, paying little attention, if any, to spelling and grammar.

During the revising stage students participate in a conference regarding their initial draft. Conferences can occur between students, in small groups, or with teachers. After the conference the student reflects on what has been said and determines how or if a revision will take place. An editing phase follows whereby students attend primarily on the mechanics of writing. This is followed by the publishing phase, which can consist of informal sharing or more formalized products in the form of papers, books, or articles for the school newspaper.

Throughout the writing process skill instruction occurs on a routine basis. Mini-lessons are frequently provided based on the writing needs of individuals or small groups of students. This instruction is coupled with conferencing whereby the teacher pays particular attention to content while asking the students reflective questions that pertain to their product. Through these discussions products are strengthened, prompting students to further revise and edit their work.

The process approach to writing has also been referred to as a writing workshop approach. Calkins (1994) is attributed with designing the components of the writer's workshop. She suggested that a designated time be established each day for writing and that writing modules be included. The writing modules can be arranged in a variety of ways and include components such as mini-lessons, work time, state-of-the-class reports, conferencing, share sessions, and the publication celebration (as cited in McAnally et al., 2007, p. 353).

Another approach used with students who are deaf and hard of hearing is the interactive model. This is a collaborative model and can be used across content areas. In this respect the content area teacher can determine what the purpose of the writing assignment is, and the language arts teacher can assist the student with the writing process. In this respect a history teacher might want students to record important dates related to the Civil War. Later, the assignment might be to incorporate these dates into a narrative. Through the interactive model the English teacher would then capitalize on the writing process, and assist the students in the appropriate use of the language while they completed their assignment.

WRITING STRATEGIES. Literacy programs throughout the United States have focused historically on writing curricula that were directed toward the development of lexical and grammatical expression. Early systems such as the Barry Five Slate System, Wing's Symbols, and the Fitzgerald Key were designed to assist students in their quest to master the essential elements of the English sentence (see Scheetz, 2001, for a discussion of these systems). All these early systems placed emphasis at the sentence level while attempting to provide students with a model for writing correct English sentences.

Although more recently educators have suggested that writing be used as a tool for reading and for learning, the skills are still being taught separately. Recent research in the field indicates that students who are deaf continue to experience problems with grammar even when they are given the opportunity to write with their primary focus being on purpose and meaning. Furthermore, the literature tends to indicate that without direct instruction the grammatical and lexical performance of students who are deaf will not improve significantly, and improvement that does occur will transpire only over an extended period of time. However, when students are enrolled in programs that encourage self-generated writing based on personal experiences, their opportunity to develop discourse organization and fluency increases (Schley & Albertini, 2005).

Summary

Acquiring adult literacy is a multidimensional, complex process that begins in infancy and continues well into adulthood. It is a social, cognitive process requiring language mastery as well as the ability to process and map information. By drawing from experiential and world knowledge, and mastering an understanding of the underpinnings of the language represented in text, one is able to crack the code and use print to broaden one's knowledge base. This same code is ultimately used in the writing process as individuals begin to map their ideas using a print format for expression. Through this process we generate ideas, form insights and opinions, and gather information.

Numerous articles and texts have been written addressing literacy and deafness. Theories, models, and approaches have all been explored as researchers and educators alike attempt to unlock the secret to reading success.

Teaching reading and writing to children who are deaf poses a special challenge to parents and educators. Due to the ramifications of deafness, instructional techniques must be modified to meet the needs of this unique population. Many of these successful modifications stem from the strategies developed by Deaf parents, strategies they engage in while reading to their children.

Deaf parents have been very instrumental in demonstrating that children who are deaf are not only able readers but can develop into very capable readers who possess a true love for literature. When interactive communication is accessible, and language instructors are prepared to adapt their methods of instruction, the stage is set for D/deaf children to more fully access the curriculum, thus giving them one more tool to use as they strive toward academic success.

Future educators and researchers are faced with the challenge of engaging in empirical research that will provide additional insights into the cadre of best practices in literacy. As those practices are identified and implemented, students will be afforded increased opportunities to become fully functioning literate deaf adults, rather than being left behind due to their limited access to the curriculum.

10

Cognition

Thought Processes and Intellectual Development

The intricate workings of the human mind have fascinated individuals since the beginning of time. Topics that focus on how we think, act, and behave have provided endless fodder for countless discussions and debates, prompting scientists to delve deeper into the field to discover how we learn, remember, and recall information. A substantial body of research has focused on the neurobiological underpinnings of the thinking process, while other investigations have examined the interactions that transpire in various social, emotional, and academic planes that contribute to the development and enhancement of cognition and intellectual development.

Through the centuries, beliefs regarding how we reason, perceive, or comprehend information have changed significantly, shifting from Gall's early work that attributed intelligence to head shape to Gardner's theory of multiple intelligences. Embracing a broad spectrum of study, cognitive psychology is robust, focusing on the richness and diversity of how the human mind works. By applying methods of scientific study professionals examine the mental processes vital for recalling and remembering information, producing and understanding language, solving problems, and making decisions.

Cognitive psychologists examine how we process, organize, and form perceptions, based on the information we receive through both our auditory and visual channels. In addition, they study the processes involved in identifying and classifying information as well as how our short- and long-term memories function. Cognition provides the hub for human activity. Scientific studies conducted in this field provide us with a fundamental understanding of how humans think and how they think about thinking, a process identified as metacognition. Recognized as one of the key concepts, cognitive psychology, together with philosophy, linguistics, anthropology, artificial intelligence, and neuroscience, comprise the interdisciplinary field referred to as cognitive science, a field where all the entities are committed to understanding the mind (Gardner, 1985).

Research in the field of cognitive psychology is extensive, covering topics such as perceptual processing and attention, memory and consciousness, representing and retrieving everyday knowledge, problem solving, reasoning, judgment, and decision making. Empirical studies continue to shed light on how we think, reason, and process information. In addition, advances in sophisticated technology are providing new insights into the field of cognitive neuroscience by furnishing fresh perspectives surrounding the various brain activities that accompany mental processing.

How does this research apply to the field of deaf education? Throughout history, how have individuals who are deaf and hard of hearing been perceived as "thinkers" capable of engaging in activities that require abstract thinking and higher learning skills? What do current empirical studies reveal about attention and perception, visual imagery, memory, problem solving, theory of mind, and the intellectual functioning abilities of learners who are deaf and hard of hearing?

HISTORICAL OVERVIEW

David Martin, an esteemed colleague and prolific writer, has graciously shared his research relating to cognition and deaf learners for this chapter. He begins by providing a brief history of attitudes toward individuals who are deaf and their ability to think critically, abstractly, and perform higher-order thinking skills. This chapter has been developed with excerpts from his work that discuss a rationale for cognitive intervention activities in the classroom and appropriate methodologies for intervention that have been empirically demonstrated to be effective. Additional passages have been included that examine specific threats that act as barriers to implementing cognitive intervention, criteria that educators should apply when designing or selecting cognitive-intervention programs for learners, and recommendations for action on the simultaneous fronts of curriculum and teacher education (Martin, personal correspondence, 2009).

> The history of attitudes toward deaf learners' powers of higher-level thought is a sad one until only recently. If we go back to antiquity, we see evidence that persons who were deaf were the subject of exclusion and abuse—the Hebrews, for example, were admonished not to curse the deaf. Aristotle said that the ear is the organ of instruction; thus, if one could not hear, one could not learn. When in the 17th century several European countries made some successful attempts to teach some deaf persons to use speech, they concluded that deaf persons could indeed learn—drawing the right conclusion but for the wrong reason.

Related Research

> The negative story continues still longer. In 1924–1925, the National Research Council (an arm of the National Academy of Sciences) reported that deaf persons were between 2 and 3 years "retarded" in comparison to hearing persons in their response to the Pinter Non-Language Mental Test. Then some researchers reviewed the available information on the intelligence of deaf persons, and, in spite of the sometimes contradictory results, concluded that children who were deaf had inferior intelligence (Pintner, Eisenson, & Stanton, 1941). As recently as the 1950s, other researchers attributed a "concrete" nature to the intelligence of deaf persons, stating that deafness restricts the learner to a world of "concrete objects and things," rather than any abstract thought processes (Myklebust & Brutton, 1953).
>
> In the 1960s forward progress finally occurred. Furth (1964), a highly regarded researcher outside the field of deafness, concluded that the poorer performance of deaf persons on some cognitive tests could be explained either by a lack of experience of deaf persons or by the conditions of those tests that favored a background of a spoken language.
>
> Two significant reviews of studies then drew together the mounting evidence for the equivalency of deaf and hearing persons' thinking potential. One

study by Rosenstein (1961) found no difference between deaf and hearing learners' conceptual performance when the linguistic elements present were within the language experience of the deaf learner; the important conclusion was that abstract thought is *not* closed to deaf persons. Another comprehensive review or meta-analysis of 31 research studies using more than 8,000 deaf children of ages 3 to 19 (Vernon, 1967) found that in 13 experiments deaf subjects had superior success when compared to either the test norms or control groups, whereas in 7 studies the scores were not significantly different. The important conclusion was that deaf youth perform as well as hearing youth on a wide variety of tasks that measure thinking.

With the establishment of the principle that deaf learners have the same range of cognitive potential as hearing learners (e.g., Furth, 1964, 1973; Meadow, 1980; Vernon, 1967), a number of studies occurred during the 1980s and 1990s in relation to the enhancement of cognitive development of the deaf learner. The studies have involved the use of several different programs of cognitive-strategy instruction to investigate the effect of explicit and systematic classroom focus on the teaching of higher-order cognitive strategies and their application to school subject matter. As a group (e.g., Berchin, 1989; Craig, 1987; Dietz, 1985; Keane & Kretschmer, 1987; Krapf, 1985; Martin, 1983; Parasnis & Long, 1979) these studies have demonstrated that such explicit classroom intervention with appropriately retrained teachers, appropriate methodology, and specially designed materials results in measurable positive effects on specific cognitive skills in deaf learners when compared to deaf students who do not have this classroom experience.

One example of such studies was an experiment with high-school-age deaf students (Martin & Jonas, 1986) that was designed to examine the effects of intervention using materials adapted from the Instrumental Enrichment (IE) program for deaf students. Seven IE instruments (parts-wholes, comparison, symmetry, projection of visual relationships, spatial relations, following directions, and classification) were used over a 2-year period with an experimental group of students at the secondary-level who were deaf or hard of hearing. At least twice a week the specially trained teachers incorporated a series of visual, verbal, and geometric activities into regular subject matter; helped students solve these problems; and conducted metacognitive discussions; they then discussed how the students' mental strategies within these problems would be used in subject matter. The experimental group's performance exceeded that of the control group in general reasoning, thinking habits as measured by observation, real-world problem-solving skills, and performance on the mathematical concepts, mathematical comprehension, and reading comprehension subtests of the Stanford Achievement Test (Hearing-Impaired).

The cognitive potential of students who are deaf and hearing has been demonstrated to be generally equivalent, and we must also remember that differences in cognitive style continue to exist. These differences make it all the more essential that cognitive education become a part of teacher preparation in the field; equally important is to remember that the tests used to determine the cognitive functioning of students who are deaf in many cases still lack validity and appropriateness (Marschark, Lang, & Albertini 2002), thus requiring careful attention to interpretation of results for such cognitive tests. (Martin, personal correspondence, 2009)

When embarking on a discussion of the differences in cognitive style one can begin with how visual attention develops during infancy. How this visual attention develops will be determined, in part, by the amount of access the infant has to the auditory environment. Although numerous children are receiving cochlear implants during their first year of life and are reaping the benefits of environmental sounds, others are not privy to this technology. Often, those infants who experience a severe hearing loss and are not implanted do not have access to the auditory environment that surrounds them. Therefore, they rely on their visual field to develop language and basic communication skills such as turn taking, which will provide them with a foundation for the later development of social cognition.

How does visual attention develop? What role does it play in cognitive development? The sections that follow describe how children who can hear and children who cannot reap the benefits of environmental sounds rely on their visual field as a communication tool.

DEVELOPMENT OF VISUAL ATTENTION BY CHILDREN WHO CAN HEAR AND THOSE WHO ARE DEAF

From the earliest months of life, shared visual attention becomes apparent between infants and their parents or significant caregivers. Beginning with spatial and object-based attention, it serves affective and communicative developmental functions that continue throughout the first 2 years of life (Spencer, 2000). Research indicates that during the first few months these shared parent–infant visual interactions primarily occur in face-to-face settings with the parent and child gazing at each other (Tronick, Als, & Bazelton, 1980). During these interactions adults frequently talk to their infants using the "motherese" register, thus engaging the child while forming a dyadic bond and fostering trust. These early exchanges are also thought to promote the emergence of basic communication skills while setting the stage for later language development (Carpenter, Nagell, & Tomasello, 1998). At approximately 6 months of age infants begin to acquire interest in the objects around them and decrease the amount of time they spend in face-to-face interactions. Parents frequently support this interest by describing or labeling the objects that have captured their young children's attention. However, at this young age the parent's monologue is frequently ignored as the child remains intent on what he or she is doing.

As children continue to grow, they develop the capacity to attend to the task at hand while simultaneously engaging in communication exchanges. As a result, by the time children are between 12 and 15 months of age they are capable of engaging in triadic visual attention episodes (Bakeman & Adamson, 1984; Carpenter et al., 1998). Furthermore, during this developmental stage they are able to switch their focus spontaneously between the object and their parents and are more receptive and attentive to what their parents are saying. By the time children have reached this age, triadic visual episodes provide teachable moments whereby children can acquire labels and descriptions for objects that they have found interesting.

Spencer (2000) posits that the ability of children who are deaf to develop mature triadic visual attention patterns may be critical for them due to their frequent need to change their visual focus from a communication partner, who is relating to them through visual communication, to an object. However, research conducted by Wood (1989) indicates that preschoolers who are deaf and communicate orally are significantly delayed in their ability to engage in coordinated object-person attention. In addition, they do not develop oral language until this task is mastered. Additional research conducted by Prezbindowski, Adamson, and Lederberg (1998) analyzed the visual attention skills of children who are deaf between 20 and 24 months of age. Their analyses revealed that although some of the children were enrolled in programs where sign language was used, average language development was significantly delayed. They further determined that children who were deaf were less likely to engage in triadic visual attention episodes than their hearing peers (as cited in Spencer, 2000).

Further research conducted with infants who are deaf and their Deaf mothers indicates that these 18-month-old infants are as likely to engage in triadic coordinated joint attention episodes as their 18-month-old hearing peers (Meadow-Orlans & Spencer, 1996). However, this finding does not hold true for infants who are deaf who have hearing mothers or hearing children whose parents are deaf. Waxman and Spencer (1997) attribute this finding to the visual and tactile attention-directing behaviors used by Deaf mothers that are frequently not employed by hearing mothers of deaf children.

Additional research conducted by Spencer (2000) indicates that hearing status alone is not associated with the developmental patterns of visual attention during the infant-toddler period. Infants who are deaf who are born to Deaf mothers engaged in significantly longer periods of coordinated joint attention episodes, and the impetus for these extended periods of time can be attributed, in part, to the amount of time young children devoted to watching their mothers sign. Further analysis suggests that when mothers are sensitive to their children's personalities and make use of visual-tactile attention scaffolding signals, their infants are provided with a rich environment that lends itself to the development of visual attention skills during this critical period.

Through these early interactions, turn taking is learned, objects are labeled, concepts are formed, and language begins to flourish. The first few years are critical to a child's physical and cognitive development. By exposing children to a multiplicity of experiences, their individual personalities are formed and shaped, and they are provided with their cognitive foundation. Once established, preschoolers are equipped to embark on their educational journey, where they will learn how to solve problems, think critically, and engage in social interactions.

How do young children learn? How do they retain information that they can later recall and retrieve from memory to answer questions or solve problems? What type of storage and retrieval system do students who are deaf use to retain, recall, and retrieve information? Do they develop the same strategies as their hearing peers?

Theory of Mind

The types of play children engage in when they begin to interact with each other and the impact play has on social and cognitive development are topics that have been of interest to psychologists, parents, and educators since play provides insights into these aspects of child development. Early in infancy children are drawn to one another, and it is common to see infants as young as 6 months old looking at and smiling at each other. By the time children arrive at their first birthday they begin to engage in parallel play, remaining attentive to what another toddler might be doing. However, by the time these youngsters are 15 to 18 months of age, their focus of play changes from merely being attentive to what others are doing; instead, they begin to engage in similar activities, signaling the beginning of simple social play. As they progress toward their second birthday they engage in cooperative play that is frequently organized around a theme, with each child assuming a different role. Throughout the preschool years, make-believe play becomes one avenue for promoting cognitive development.

Play also serves as a mechanism for internal reflection, assisting youngsters as they begin to gain insights into themselves, as well as others. As they play and interact with their parents and other children, they begin to realize that people have their own thoughts, beliefs, and intentions. Even at a relatively young age children realize that behavior is often intentional, designed to achieve a goal. Once children begin to grasp the concept of intentionality, they quickly begin to develop a theory of mind, a metacognitive skill that allows them to think about something in the abstract that has been removed from the immediately perceptible environment (Spencer & Marschark, 2010).

Henry Wellman (1993, 2002) ascertains that children's theory of mind moves through three phases: becoming aware of their desires, and that their desires and the desires of other people can cause behavior (by age 2); developing the ability to distinguish the mental world from the physical world (age 3); and understanding that behavior is often based on a person's beliefs about events, even when the beliefs are wrong (by age 4). This developmental transformation has been assessed by engaging the child in a false-belief task.

The most frequently used task of this nature is often referred to as the Sally-Ann task. In essence, it involves putting an object in one location in view of the child and another person. The other person leaves the room and the object is moved to a different location. The child is asked to predict where the person will look for the object when he or she re-enters the room. This task requires the child to utilize metacognitive skills to predict where the individual will look.

During the 1990s a body of research began to emerge in the literature that focused on the development of theory of mind in children who are deaf or hard of hearing. Recognizing that this metacognitive skill typically develops in hearing children between the ages of 3 and 5, professionals within the field of deaf education wanted to determine if the population they served also developed this skill set at approximately the same time, and if there were any differences in how the skill was developed. A study conducted by Courtin (2000) investigated how students who were deaf or hard of hearing would compare to those who could hear on the false-belief task. He further examined the effects of language skills and early exposure to language with respect to four groups of deaf children: signing children who had Deaf parents, signing children of hearing parents, orally trained children of hearing parents, and hearing children of hearing parents. His findings revealed that by age 6 deaf children of Deaf parents were more likely to succeed on the task than the other two groups of children who were deaf or the hearing children. Although Courtin's results indicate that one's inability to hear sound and spoken language do not impede the development of theory of mind, he states that the increased scores exhibited by those who communicated through sign could be influenced in part by the eye gaze exhibited by the examiner, possibly influencing some of the participants' responses. However, additional studies conducted by Schick, de Villiers, de Villiers, and Hoffmeister (2007) as well as earlier research conducted by Moeller and Schick (2006) and Wellman and Liu (2004) reveal that children with hearing loss who have delays in language development also exhibit delays in this metacognitive skill.

Spencer (2010) has indicated that theory of mind appears to develop in a parallel manner for children who can hear as well as those who cannot when three factors are in place. First, language must be accessible to children beginning in infancy; second, language must be produced during supportive interactions; and third, children must acquire language skills at a pace that will allow them to become involved in those activities that will promote cognitive development (p. 421).

Theory of mind is only one area through which adults are provided with a window of opportunity to observe social, cognitive, and linguistic development. Other areas that have been studied extensively are the processes that are required for individuals to store information in both their short-term and their long-term memory, and how we store visual as well as spatial information.

MEMORY SYSTEMS: STORING VISUAL AND SPATIAL INFORMATION

For over three decades research has been conducted to identify the set of processes that we use to maintain and rehearse information that comprises our conscious thoughts. Beginning with the information-processing approach to memory, formalized by Waugh and Norman (1965) and continuing with the modal model (also referred to as the information-processing model) proposed by Atkinson and Shiffrin (1968), three different types of memory storage were identified.

Depicting a model with chronologically arranged stages, Atkinson and Shiffrin (1968) postulated that information can be kept in three different types of memory storage: sensory memory, short-term memory, and long-term memory. In essence, sensory memory initially receives the incoming stimulus and retains it for a very brief amount of time. The incoming stimulus then proceeds into one's short-term memory where a series of complex processes enable us to hold and rehearse information.

Short-term memory (STM) or working memory (WM) has become the focal point for copious research studies relating to the complex cognitive processes involved in reading and problem solving. WM provides a "workbench" where we can temporarily store and manipulate information that is pertinent to solving the task at hand. During the first decade of the 21st century, numerous articles documented a significant relationship between the size of STM capacity for linguistic material and language abilities (Boutla, Supalla, Newport, & Bavelier, 2004). Originally perceived as a temporary holding and recycling buffer for information, STM is now recognized as an intricate system used to process information stored in our consciousness.

Since the inception of the early processing models, investigators have continued to propose increasingly complex models demonstrating the richness and variety of STM processing (Robinson-Riegler & Robinson-Riegler, 2008). One of the most popular of these models is Baddeley's (1986) model of WM. Described as a number of closely interacting subsystems working together to support numerous higher-level thinking processes, three of these subsystems merit further discussion: the articulatory loop, the visuo-spatial sketchpad, and the episodic buffer.

The Articulatory Loop

Baddeley's (1986) WM model describes the articulatory loop as a mechanism for actively retaining information on a temporary basis. This process is accomplished through the use of two subcomponents: the phonological store, which retains the information temporarily, and the articulatory process, referred to as the subvocal rehearsal mechanism, which allows for the rehearsal of information (Robinson-Riegler & Robinson-Riegler, 2008). Although the term *subvocal* implies a mechanism that is based solely on audition, it extends to any form of language that is articulated. Hence, both ASL and speech that are produced using visual and auditory modes can be used to rehearse information. A substantial body of research indicates that hearing people use a speech-based coding system to rehearse and recall information and that this process plays a central role in the processing of information (Baddeley, 1986, 1990; Baddeley & Hitch, 1974; Conrad, 1964; Shiffrin, 1999). Referring to this phenomenon as using "an inner voice," researchers have determined that hearing individuals rely on a phonetic code in short-term memory situations when they are presented with lists of printed words. Studies further indicate that when presented with words that are similar in sound, the task of remembering them becomes more difficult than when they are presented with different-sounding words. Similar research has been conducted with prelingually deaf individuals to determine what primary language-coding system they rely on for the temporary retention of written words.

Research: Short-Term Memory Encoding by Students Who Are Deaf or Hard of Hearing

Studies in this domain have presented a complex picture indicating the heterogeneity of the deaf population with respect to how and if they use phonological coding to represent and mediate information in their WM (Miller, 2007). Although some prelingually deaf individuals mediate information phonologically (Charlier & Leybaert, 2000; LaSasso, Crain, & Leybaert, 2003; Leybaert & Lechat, 2001; Miller, 2002), this strategy does not appear to be used by the majority. Unlike their hearing counterparts who typically rely on their phonological code to maintain spoken or written information in their WM, individuals with prelingual deafness tend to develop strategies that are not rooted in spoken language (for a review, see Musselman, 2000).

Miller (2007) reports findings from different lines of research that describe the discrete factors that may influence the strategy or strategies used by individuals who are deaf to maintain and process information in their WM. These include the primary mode of language (spoken or sign language), the mode in which the information is presented (orally, visually, or manually), and the type of information that the person is asked to retain. Furthermore, an additional body of research suggests that when this population is asked to process spoken language, they rely on a multimodal encoding process. This process includes the ability to recode spoken words into their WM using residual hearing, visual cues, fingerpselling, and/or exposure to print (Dodd, McIntosh, & Woodhouse, 1998; Harris & Beech, 1998; LaSasso, Crain, & Leybaert, 2003; Padden, 1991).

Contemporary research within the field of deaf education has also examined the role of sign language with respect to how it is used in WM to retain and process information. Research conducted by Wilson and Emmorey (1998, 2003) suggests that Deaf native users of ASL use a "phonological loop" in sign language that is parallel in structure to the phonological loop for speech used by hearing individuals. In a series of studies, they report that WM for ASL is sensitive to irrelevant signed input that corresponds to the effects of irrelevant auditory input on WM for speech. This finding supports earlier research conducted by Bellugi, Klima, and Siple (1975) and Hanson (1982) who report that performance in recalling lists of ASL signs is hampered when interim signs are produced that have similar handshapes or locations—two of the phonological parameters of ASL.

Investigations have also been conducted regarding word length and recall from WM for both speech and ASL. Studies conducted using articulatory suppression tasks have provided additional insights into the role that the "inner voice" plays in WM. These tasks involve giving persons a list of specific words and asking them to remember them while also asking them to say something nonsensical, such as "la, la, la." while they are simultaneously trying to rehearse (or remember) specific words. Evidence suggests that this procedure makes the retention of information in WM far more difficult. Studies in articulatory suppression have also been conducted to determine if any differences occur when the incoming word being produced (short or long), or if the mode through which the word is produced (sign or speech) impacts retention. Findings indicate that the effect on word length is similar, regardless of the length of the word or the mode in which it was produced.

In a study with prelingually deaf individuals who use ASL to communicate, participants were asked to engage in a manual task—that is, producing the number 8 while simultaneously rehearsing specific signs. Results indicated a disruption in the WM regardless of the length of the sign that was presented. This result further supports previous studies that have investigated the effect of articulatory suppression on speech (Wilson & Emmorey, 1997). This result additionally supports prior research showing an articulation mechanism that immediately encodes incoming information in the language that one primarily uses for processing information.

Although Wilson and Emmorey (2003) report that the structure of WM for language develops in response to language input regardless of the modality that is employed through sign or speech, they also suggest key differences between WM for signs and for speech. They posit that this finding can be attributed to the differing information-processing capabilities of the visual and auditory modalities (p. 97). In essence, it appears that individuals who are deaf use spatial coding to represent the serial order of signs—a feature that has no parallel in WM for speech.

The Visuo-Spatial Sketchpad

According to Baddeley (1986) the articulatory loop is one of the key components in WM. The loop is comprised of two components: a phonological store that holds memory traces in acoustic or phonological form that fades in a few seconds, and an articulatory rehearsal process analogous to subvocal speech. A second key component or subsystem is the visuo-spatial sketchpad. Working independently of the other subsystem it is responsible for storing and manipulating visual and spatial information, a process that is critical for performing a range of cognitive tasks. Based on research conducted by Della Sala, Gray, Baddeley, Allamano, and Wilson (1999), the two functions are viewed as separate entities. The visual processing component is responsible for remembering the appearance of an object while the spatial process is delegated to remembering the positional sequence that relates to the distance, direction, and order with which an object is presented.

Several empirical studies have provided a wealth of information on the capacities and properties of the visuo-spatial WM (see Awh & Jonides, 2001; Baddeley & Hitch, 1974; Logan, 1978; Logie, 1995; Oh & Kim, 2004; Smith, 1996). Working as a subsystem of WM, it serves the function of "integrating spatial, visual, and possibly kinesthetic information into a unified representation which may be temporarily stored and manipulated" (Baddeley, 2003, p. 200). Functioning in a different capacity from the phonological loop, it provides a system for engaging in everyday reading tasks, enabling the reader to maintain a representation of the page and its layout while facilitating such tasks as moving the eyes accurately from the end of one line to the beginning of the next.

Research: Use of Visuo-Spatial Memory Between Deaf Signers and Non-Signers

Research that focuses on how the STM or WM functions in children who are deaf has generally confirmed that individuals who are deaf and those who can hear may encode information in different ways, depending on the type of information and the way that it is presented. People who can hear tend to rely on verbal-sequential coding that is thought to be phonological, articulatory, or acoustic in nature; people who are deaf have been assumed to rely more heavily on visuo-spatial short-term memory codes (Marschark & Mayer, 1998). Findings reported by Bellugi et al. (1990) report that children who are deaf and sign can discriminate among faces under different conditions of special orientation and lighting better than their counterparts who can hear. Further studies conducted by Bettger (1992) and Bellugi and Emmorey (1993) have determined that the ability to discriminate among faces continues into adulthood. These studies prompted additional research by Emmorey, Kosslyn, and Bellugi (1993) to investigate other visuo-spatial skills that are evident in deaf and hearing signers that might not be as apparent in nonsigning hearing individuals. Emmorey et al. determined that both deaf and hearing sign-language users demonstrate an enhanced ability to generate relatively complex images that include visual imagery and facial discrimination.

Further research conducted by Cattani, Clibbens, and Perfect (2007) suggest that sign-language use improves visual memory. Signing individuals display better memory performance for abstract shapes than nonsigning individuals, and sign-language users exhibit enhanced skills with respect to visual-location memory for special items. This finding supports previous research conducted by Arnold and Mills (2001) and Proksch and Bavelier (2002). These findings are primarily attributed to the use of sign language rather than being ascribed to the physical condition of deafness.

Blatto-Vallee, Kelly, Gaustad, Porter, and Fonzi (2007) have also examined how students who are deaf and those who can hear use visuo-spatial schematic representation while attempting to solve mathematical problems. Distinguishing between visuo-spatial "schematic" representations that encode the spatial relations compared with the visuo-spatial "pictorial" representations that encode the visual appearance of the objects described in a problem, they determined that the students who could hear performed significantly better at all educational levels than their peers who were deaf (p. 432). This finding was attributed to the fact that the participants who could hear utilized visuo-spatial schematic representation to a greater extent than did the participants who were deaf. However, when utilized by students who were deaf the schematic was recognized as a strong predictor of their ability to solve mathematical problems.

Studies such as these and those previously described delineate the differences that exist as well as the similarities that are present between the skills and knowledge bases of deaf and hearing individuals (Marschark & Everhart, 1999). These differences seem to be most striking in children who are deaf who have hearing parents. It is well documented in the literature that deaf children of hearing parents frequently reside in family units where effective modes of communication are weak if not altogether almost nonexistent. This fact significantly impacts children who are deaf in their early developmental years, leaving them less prepared to engage in social and educational interactions when they arrive at school. Consequently, many require cognitive intervention so that they can more fully participate in the academic challenges that await them.

In the sections that follow, David Martin (personal communication, 2009) sheds light on the need for cognitive intervention by providing insights, information, and recommendations regarding how to enhance the learning environment for students who are deaf and hard of hearing.

Why Implement Cognitive Intervention?

Since the establishment of the equivalency of deaf and hearing learners' cognitive potential, the rationale for intervention is clear. However, careful planning must occur to guarantee a place in the school curriculum for systematic and explicit instruction in cognitive strategies for that potential to be realized. The rapid expansion of knowledge today means that all young people (deaf or hearing) must have preparation in how to locate, evaluate, and create knowledge, rather than only to memorize knowledge that may change next week or next year.

A Method

A number of different cognitive intervention programs are available to committed teachers; some require special training and materials. One method would be the one referred to in the Martin and Jonas (1986) study. Using paper-and-pencil exercises, students solve problems on the cognitive themes referred to in the study, with assistance (mediation) from the teacher or a peer; then have metacognitive discussions to make clear the mental processes just used; and then discuss applications of each cognitive strategy to subject matter or outside-school life. Only two adaptations for deaf learners seem to be required in this method, which was originally designed for hearing students: somewhat slower pacing to give adequate time for processing some completely new strategies, and careful explanation of cognitive terms that may be known to hearing learners but perhaps not yet to deaf learners (e.g., terms for such processes as comparison, classification, sequencing, organizing, etc.). In addition to instruction in this area in a classroom in which sign language is the medium of communication, accepted signs already exist in ASL for all these conceptual processes; thus, the use of manual communication poses no barrier to cognitive interventions of this kind.

Barriers

However, two significant barriers to this implementation do exist in the early 21st century world of education in the United States, and each must be overcome if higher-level thinking strategies are to become part of the repertoire of deaf (and hearing) learners. The first of these is the widespread emphasis (some would say overemphasis) on standardized testing as mandated by state and federal legislation. Teachers are, understandably, feeling great pressure to "cover" the curriculum and to prepare students for the tests, with the result that many teachers believe that, although cognitive-strategy instruction might be desirable, they and their school administrators see no relationship between the tests and cognitive strategies. This view is unfortunately shortsighted because the cognitive strategies are what will endure in an individual's life, long after the facts tested on an examination have faded; and, ironically, cognitive strategies can actually assist with student success in such examinations in procedures such as decision making (e.g., on multiple-choice items), thinking through a problem before responding (e.g., on short-essay items), planning, and so on. We would not attempt to make the case for cognitive education solely on the basis of helping students succeed on standardized tests, but that enhancement is clearly a by-product of cognitive instruction.

The second barrier is a controversy among some educators as to whether cognitive strategies are specific within each subject-matter domain versus generic across different subject matters. For instance, a question would be, Is classification in biology actually different from classification of events in a study of history? This controversy is resolved by recalling that the fundamental process of, for example, classifying is one general mental process and sequence, even though its application to different subjects may vary. Thus, the case appears to be clear for generic cognitive-strategy instruction, with the teacher helping the students to make the appropriate applications to whatever subject is at hand.

Selecting a Cognitive Intervention Program

If an educator of students who are deaf and hard of hearing is willing to make the commitment to systematic cognitive instruction across the curriculum with an emphasis on explicit thinking strategies, the selection of a program to use is then a next step. Among the hard questions to ask about any given program would be the following:

1. Does the program have a strong theoretical base?
2. Has the program been well researched?
3. Has the program been found to produce positive outcomes? For many kinds of students?
4. Does the program avoid the promise of a quick fix (i.e., does it recognize that changing one's thinking habits is a deep and iterative process involving explicit attention and time)?

5. Does the program require a commitment to teacher development in its methodology?
6. Is the program comprehensive in the sense of focusing on cognitive skills that apply to a variety of subject matter rather than just to one academic discipline?

An affirmative answer to each of these six questions would establish a firm case for adopting or adapting a particular cognitive-strategies program for one's classroom.

Professional Actions

If we are serious about recognizing the importance of higher-level thinking strategies for learners, six actions are now essential:

1. Programs of professional development in cognitive education for currently practicing teachers must be initiated to prepare them to meet the needs of students who are deaf who are already in their classroom.
2. Teacher-education faculty members in university teacher preparation programs must become attuned to the underlying cognitive dimensions of their subjects, and of the entire process of teaching, as they prepare the next generation of teachers.
3. Teacher education curricula must include supervised practice in the teaching of critical and creative thinking during practicum experiences in the presence of master teachers who are themselves strong models of teaching thinking.
4. The underlying cognitive dimensions of the regular school curriculum must be made explicit for both teachers and students to be aware of and apply higher-level thinking in every subject-matter context, as opposed to only factual understanding.
5. Educators of students who are deaf and hard of hearing must recognize that the clear majority of these students are now educated in inclusive settings, making it all the more important for teachers in these settings to know how to address the cognitive characteristics of learners who are deaf and then work with them. This point extends to the preparation of any teachers who are expected to have a diverse population of students in their classrooms, some of whom will have special needs, but to remember to maintain the same expectations for all students, both hearing and deaf, in terms of cognitive achievement.
6. Research must continue to investigate both the variety of ways of helping students who are deaf achieve their cognitive potential, and the differences in cognition among this diverse group of students in today's classrooms: profoundly or severely deaf with cochlear implants, profoundly or severely deaf without cochlear implants, moderately deaf with aided hearing, moderately deaf without aided hearing, and other combinations of characteristics that would include whether or not any of the variety of deaf learners' preferred mode of communication might be ASL, pidgin sign, simultaneous communication, speech, or combinations of any of these approaches. All these students, however, regardless of their individual combination of characteristics, are capable of acquiring higher-level cognitive strategies that will serve them throughout their lives.

In conclusion, today's students will become adults well into the 21st century and are faced with a different world than the one that many of today's educators experienced as students themselves. Knowledge is increasing at a geometric rate; electronic communication rules one's life in many ways; rapid interaction among individuals is possible and expected; and entirely new social patterns and relationships are evolving and being invented. However, students who become adults after having had experiences in developing, using, and seeing the applications of the cognitive underpinnings of school learning, social life, family life, and work life will have a distinct advantage over those who have not had such experiences in their abilities to comprehend and thrive in the world as a whole. (Martin, personal communication, 2009)

INTELLECTUAL FUNCTIONING: COGNITION AS IT RELATES TO INTELLIGENCE TESTS

Intelligence tests play a vital role in the assessment of individuals who are deaf for several reasons. They are used to guide in the development of IEPs, they assist in determining educational program placement, and they are utilized to monitor progress. The origins of intelligence testing can be traced to Paris, France, in the early 1900s and the work of Alfred Binet. Designed to measure the same mental functions that contribute to classroom attention, the processes revolved around mental abilities such as memory, attention, comprehension, discrimination, and reasoning.

The first intelligence test was normed on a group of 50 children ranging in age from 3 to 11 and thought to have normal intelligence. After norms had been established, children suspected of being mentally retarded were given the test. Their performance was compared with children from the norm group of the same chronological age. Those students, performing significantly below their intellectually normal agemates, were viewed as incapable of entering the regular classroom and were assigned to a classroom for mentally retarded individuals. The scale was refined twice, the second time in 1911.

The next significant event in the development of intelligence tests occurred in 1916 when Lewis Terman of Stanford University published an extensive revision of Binet's 1911 test. The revision became known as the Stanford-Binet and remains very popular. Within this revised test, Terman expressed a child's level of performance as a global number, called an intelligence quotient (IQ). In addition, this instrument was normed on 400 American children, ages 4 through 19, from a variety of backgrounds. The directions Terman provided for administering the items were clearer and more detailed than Binet's, thus rendering it a more reliable and useful instrument (Edwards, 1979; Seagoe, 1970). From the onset, Binet's and Simon's test items were devised to differentiate between children who could profit from normal classroom instruction and those who would require special education. In essence, they were designed to predict classroom success.

What Intelligence Tests Measure

Early in the 1900s when intelligence tests were beginning to be administered, the British psychologist Charles Spearman noticed that children given a battery of intelligence tests tended to rank consistently from test to test. It became evident that some children scored well on some tests but performed poorly on others. Spearman explained this pattern by saying intelligence was made up of two types of factors: a general factor (*g*) that affected performance on all intellectual tests and a set of specific factors (*s*) that affected performance only on specific intellectual tests. Although Spearman's research was done in 1904, contemporary intelligence tests are still designed to provide the examiner with specific and general measurements of intelligence.

Additional Views

Contemporary psychologists, such as David Wechsler (1974), have emphasized that "intelligence is not simply the sum of one's tested abilities" (Gage & Berliner, 1988, p. 169). According to Wechsler, intelligence is the global capacity of the individual to act purposefully, to think rationally, and to deal effectively with the environment. This definition, which is endorsed by many psychologists, further states that the tests are designed to predict the person's global capacity to perform effectively on academic tasks in a classroom environment.

Although people display intelligent behavior outside the classroom situation, to assess total intelligence would require test instruments that are extremely subjective. Two contemporary psychologists, Robert J. Sternberg (1985) and Howard Gardner (1983) believed that the arena of intelligence testing should be expanded to include assessments that examine how well individuals can apply their intelligence to a variety of settings. They both stressed that intelligence is multifaceted and cautioned society against focusing on the results of IQ tests to the exclusion of other worthwhile behaviors. Reuven Feuerstein (1980) extended this thinking to include the proactive processes of mediation so as to increase the intellectual potential of any individual, no matter where she or he was at the moment of intervention.

Limitations

When examining intelligence tests and attempting to gain a perspective on their usefulness, four issues warrant special consideration. First, the appraisal of intelligence is limited by the fact that it cannot be directly measured. Second, one must be aware that the intelligence we test is a sample of intellectual capabilities that relate to classroom achievement better than they relate to anything else. Third, educators must keep in mind that no intelligence score is an absolute measure; it is merely an estimate of how successfully a child solves certain problems as compared with his or her peers. Fourth, because these tests are designed to predict academic success, anything that occurs in the classroom to enhance learning can have a positive effect on intelligence test performance.

Description

One of the intelligence tests frequently administered to individuals who are deaf is the Wechsler Intelligence Scale for Children-Revised (WISC-R, 1974). It is one of three individual intelligence tests devised by David Wechsler that are currently in use. The other two are the Wechsler Preschool and Primary Scale of Intelligence (1967) and the Wechsler Adult Intelligence Scale-Revised (1981).

The WISC-R can be given to children ages 6 through 19. It is comprised of 12 subtests equally divided between a verbal scale and a performance scale. Table 10.1 provides a chart indicating the names of the subtests and the sequence which they are given.

The WISC-R yields three summary scores: a verbal IQ, a performance IQ, and a full-scale IQ. The mean of the test is 100, and the standard deviation is 15. In addition, 99.72% of all IQ scores fall between 55 and 145 (these scores represent 3 standard deviations below and above the mean).

The items for each subtest range from easy to difficult, thus accommodating the 6- to 16-year-old range and the full range of intellectual ability that can be seen at any age. The test questions are designed to reflect general knowledge and experiences that are common to practically all children.

TABLE 10.1 Weschler Intelligence Scale for Children–Revised

List of Subtests in Order of Sequence Given	
Verbal	**Performance**
1. Information	2. Picture Completion
3. Similarities	4. Picture Arrangement
5. Arithmetic	6. Block Design
7. Vocabulary	8. Object Assembly
9. Comprehension	10. Coding
11. Digit Span	12. Mazes

Although the Wechsler Intelligence Scale for Children-Third Edition (WISC-III) appears to be one of the most widely used when testing children who are deaf, other assessments have also been used with this population. Ulissi, Brice, and Gibbins (1989) report that when children who are deaf are assessed using the Kaufman Assessment Battery for Children (K-ABC), they obtain IQs in the normal range when compared with hearing children. A further review of the literature indicates varied results when examining how individuals who are deaf perform on other nonverbal intelligence tests when compared to their counterparts who can hear (Maller, 2003).

Intellectual Testing and Deafness

When reviewing the performance data compiled on individuals who are deaf, it is wise to view the findings in light of the following questions (Maller, 2003, p. 451): Is the sample representative of individuals who are deaf? Does the sample include individuals who have additional, unidentified disabilities? Do those taking the evaluation understand the directions and the questions? Due to the ramifications of deafness, do the items hold a different meaning based on experiential deprivation or different opportunities to learn the material?

When reviewing the literature on the intellectual functioning of individuals who are deaf with no secondary disabilities (Vernon, 1968, 2005), and comparing it to the data collected on individuals who can hear, the research findings consistently reveal that the IQ distribution between those who are deaf and those who can hear is nearly identical (see Braden, 1994, for a review). Akamatsu, Musselman, and Zwiebel (2000) have reported similar findings based on a longitudinal study of Canadian high school students who were deaf with nonsyndromic, hereditary deafness. The results of their study revealed that the IQs of the students who were deaf were equal to or higher than those of their peers who could hear (Akamatsu et al.).

Related investigations also indicate that children who are Deaf of Deaf parents score significantly higher on performance IQ tests than children who are deaf who are raised in families with parents and siblings who can hear (Conrad & Weiskrantz, 1981; Kusche, Greenberg, & Garfield, 1983; Sisco & Anderson, 1980; Sullivan & Schulte, 1992; Zwiebel, 1987). More recent studies indicate considerable variability in nonverbal IQ test scores. This finding is thought to be attributed to the types of tests involved and the greater heterogeneity of children who are deaf relative to children who can hear (Maller, 2003; Marschark, 1993). Children who are deaf are born into a multiplicity of family units. Although the majority of these children are surrounded by those who can hear and use speech to communicate, only a few are privy to the ease of communication access from birth. Faced with early and continuing communication barriers, children who are deaf and nurtured in hearing families are generally privy to less information while oftentimes relying on their visual perception to create meaning from what they observe. Antia, Stinson, and Gaustad (2002) argue that because of these early environments children who are deaf who are raised in hearing families are frequently faced with "unfamiliar situations." Consequently they may find they do not have the problem-solving skills or strategies that will prepare them to resolve these dilemmas.

A plethora of studies pertaining to deafness and intellectual functioning have shed myriad insights for the field, while also raising at times some pointed and noteworthy questions. Although several of these questions revolve around the topic of language and the barriers that can be created by deafness, others question the effect of the different patterns of early socialization. Researchers continue to examine verbal intelligence tests in light of whether they are culturally fair for this population. Other researchers have identified serious flaws in the construction and expression of a number of standardized tests in terms of their accessibility for test takers who are deaf; such flaws are understandable in view of the fact that most standardized tests are developed by hearing persons with hearing test takers in mind. (See Mounty & Martin, 2005, for a detailed analysis of this problem area and some strategies that need to be employed in order to make tests fair and accessible to test-takers who are deaf.)

Educational environments continue to be explored, and the possible need to develop strategies for visuo-spatial learners is receiving increased attention. Educators continue to search for ways to adapt their instructional methods, thereby enhancing the overall cognitive development and academic achievement of students who are deaf and hard of hearing. By promoting curricula that foster the incorporation of metacognitive skills, students are being exposed to strategies that will improve their reasoning abilities, promote creative and critical thinking, and encourage abstract thought.

Developing Metacognitive Skills

According to Al-Hilawani (2000), "the concept of metacognition embraces higher-order thinking processes that include recognition, discrimination, judgment, and cognitive restructuring of events." Costa (2001a) describes metacognition as the process of being conscious of our own thinking and problem solving during the acts of thinking and problem solving. A historical review of the literature depicts individuals who are deaf as concrete thinkers (Myklebust, 1964), who tend to rely on visual/perceptual skills (Zwiebel & Mertens, 1985), who are not as proficient in solving problems, forming conclusions, and engaging in spatial reasoning (Jonas & Martin, 1984) as their peers who can hear. Research conducted by Luckner and McNeill (1994) noted that students who are deaf or hard of hearing do not perform as well as students who can hear on problem-solving tasks, due to the fact that problem-solving skills are not taught; however, they determined that the gap narrows with age. Further research conducted by Schirmer and Woolsey (1997) determined that when given a template of questions designed to promote abstract and critical thinking, readers could be encouraged to engage in higher level thinking skills.

During the 1980s another body of research began to take shape and evolve, based on the work of Reuven Feuerstein. David Martin and other colleagues began to investigate and apply a cognitive-skills program identified as Instrumental Enrichment (Feuerstein, 1980). This research shed additional insights into the cognitive functioning abilities of individuals who were deaf.

FEUERSTEIN'S VIEW OF COGNITIVE GROWTH

Feuerstein, an Israeli psychologist, asserts that cognitive growth occurs due to mediated learning experiences. Postulating that learning takes place through incidental and planned interactions that occur in the environment, he contends that we also benefit from mediated learning. Mediated learning is defined as "learning which is assisted by an adult who focuses, sharpens, elaborates, emphasizes, provides cues, and corrects as he or she tries to get the learner to understand and solve a problem" (Gage & Berliner, 1988, p. 104).

For children to possess the structural ability to adjust and adapt to life situations, they must achieve a level of cognitive competence (Scarr, 1981). In this context, structure refers to the cognitive/intellectual and affective schemes that enable individuals to adapt to novel situations. Feuerstein states that construction of these schemes is affected by two modalities of learning: direct learning experiences and mediated learning experiences. Through the constant bombardment of direct stimuli, individuals respond and their behavioral repertoire is expanded. In mediated exposure, direct experience with environmental stimuli is transformed through the intermediary actions of an "experienced, intentional and active human being" (Feuerstein, 1979 p. 110).

Feuerstein further contends that through mediated learning, the individual is later able to benefit from direct experiences, which not only enhance learning but also are essential for continued direct exposure to it. He suggests that this type of learning is a prerequisite for the child to independently and autonomously make use of environmental stimuli. By engaging in such activities, the child is able to develop a positive attitude toward thinking and problem solving, enabling him to organize the stimuli in the world around him. Through a repertoire of actions, the mediating agent organizes and orients the phenomenological world for the child. Appropriate learning sets are transferred to the child by the caring person, and cognitive growth occurs.

Within the framework of cultural deprivation, Feuerstein has stressed that some segments of all societies impose a lack of intergenerational transmission. Culture is viewed as being normally established and shaped through the intergenerational transmission of ideas. It is not appropriate to say that the culture found in certain ethnic subgroups deprives its members of the ability to learn cognitively; rather, Feuerstein states that the culture is not responsible for lags in cognitive development but the lack of significant mediational learning taking place within that culture is responsible.

Initially developed as a supplement to the curriculum, the Instrumental Enrichment program incorporates mediated learning experiences for culturally disadvantaged groups of individuals. Initially developed as a supplement to the curriculum, the program was designed to engage children in a series of increasingly difficult tasks structured to develop and enhance cognitive skills (Martin, Rohr, & Innes, 1982, as cited in Schirmer, 2001). According to Martin (1983) among the objectives of Instrumental Enrichment are the improvement of spatial reasoning, manipulation of multiple sources of information simultaneously, and understanding cause-and-effect relationships. Fourteen "instruments" or sets of cognitive tasks comprise the program, which is aimed at students of ages 9 through adult; a recently developed version of the program for young children of ages 3 to 8 is comprised of 10 instruments; they consist of curriculum guides and largely, although not exclusively, paper-and-pencil exercises that are intended to be used several times weekly in the classroom in 1-hour increments.

Research conducted by Martin and Jonas (1986) indicated that, when given problem-solving situations, students who were deaf who enrolled in the Instrumental Enrichment program were able to produce more responses to solving these situations than students who were not enrolled in the program. Further studies by Martin (1995) revealed that when Feuerstein's approach was implemented and students who were deaf were encouraged to reflect on their thinking and reasoning processes, they were better equipped to transfer their acquired cognitive skills to real-life situations and curricular settings (Al-Hilawani, 2001). Conducting a 2-year pilot study at the Model Secondary School for the Deaf at Gallaudet, Martin (1984) determined that students engaged in the program demonstrated improvement in problem solving, nonverbal logical thinking, abstract thinking, reading comprehension, and mathematical computation. This set of findings has been further documented in studies conducted by a number of other researchers within the field of deaf education (Haywood, Towery-Woolsey, Arbitman-Smith, & Aldridge, 1988; Huberty & Koller, 1984; Johnson, 1988; Keane & Kretschmer, 1987).

Instrumental Enrichment is designed to serve as a supplemental curriculum, separate from but integrated within the content areas. Other approaches have been developed that focus on incorporating thinking skills across the curriculum. Although the goal is not to provide an exhaustive or in-depth explanation of any of these approaches, the intent is to highlight the principles underlying the various approaches.

INCORPORATING THINKING SKILLS ACROSS THE CURRICULUM

When reviewing the literature on thinking skills, several other individuals have also made significant contributions to the field. The list includes but is not limited to the writings of Feuerstein, Rand, Sternberg, Ennis, Coleman, Swartz, Beyer, Paul, Kallick, and Costa. Costa and Kallick (2000) provide the reader with 16 habits of mind that when employed present human beings with a disposition for behaving intelligently when confronted with problems.

Costa (2001b) emphasizes that "employing habits of mind requires a composite of many skills, attitudes, cues, past experiences, and proclivities" (p. 80). He further describes the 16 habits of mind that individuals engage in when responding intelligently to problems. Indicating more than 16 ways in which people display intelligence, Costa and Kallick (2000) view the list as a starting point for the collection of additional attributes. Costa believes that it is important when teaching students to provide them with information; however, it is even more critical to furnish them with habits of mind that they can draw upon when they need to solve a problem. The following 16 habits of mind can be used across the curriculum to solve problems in a multitude of content areas:

1. ***Persistence***—sticking with a task until it is completed
2. ***Managing impulsivity***—thinking before they act
3. ***Listening to others with understanding and empathy***—listening is a very complex skill, requiring the ability to monitor one's own thoughts while attending to someone else's words
4. ***Thinking flexibly***—the ability to draw upon a repertoire of problem-solving strategies; knowing when to be broad and global in their thinking and when to apply detailed precision
5. ***Thinking about our thinking***—metacognition—developing a plan of action, keeping that plan in mind, and evaluating the plan upon its completion
6. ***Striving for accuracy and precision***
7. ***Questioning and posing problems***—learning how to ask questions to fill in the gaps between what they know and what they do not know
8. ***Applying past knowledge to new situations***—learning from past experiences
9. ***Thinking and communicating with clarity and precision***—striving to communicate accurately in both written and oral/signed form
10. ***Gathering data through all senses***
11. ***Creating, imagining, and innovating***—develop the capacity to conceive of different problem solutions by examining alternative possibilities from many angles
12. ***Responding with wonderment and awe***—having a passion for solving problems independently
13. ***Taking responsible risks***—viewing setbacks as interesting, challenging, and growth-producing

14. ***Finding humor***—being able to laugh at situations and at themselves
15. ***Thinking interdependently***—learning to work cooperatively in groups
16. ***Learning continuously***—seizing problems, situations, tensions, and conflicts. (Costa, 2001b, pp. 81–85)

They view all of these circumstances as valuable opportunities to learn.

By establishing these habits of mind as a foundation for classroom instruction and interaction, students can draw upon them as they gather information, organize, analyze, integrate, and evaluate new information. Students, who are deaf, like their peers who can hear, need to be provided with a framework and strategies for solving problems. By being exposed to core thinking skills that include classifying, categorizing, analyzing, summarizing, hypothesizing, and applying facts and principles to new situations, they will be better equipped to think critically and creatively.

Summary

The issues and theories surrounding cognition and intellectual functioning are complex and far reaching. Recognizing that language and experiential differences exist between individuals who can hear and those who are deaf, strategies must be developed and implemented that address these differences while tapping into the cognitive potential dwelling within each of these unique individuals. By viewing these differences in a positive light rather than in the shadow of deficiencies and shortcomings, methods of testing and teaching can be developed that will further meet the needs of this unique population. When this process takes place, a tremendous potential will become available for reducing the intellectual/academic achievement gap for learners who are deaf.

Ultimately, practitioners in the field must assume the responsibility for employing such strategies as Costa and Kallick's habits of mind. They must put aside age-old disputes over mode of communication, become active researchers and listeners, and apply past information to new situations. By gathering data, thinking flexibly, and gathering new insights into how language modality and experience influence learning and cognitive strategies, today's professionals will be better prepared to meet the needs of this and future generations of students who are deaf. Only by changing our focus can we hope to open minds, encourage our students to think, and begin preparing them for the next century.

11

Personal, Social, and Cultural Development

Forming an Identity

The global landscape has changed dramatically over the past several decades. Consequently, the social context where interpersonal interactions transpire is more complex. Individuals involved in these exchanges represent a diverse and multifaceted population who further embody a wide range of societal and cultural forces. At these critical junctures our identities are formed, shaped, and constructed while a heightened awareness of one's sense of self is ultimately brought to a new level of consciousness. Through our interactions with others we begin to determine what we do and do not believe, what we stand for, and who we are with respect to other members of society. As Josselson (1994) has so aptly stated, "identity represents the intersection of the individual and society, in framing identity, the individual simultaneously joins the self to society and society to the self" (p. 12).

The Western world is comprised of a multilayered society representing a tapestry of cultures that share their values, traditions, and beliefs with their offspring. As infants enter the world they are initially shaped by their surroundings. Relying foremost on the family constellation and social environment, the child begins to form a sense of self. Later, as children embark on the path of formalized education, their sense of identity continues to transform as they encounter cultural diversity, academic challenges, personal success and defeat, and inclusion or exclusion from group membership. These interactive events ultimately contribute to the overall socialization and formation of the child's self-concept. Through a lifetime of both experiencing and reflecting on life events, the complex self perpetually forms, always maintaining some degree of fluidity, in the face of new experiences.

The construction of one's identity has been studied by psychologists, sociologists, and social psychologists. Viewed from both a developmental and an environmental or ecological model, the formation of a positive self-concept has unequivocally been determined to be an integral component when individuals describe their satisfaction with life.

How do individuals who are deaf develop their identities, and form their self-concepts? How do the family unit, educational environment, and mode of communication influence the deaf person's sense of cultural, familial and social belonging? Furthermore, how do the individuals who are deaf mediate between hearing and Deaf cultures while maintaining their personal sense of identity?

SHARING CULTURAL VALUES AND BELIEFS: IMPACT ON SELF-CONCEPT AND IDENTITY

According to the National Institute on Deafness and Other Communication Disorders (NIDCD, 2010) about 2 to 3 out of every 1,000 infants born in the United States enter this world with varying degrees of hearing loss, from mild to profound. Some children are born with a hearing loss, and others will lose their hearing at various stages of development. As they enter this world and become part of the family unit, less than 10% of them will be raised by one hearing and one Deaf parent, and even fewer by two Deaf parents. In fact, the majority will be raised and nurtured by parents who can hear or are hard of hearing. This defining characteristic coupled with their family's ethnic, racial, and cultural backgrounds will all be instrumental in contributing to their initial perceptions of who they are, how they will communicate, and what the term *deafness* implies. Through these interactions, young children become engaged in observing and responding to others, and it is through these interactions that the social construction of the self begins to emerge (Crocker & Quinn, 2000). The degree of integration into the family structure is based on the parents' background knowledge and their understanding of the ramifications of deafness, coupled with their communication beliefs and their views and attitudes regarding what it means to be deaf. These factors, in conjunction with the outward expression of opinions conveyed by extended family members will contribute to and determine the cultural underpinnings of the child's upbringing.

It is well established within the field of deaf education that when children who are deaf are raised in families with adult Deaf role models and communication exchanges occur in ASL, the child will in all likelihood become immersed in Deaf culture. These children frequently develop a strong affinity for the language and the community while developing a strong Deaf identity. Later, if they attend a school for the deaf their affiliation with the Deaf community has a proclivity to be strengthened as they develop friendships with their peers. The bonds established through these friends typically remain with them throughout their lifetimes. Often these individuals maintain a monocultural perspective until they arrive at young adulthood when they enter postsecondary institutions or join the ranks of the workforce. Although these children represent a very small percentage of the Deaf population, as they grow and develop they will play a vital role in the Deaf community by sharing and passing down beliefs, values and, traditions to both those inside and outside the community.

Those raised in this environment will typically embrace the values cultivated by the Deaf community, including companionship, folklore, art, shared experiences, and a common history. They are proud of being Deaf and primarily socialize with other Deaf individuals, communicating through a language that they both cherish and revere. In this respect the term *community* can be used to epitomize individuals who ascribe to any one or a combination of the following attributes: linguistic parameters, social networks, or merely residing in a geographic area without any clearly defined social relationships. According to Senghas and Monaghan (2002), to gain an understanding and appreciation for the complex nature of Deaf communities it is critical that one attain an understanding and a sensitivity of how group members view themselves and use and think about language.

When infants who are deaf are born into hearing families they frequently enter environments inhabited by caregivers who have had no previous exposure to children who are deaf. These parents are typically influenced by medical professionals and educators who may view deafness from the perspective of a medical model. As a result, they are often encouraged to seek treatments, such as cochlear implants, that will provide their child with the optimum opportunity to access environmental sounds while accessing the language and communication mode used within the home. Typically family members who can hear embrace an oral means of communication and want to expose their children who are deaf to values cherished by hearing society. Subsequently, the majority of these children are raised primarily with hearing community values that emphasize the importance of speech and clearly spoken communication exchanges.

Initially exposed to a hearing identity, most will attend included programs where each will remain the sole student who is deaf in the public school setting. Depending on the mode of communication used, some will rely on speech reading and speech to communicate while others will access their education through support services provided by sign-language interpreters or other types of communication facilitators. As a result, throughout their tenure in the educational setting they may remain unaware of a Deaf identity, culture, or community, thus maintaining a static hearing identity until they reach adolescence or adulthood. While some individuals who are deaf succeed in this environment, others become frustrated with communication and struggle while trying to master academic content.

Another group of individuals who are deaf have achieved a bicultural identity. Typically characterized as those who functional bilingually in spoken and signed communication, these individuals recognize the strengths and weaknesses of both hearing and Deaf people and are comfortable identifying with both cultures (Cornell & Lyness, 2004). They have achieved an inner security and serenity with being Deaf and are comfortable navigating between both cultural groups (Fischer & McWhirter, 2001).

Within this group, there are some Deaf adults, with an established Deaf identity, who elect to get cochlear implants for themselves or their Deaf children. Recognizing the benefits of being able to engage in conversations with members of both the hearing and Deaf communities, they are equipping themselves and their children with a skill set that will maximize their ability to ease into hearing environments while maintaining their Deaf cultural affiliation (Leigh, 2010). Cognizant of what cochlear implants have to offer, these adults look for avenues for themselves and their Deaf children to reap the auditory benefits that implants can provide, thus benefiting from what each cultural linguistic group has to offer.

For some, developing a bicultural identity can involve a long and reflective process. When adolescents have developed a strong affiliation with either hearing culture or Deaf culture, they may experience conflicts as they struggle to define their role between and within the two cultural groups. Some arrive at adulthood having been immersed in a hearing cultural perspective. When they encounter culturally Deaf individuals for extended periods of time they may begin to question where they belong (Fischer & McWhirter, 2001; Glickman, 1993).

Likewise, those submerged in Deaf culture due to their parental or familial cultural affiliation may find, as a result of their educational experiences, that the larger hearing culture affords them infinite opportunities. For some, the desire to form an allegiance with members of the hearing community, thereby benefiting from what they have to offer, can create feelings of angst and betrayal that stresses their affiliation with the Deaf community. Struggling to determine where they belong, they may remain immersed in the Deaf culture while maintaining a negative view of the hearing culture (Glickman, 1993). While this presents a challenge for some, for those who assimilate into a bicultural sense of community it is not an issue.

A substantial body of literature examines the cultural identities of individuals who are deaf, how one's cultural identity relates to self-concept and self-esteem, and what effect mode of communication has on the child's formation of his or her identity. The effects of parental-child relationships have been examined, educational experiences explored, and interviews conducted. In a study conducted by Bat-Chava (2000), questionnaires were administered and individuals were interviewed to discern their identities (Culturally Deaf Identity, Culturally Hearing Identity, or Bicultural Identity) and how these identities relate to their self-esteem.

Comments from these interviews capture the insights and opinions of individuals identifying with each of the three categories. Excerpts reflecting each of the three established identities are included in the following sections. It is critical when reading the discourse to recognize that these are individual responses, reflective of each of the individuals who responded. As such, they cannot be viewed as an overlay that is representative of each member who might affiliate with that group.

Culturally Deaf Identity: Mark

At the time of the interview Mark indicated that he is the child of Deaf parents and has a Deaf sibling. He initially attended an oral residential school for the deaf and later attended Gallaudet University. He was raised in a culturally Deaf environment and remains so today. He now teaches ASL at an interpreter training program. His comments follow:

> "Having to read lips in school was really frustrating; it was a traumatic experience. . . . Not until I finished school did I understand that oralism was good for communicating with the hearing . . . [it is important] for survival . . . so hearing people can help you."
>
> "Growing up, I used to go to deaf church with my family, picnics, and other events. Most of the time we'd socialize with other deaf people. . . . As an adult I have more deaf friends than hearing, maybe 75% and 25%. . . . Deafness was given to me by God; why fight it? Why object to it? Why deny it? It's my life; I'm deaf, that's it. I'm happy with who I am." (Bat-Chava, 2000, p. 425)

Culturally Hearing Identity: Oliver

Oliver reflects the attributes of a culturally hearing person. He was born profoundly deaf into a family that stressed oralism. Throughout his academic life he attended hearing schools and is currently employed as an engineer. He relies on speech and speechreading to communicate. These are his comments:

> "Sign language, I don't believe in it . . . I'm as uncomfortable with sign language as someone else. I don't understand it and I don't think it's necessary for myself, for my situation. . . . Lipreading is great, it really helps me. . . . Being part of the deaf world scares me. I don't agree with the philosophy of institutions like Gallaudet because I don't agree with a total deaf environment."
>
> "If you could take a pill and become hearing, would you do it?" He responded, "Of course! That's a ridiculous question; of course I would do it!" (Bat-Chava, 2000, p. 425)

Bicultural Identity: Amanda

Amanda was raised in a hearing family. She attended oral deaf and hearing schools until she graduated from high school. Her postsecondary degrees were earned at the National Technical Institute for the Deaf. Holding two master's degrees, she currently works in a human services agency with clients who are deaf. She recommends that ASL be used for instructional purposes. She made the following comments:

> "[Deaf students should have] as many deaf teachers as possible and hearing people skilled in ASL. . . . Do I think that it is important to speak clearly and to read lips?

Maybe. Sometimes yes and sometimes no. . . . It's easier to use speech in the hearing world; on the other hand, there are more important things to be concerned about than talking; speech is important, but it should not become the raison d'etre of deaf education."

"I started to socialize with deaf people and I was really in the deaf experience, in the deaf world. . . . It feels more normal for me, more natural. . . . There is nothing negative about being deaf in and of itself. What's negative is other people's treatment of deaf people. People should focus on abilities, on health and strengths, rather than on inabilities." (Bat-Chava, pp. 425–426)

SCHOOL SETTINGS: INFLUENCE ON CULTURAL PERCEPTIONS

Although identity begins to form and take shape during infancy and early childhood, identity is further framed and defined throughout the academic years as children form friendships, draw boundaries, experience inclusion as well as exclusion, while interacting with their peers. During the elementary school years children develop a sense of their psychological self as well as their valued self. Beginning in first or second grade the child uses self-descriptors such as "smart" or "dumb" as a way of identifying who they are. By the time a child arrives at fifth grade he or she is using phrases such as "I'm smarter than most other kids" or "I'm not as talented in art as my friend" to describe who they are (Rosenberg, 1986; Ruble, 1987, as cited in Boyd & Bee, 2009).

As they enter middle childhood they begin to develop perceptions of how well they can use their skills and abilities within a variety of different areas. During this time feelings of self-efficacy become ingrained in one's mind-set. While making social comparisons with their peers, children begin to gain and form insights into how well they can accomplish tasks with respect to their role models. Later, when they arrive at adolescence they begin to form their self-concepts based on their perceptions of who they are within the various roles they play. At this developmental juncture they start to differentiate the way they respond in their various roles. For example, they become aware of how they relate differently when they are in the role of a student, a friend, or relating to their parents as a son or daughter. In each of these roles they begin to see themselves somewhat differently (Boyd & Bee, 2009).

The adolescent period is marked by young people transitioning as they attempt to fashion an identity that is different from childhood but not quite into adulthood. During the early part of this stage the child is faced with problems surrounding independence, emancipation, and freedom from the family. It is at this social juncture that "fitting in" with peer groups becomes increasingly important. School settings provide adolescents with a social environment whereby they learn about social rules and acceptable patterns of interaction (Israelite, Ower, & Goldstein, 2002).

Throughout adolescence teens fashion their self-concepts by comparing themselves both internally and externally within the constructs of academic performance. This occurs internally when one establishes a self-generated ideal and then compares his or her individual performance to it; it takes place externally when teens compare their successes to those of their peers (Bong, 1998). Preconceived competencies in one domain frequently affect how a teenager views his abilities in other areas (Cheng, Xiaoyan, & Dajun, 2006). Social self-concepts further serve as predictors of behaviors with respect to how adolescents view their abilities to engage in distinct and varied social situations. The majority of students who have internalized positive self-concepts typically maintain satisfactory relationships with their family members and rely on their support throughout adolescence. However, many of the teens who are estranged from their families generally perceive that they are less competent in the art of engaging in daily exchanges that are required for satisfactory give-and-take involved in establishing and maintaining fulfilling family relations (Swaim & Bracken, 1997).

During adolescence friendships and peer groups play a significant role in the developmental process. Teens typically choose friends who are committed to the same activities which they enjoy participating in and with whom they are comfortable sharing their inner feelings and secrets. Many utilize electronic communication devices to establish and maintain their friendships. Socializing within virtual communities such as MySpace, and Facebook allows interaction through online instant messages and e-mail while establishing a variety of social networks (Foehr, 2006).

During this developmental period teenagers seek out groups that mirror their values, attitudes, behavior, and identity status (Akers, Jones, & Coyl, 1998; Mackey & LaGreca, 2007; Urberg, Degirmencioglu, & Tolson, 1998). As they transition from middle school to high school they begin to identify with groups that contribute to the shaping and reinforcement of their own identities. By labeling others and oneself as members of a particular group, boundaries between personal friends and foes are established as teens ultimately determine where they belong and what their beliefs are.

Although peer groups play a vital role throughout this developmental period, another hallmark that characterizes this stage is the transition from same-sex friendships to romantic relationships. Those who feel competent in their relationships with parents, peers, and friends will find this transition easier as they strive to form opposite-sex friendships and romantic relationships (Thériault, 1998). Teenagers, at a young age, develop a sense of what it means to be "in love," and they prefer to both date someone they are in love with and end relationships if they feel they have fallen "out of love." Dating throughout this period provides young adults with opportunities to explore and crystallize their feelings, which further defines their sense of identity as they move toward adulthood.

What impact does the school environment have on the development of one's identity, self-concept, and self-esteem as well as feelings of acceptance and belonging to peer groups when the individual is deaf or severely hard of hearing? What opportunities do these students have to interact within this social milieu? How do students who are deaf form their sense of identity within the various academic settings?

Socialization Experiences in Mainstream/Included Educational Settings

It is well documented in the literature that mainstream educational settings vary tremendously in the way they serve students who are deaf and hard of hearing (Marschark, Young, & Lukomski, 2002). Some students are fully included in hearing classrooms, accessing their education through sign language interpreters and assistive devices; others interact with their hearing peers on a more limited basis, primarily having contact with them while engaged in nonacademic subjects. In these academic settings the ease of spoken communication is valued, appropriate social skills are expected, and academic achievement is anticipated, all within the confines of the dominant social culture that maintains fluid expectations for its members.

Although there is tremendous diversity within the school-age population comprised of students who are deaf and hearing, many of them frequently face challenges in social development that their peers who can hear are spared (Bain, Scott, & Steinberg, 2004). Often they arrive at school lacking an understanding of the social expectations, mores, and rules considered optimal to access the social mainstream of their educational environment. To be fully integrated in these settings students must be able to access both formal and informal communications with their peers and teachers, while establishing peer relationships and participating in extracurricular activities (Stinson & Foster, 2000). It may become a challenging if not altogether daunting task for those who are deaf or hard of hearing. Entering a milieu monopolized by those who can hear who have had limited, if any, exposure to individuals who are deaf, they are frequently met by a segment of society that has preconceived ideas of what it means to be deaf. These perceptions are often based on erroneous information and when coupled with barriers to communication they can have a tremendous effect on the social climate that resonates throughout the school.

One of the key philosophical tenets supporting the concept of inclusion is that students coming from diverse backgrounds, including those with disabilities, are given the opportunity to become full members of the school community. This is based on the assumption that when students are placed in classrooms with support services they will have equal access to the academically rich curriculum afforded those students without disabilities (Angelides & Aravi, 2006/2007). Theoretically, the provision of support services was intended to reinforce classroom assimilation, thereby encouraging social acceptance of students who are deaf and hard of hearing by their hearing peers while affording increased opportunities for hearing–deaf peer interaction (Israelite, Ower, & Goldstein, 2002; Stinson & Kluwin, 2003). However, if and when these interactions occur, they are frequently stilted, limited in duration, and typically lack the depth and detail characteristic of peer discourse.

Since the mid 1970s the trend for educating students who are deaf has shifted from residential and special day school settings to those promoting mainstream/inclusion settings. Several studies have been conducted to investigate the effect this environment has on identity formation for students who are deaf and hard of hearing. This research has examined peer relationships, school atmosphere, deaf students' perceptions of being in included settings, and the impact it has on one's identity (see Leigh, 2009, for an in-depth discussion of these topics). At the heart of all this research lies one of the major ramifications of deafness: the effect it has on communication access and the ability to communicate with others. The implications for communication access are profound and far reaching, impacting identity, socialization, and feelings of self-worth.

Students who are deaf and hard of hearing entering the mainstream will access their education and socialize with their peers through different communication pathways. Some will arrive with cochlear implants and espouse an aural/oral approach; others communicate through sign language; still others will embrace sign-supported speech. Each mode of communication can present its own set of unique challenges influencing the social exchanges and ultimately contributing to the shaping of the person's identity.

Numerous studies have been conducted that demonstrate the importance of intelligible speech while engaging in conversations with peers who can hear (Bat-Chava & Deignan, 2001; Musselman, Mootilal, & MacKay, 1996; Stinson & Antia, 1999; Wheeler, Archbold, Gregory, & Skipp, 2007, as cited in Leigh, 2009). Furthermore, accounts describing the experiences of individuals who are deaf who use speech to communicate have been captured in *Voices of the Oral Deaf* by Reisler (2002). Throughout Reisler's book 14 role models describe their experiences while attending public schools and interacting primarily with hearing individuals. These anecdotes provide a snapshot of both their feelings of frustration, as well as their sense of accomplishment, and are intended to provide insights into their experiences in mainstreamed/included settings.

> "Seventh grade, however, was really tough. Here I was mainstreaming for the first time and many of my classmates had never even met a deaf person before and they were confused about my speech. They didn't know what to make of me . . . the reaction was, 'Oh my God, she's deaf!'

"Seventh grade was the first and only time that I was embarrassed to be deaf and wished that I could be hearing so I could be like other people. I had a hard time being accepted and I didn't do as well academically. . . . I pretended to be hearing. . . . I wore my hair down all the time to hide my hearing aids and never talked in class. When a teacher called on me, I'd shrug and say, 'I don't know,' because I didn't want to talk in front of others." (Buehl, 2002, p. 8)

"I remember second grade being pretty difficult. I was at a new mainstreamed school and very unsure of how I'd do and how I'd fit in. I remember classmates looking at hearing aids and always asking me, 'What are those? And 'What's that in your ears?' Kind of typical questions. Swimming really helped me fit in. . . . Swimming gave me confidence. . . . I had an interesting experience when I went to Romania . . . for the World Championships for the Deaf. I saw it as an opportunity to swim, travel and see a bit of the other side of deaf life—the 'signers.' It was really eye-opening to me, because the signers wanted me to be one of them. . . . I just never felt any particular pull to joining the signers, to becoming 'one of them.' I was the only hearing-impaired student in my high school, but I never felt a need to join the signers." (Float, 2002, pp. 26–31)

"By the time I was entered seventh grade, the school system provided me with an itinerant teacher—an educational specialist in hearing loss. . . . On the one hand I was grateful to have her help. I finally had a cushion, someone to help buffer some of the stress of going to a competitive and academically challenging public school with a hearing loss. On the other hand, I hated being singled out, being different and having to deal with this deficiency. I think I felt this way intensely because I didn't have friends who were hearing impaired or any role models." (Ginsburg, 2002, pp. 36)

"I'd had almost no contact with the world of deafness, and most of the few deaf people I did encounter were as mainstreamed as I was, until sometime in the early '80s. . . . I'm not really that interested in deafness—it does not define me—but I've discovered that I am very interested in encouraging other parents who want to give their deaf children that great thing my parents gave me as a deaf person: spoken language, and thereby direct access to the wide world." (James, 2002, p. 59)

"I didn't always know where those parties were and was never in the loop on teenage social gossip, because I found it extremely difficult to understand the feverish, energetic teenage dialogue bouncing off the walls of Hastings High School. In fact, I never knew there was such a thing as a 'party' (in the high school sense without adult supervision, if you can get my drift) until eleventh grade, when a friend brought me to my first meadow party." (Janger, 2002, p. 63)

When students who are deaf and hard of hearing receive their education in mainstreamed/included settings they are challenged by the rigors of the curriculum afforded those enrolled in general education classrooms. However, they are frequently denied the social experiences that serve to promote emotional and psychological well-being. It has been suggested that students who are deaf attending these programs are often excluded from activities enjoyed by their hearing peers, thus limiting their access to the full array of educational and social opportunities provided by the general school environment (Israelite et al., 2002; Kinsella-Meier, 1995; Stinson, Whitmire, & Kluwin, 1996). Sensing rejection from their hearing peers, solitary deaf students often experience feelings of isolation and emotional turmoil as they seek to gain peer acceptance (Oliva, 2004). Although some students report that their mainstream experiences were worthwhile, several describe the pain they experienced attempting to achieve a sense of equality and internal validation with respect to their hearing peers (Leigh, 2009; Leigh & Stinson, 1991; Oliva).

Further insights can also be gleaned from reading accounts of Deaf individuals who were raised with little or no knowledge of other individuals who are deaf and no exposure to the Deaf community. Tom Humphries (Padden & Humphries, 2005, pp. 144–146), a renowned author and respected Deaf professor, has described his experiences and his initial reaction to the Deaf community, after being raised in a hearing family, as a "hearing person who didn't hear." Attending public schools where he was the only student who was deaf, he was unaware of Gallaudet University and was totally unprepared for what he would experience once he enrolled and arrived on campus. His feelings of discomfort when he initially arrived on Gallaudet's campus are clearly articulated in the following:

> "What he noticed first was that the other students seemed to have a familiarity and an ease with each other that he did not have and at the time could not imagine ever having. . . . The most daunting realization of all was that he was living among a group of people who shared a history he did not know and who in turn knew little about how he had grown up and lived as a deaf person. . . . He did not know that there was a social network of Deaf families and Deaf communities. . . . He could not figure out how to manage a signed conversation, where to look and what to say first. . . . Worse, he had to admit he was feeling uncomfortable in this environment. He was surprised at his reaction at being in the company of other deaf people. In his hearing family and community, he had always been taught that he was special, that no other deaf person was like him, and that it was undesirable to be like other deaf people. . . . His view of sign language was especially strong. He thought it was inadequate and of little use in an English-speaking world. Yet he soon realized that his view of himself contradicted those of the Deaf people around him. . . . they delighted, even celebrated, those things that made him uncomfortable." (Padden & Humphries, 2005, pp. 144–146)

Later, as he continued to socialize, interact, and learn ASL while simultaneously becoming familiar with Deaf culture, he began to feel comfortable with his new identity as a Deaf person. He further reiterates that he felt "included in a way that he hadn't felt back home among his hearing family and community. In fact, he began to feel quite angry at his own older attitudes and misguided ideas about Deaf people and ASL" (Padden & Humphries, 2005, p. 147).

Socialization Experiences in Residential and Day School Settings

Although the majority of students who are deaf and hard of hearing are educated in mainstream settings, approximately 26% are educated in residential and specialized day schools (Gallaudet Research Institute, 2006). In these settings, students have access to a Deaf peer group, Deaf adult role models, and with the exception of oral programs, the ease of communicating through sign language. Researchers within the field suggest that schools for the deaf provide more than just an education for those who attend (Hadjikakou & Nikolaraizi, 2007); moreover, these environments are considered the locus of sign language and Deaf culture (Hadjikakou & Nikolaraizi; Maxwell-McCaw; 2001; Supalla, 1994).

Rachel McKee (2001) has collected stories from Deaf people in her book *People of the Eye: Stories from the Deaf World.* These narratives furnish readers with glimpses into the world through the eyes of those who are Deaf while providing additional insights into the complex cognitive and social construct of deafness. The first are excerpts from Della, born into an all Deaf family; she makes the following comments:

> "I was born Deaf, like my parents and my two younger sisters. My father's parents and all of his relatives are Deaf. . . . Because there are no hearing people in my family, I didn't have much experience of hearing people as a young child. . . . at Deaf school, all the pupils signed and it was easy to communicate. Everyone helped each other by surreptitiously explaining when someone didn't understand. . . . I was always explaining to the others in sign language what the teacher had said. . . . You see, I had a big advantage at school. I absorbed a lot of information from talking with my family. . . . I think the students enjoy having Deaf house-parents because it's a chance for them to talk about all sorts of things with a Deaf adult. Many of them have big gaps in their life education—things that you would expect kids of that age to have picked up, but somehow they haven't. . . . some of the kids don't feel confident about going to McDonald's and knowing how to order food. . . . One area, for example, is knowing the boundaries between what they're allowed to do and not allowed to do—what is acceptable behavior. Many of them aren't aware of basic manners—like how to talk appropriately to people in different situations, when it's not ok to swear, all those social skills." (Buzzard, 2001, pp. 162–167)

The second story is one told by Douglas. He was born hearing, and within the first 2 years of his life he lost his hearing due to a blood disorder. He describes leaving his family and attending a residential school:

> "The first day I was pretty scared because there were a lot of Maori children and they seemed so different to me. As time went on, I got used to being there with the other Deaf children. I really enjoyed being at school for the sports, and all the different things we kids got up to together. . . . we'd play Tarzan on this lovely tree. . . . or play hide-and-seek, or the flying fox—our favorite thing. Going home with my grandparents for the weekends, by comparison, was very quiet. . . . I was eight when I moved to a regular school. . . . [T]here were seven other Deaf at the school and two of them had Deaf Parents . . . the Hunts, were from England. I really liked talking to them because they could sign fluently. . . . They took me out to the Deaf Club where I met lots of Deaf people. The adults signed a lot different: it was so clear and easy to understand. I felt at home with them straight away. . . . I went back to Kelston Deaf school. . . . I boarded there until I was 11. . . . [Later] I became a day pupil, but I got really homesick for school and begged Mum to let me go back as a weekly boarder. I wanted to be with my Deaf friends at school Monday to Friday and only come home for the weekends." (Croskery, 2001, pp. 118–120)

Several other authors have shared similar experiences when describing their experiences of what residential schools mean to them, their identities, and their sense of community and culture. In *Understanding Deaf Culture: In Search of Deafhood,* Paddy Ladd (2003) also recalls how residential schools are frequently viewed by those who attend them. The importance of communication, peer groups, and older Deaf role models are frequent themes throughout these narratives.

> "The pupils . . . who traveled home every day really wanted to stay at the school like those who were boarders. They were happy just signing away with the others for the rest of the night, but were made to get on off home. . . . When they came back next morning, they were frantically signing away to make up for lost time! Home was all right, but boring, I was excited to get back to school." (Ladd, 2003, p. 299)
>
> "It is especially important . . . for the very youngest children . . . when they might be psychologically nervous/uncertain about being Deaf to see other children like themselves helps them to feel good about themselves. They start to *realize that they are kin*, start to jostle and play. Safety in numbers, you might say. That's the start of communication, the start of friendships. That's the first re-assurance. (Ladd, 2003, p. 300)

These narratives epitomize the feelings of many who have attended schools for the deaf. Becoming a social haven where Deaf students can communicate freely, these facilities have provided environments where students can experience full participation in social and athletic events, share in each others' successes and failures, and have contact with Deaf adult role models. Through these interactions individuals who are deaf begin to acknowledge their identity as a Deaf person, feelings of belonging are awakened or strengthened, and a sense of community is formed.

Deaf individuals can develop this sense of community at various times in their lives. Although some are granted entry as part of their birthright, coming from a lineage of Deaf family members, others must make a commitment to the language, values, and beliefs before group affiliation is acknowledged by those already recognized as members of the community. Those comprising the group are as diverse as the pathways they used to achieve group membership and acceptance. Representing individuals from all walks of life, they share a rich heritage and language and are unified by their experiences living their lives as Deaf individuals. Through the development of their individual identities, they have formed their self-concepts and feelings of self-esteem.

Developing a Self-Concept and Feelings of Self-Esteem

Self-concept has been defined as our perceptions of ourselves that are derived from our social environment. Self-concept is believed to provide the culminating force in directing our behavior (Byrne, 1984; van Gurp, 2001). One's self-concept is multifaceted and comprised of internally consistent, hierarchically organized concepts (Shavelson, Hubner, & Stanton, 1976). Developing out of social interactions with others, it is dynamic and changes with experience. One aspect of self-concept is the basic need for self-esteem (van Gurp, 2001).

An individual's self-concept is multidimensional in nature and is comprised of both academic and nonacademic components. One's academic self-concept is shaped by how one perceives his or her academic skills in comparison to those of one's peer group; one's social self-concept develops as one makes a comparison between self and those groups one holds in high regard. In essence, self-concept can be defined as how we view ourselves, and self-esteem is how we feel about this perception in relation to others.

Susan Harter (1990), a developmental psychologist, has conducted extensive studies with respect to the development of self-concept and self-esteem. She maintains that self-concept can be characterized through five domains: scholastic competence, athletic competence, physical appearance, peer social acceptance, and behavioral conduct. Harter has postulated that children's self-concepts show increasing differentiation and integration with age. Her research reveals that children between the ages of 4 and 7 are unable to differentiate between cognitive and physical competence; however, children between the ages of 8 and 12 can distinguish between mathematical and reading competence.

Harter further supports the premise that children develop an understanding of themselves based on the various roles and membership categories that define who they are. Her findings are significant when examining how school-age children develop their sense of self within the various settings. With respect to self-esteem she portends that it is tremendously impacted by two major influences. First, there is a direct correlation between the comparisons children make between their ideal selves, their actual experiences, and what they consider to be important or of value. Although a child may excel in academics, sports, or other extracurricular activities, these attributes in and of themselves do not hold value; rather it is the child's perceptions of the worth of a skill that will have a direct bearing on self-esteem. The second major influence is attributed to the overall support children believe they are receiving from the significant people in their lives. This includes feeling that they are liked and accepted by their family members and friends who have similar likes and skills (Boyd & Bee, 2009, p. 282).

Children who are deaf and hard of hearing fashion their self-concepts and their self-esteem in parallel with hearing children. Beginning in infancy and continuing through adulthood, their family units, school experiences, and the values they cherish will all contribute to their feelings of self-worth. Throughout their lifetimes each will develop a self-image, a concept of what their ideal self should entail, and feelings of self-esteem. Those who feel accepted and are comfortable with who they are and what they have accomplished will develop a higher self-concept and a more positive view of the world than those who feel rejected. What does the research reveal about individuals who are deaf and hard of hearing? Where do they fall on the continuum regarding feelings of self-worth?

RESEARCH WITH STUDENTS WHO ARE DEAF AND HARD OF HEARING: A GLIMPSE INTO SELF-CONCEPT AND SELF-ESTEEM

Feelings of love and acceptance are conveyed through communication that originates in the family and is later experienced within the confines of the educational setting and society. The initial role the family plays and the quality of family involvement directly impacts the child who is deaf, playing a critical role in the developmental process. When children sense they are valued members of the family and are included in daily conversational exchanges, the stage is set for them to develop as psychologically healthy deaf children who are communicatively competent (Luckner & Muir, 2001).

All children want to feel they are valued members of the family unit; this is conveyed by including them in the conversations that transpire at family gatherings, regardless of whether it is merely sitting around the table for daily meals or attending family reunions when extended family members join together. It entails answering their questions, including them in the conversation, asking for their preferences and opinions, and treating them as equal members of the group. This is accomplished by listening to what they have to say and ensuring that they are privy to all the comments and ancillary conversations that contribute to the filial experience.

Children and adults who are deaf have shared their feelings of frustration and disconnect with family members when they do not have access to communication with immediate family members (Breivik, 2005; Cerney, 2007; Ladd, 2003; Lane, Hoffmeister, & Bahan, 1996; McKee, 2001; Sheridan, 2008). Comments describing feelings of loneliness, isolation, disconnection, and separation from family members are evident throughout the literature. However, when open communication occurs, children who are deaf are provided with the same conduit for exchanging information that is experienced by children who can hear. This, in turn, provides children who are deaf with a milieu whereby feelings of being included in the family are promoted while simultaneously fostering feelings of independence and self-actualization (e.g., Eriks-Brophy et al., 2006; Leigh, 2009).

When parents make the decision to learn sign language they convey to their children a willingness and commitment to communicate with them using the language preferred by Deaf adults. This in turn may also indirectly validate that deafness and sign language are both acceptable attributes possessed by the child. Parents who select a spoken language option to communicate with their children are also making a substantial commitment. While attempting to prepare the child for the hearing world, these parents invest time and ongoing effort to ensure that the child feels included and can access all aspects of spoken exchanges. Research indicates that when mutual communication exchanges occur, whether orally or through sign language, the stage is set for children to begin life with positive feelings of belonging and acceptance, both critical elements to the formation of one's self-concept and self-esteem (Hintermair, 2006; Leigh, 2009; Wallis, Musselman, & MacKay, 2004).

Children who are deaf, along with those who can hear, segue into the educational arena where they will begin examining how they compare academically, physically, and athletically with their peers. Their perceptions of these comparisons, the self-imposed value they place on them, combined with their ability to form close friendships and feel socially accepted, will all contribute to their feelings of self-worth or self-esteem. Research findings examining self-esteem in school-age children who are deaf indicate that deaf peer groups play a significant role, particularly when students are enrolled in mainstreamed settings. Kluwin (1999), Stinson and Kluwin (2003), and Yetman (2000) all report that self-esteem among students who are deaf is not necessarily affected by their hearing peers' level of acceptance of them if there is a deaf peer group with whom these students can make comparisons. This supports previous research findings reported by Coyner (1993) and Bat-Chava (1993, 1994) that indicate if individuals who are deaf relate to Deaf role models, assume a Deaf identity, and perceive a high degree of acceptance from their deaf peer group, their self-esteem will not be affected by a low level of acceptance conveyed by their hearing peers. However, when there is not a deaf peer group to belong to and compare with, isolated students who are deaf, alone in the mainstream, often comment on the emotional turmoil and social difficulties they experienced as they struggled to be fully accepted by their hearing peers.

Kluwin, Stinson, and Colarossi (2002) reviewed 33 studies of the social processes and outcomes of students who are deaf and hard of hearing attending classes with their peers who can hear in mainstream educational settings. All of the studies examined various aspects of four major topics: social skills/social maturity, social interaction and participation, social acceptance, and affective functioning. Social skills/social maturity is defined by Meadow-Orlans (1980, 1983) "as those behaviors that are associated with performing competently, functioning independently, relating well to others, and acting responsibly" (1983, p. 827). Of the four studies reviewed, the results suggest that middle school hearing peers may be more socially mature than their deaf peers, but these differences become apparent only when the teachers were conducting the evaluations.

With respect to social interaction and participation, 12 observational studies of interaction were reported, with a large percentage of them conducted during the 1980s in Dallas, Texas. These studies reveal a fairly consistent pattern with respect to the interactions that occur between peers that can hear and those who are deaf. As one would expect, students who are deaf have a tendency to interact more frequently with their deaf classmates, preferring to engage in conversations with like peers rather than with their hearing classmates. The third group of studies examined social acceptance between peers who are hearing and deaf. The first set of studies was conducted using peer ratings; the second set utilized self-ratings that the students who were deaf completed with respect to their perceived quality of their peer relationships.

Kluwin et al. (2002) summarized these studies in the following way: With respect to peer-rated acceptance, three of the four studies indicated that peers who could hear accepted students who were deaf in mainstreamed classes; however, the extent of contact and gender may have had some bearing on the results of these studies. In the fourth study the findings revealed that students who were deaf were not as accepted as the students who could hear. With respect to their perceived quality of peer relationships, the adolescents frequently surmised that they liked "them alright, but I'd prefer my own kind if I have a choice" (p. 208).

The fourth group of studies examined affective functioning. According to Gresham and MacMillan (1997) affective functioning refers to personal dispositions of individuals. With regard to the students who were deaf and hard of hearing who were enrolled in mainstreamed settings, the dimensions that were studied included loneliness, perceived social competence, and self-image. The studies that were reviewed indicated that for those students who were deaf and receiving their education in mainstreamed settings, there were no general differences in self-perceived image or self-esteem. Overall, the studies suggest that although students in mainstream programs may not fully interact or enjoy their experiences with their peers who can hear, the effect of these encounters is not necessarily detrimental to their feelings of self-esteem. Rather, feelings of self-esteem depend primarily on the student's individual characteristics and how well they are matched to the program that they attend (Kluwin et al., 2002).

Research conducted by Schmidt and Cagran (2008) has also investigated the effect included settings have on the development of one's self-concept. They compared seventh-grade students with varying degrees of hearing loss with their hearing peers by examining three domains: general self-concept, social self-concept, and physical self-concept. Their findings revealed that integrated students had a higher academic self-concept than a social self-concept; however, the researchers also discovered that the integrated students demonstrated a higher physical self-concept than their hearing peers.

With respect to their academic and social self-concepts, one can surmise that when appropriate support services and the necessary accommodations are made available, students have access to the curriculum, thus setting the stage for individual accomplishment and the formation of a positive self-concept. However, due to the communication problems frequently created by their hearing loss and the resultant obstacles that become even more significant when students who are deaf and hard of hearing try to engage in social exchanges with their hearing peers, social relationships may not form, thereby negatively impacting one's self-concept.

An unexpected finding of the Schmidt and Cagran (2008) study indicated that the integrated students with a hearing loss demonstrated a higher physical self-concept when compared to their peers who could hear. Although the reasons for their increased satisfaction with their physical appearance were not explored, Schmidt and Cagran contend that it is probably due to the fact that when students with a hearing loss compare their physical appearance with those of their hearing peers, they perceive similarities in their looks, dress, and overall appearance, thus feeling they are part of the group. One can further posit that they are satisfied with how they look and accept themselves as they are.

Within the body of research on self-concept and self-esteem among students who are deaf and hard of hearing is a group of studies that have explored friendships between students who can hear and those with a hearing loss. This research has examined the impact of speech intelligibility, loneliness, and a sense of coherence when children who are deaf and hard of hearing receive their education in individual (one student who is deaf or hard of hearing in an included classroom of all hearing students) and group-inclusion (special classes within regular school settings) (Markides, 1989; Most, 2007; Most, Weisel, & Tur-Kaspa, 1999; Stinson & Antia, 1999). These studies reveal that students must exhibit a high level of speech intelligibility in order to establish friendships with hearing students. Markides reported that although 27% of students who are deaf and hard of hearing reported having a hearing friend, only 3% of the hearing children reported that they had a friend who is deaf or hard of hearing. This finding indicates that the perceptions of what denotes friendship might vary between the two groups.

Most (2007) explored the relationship between included settings and speech intelligibility to determine socioemotional experiences of students who were deaf and hard of hearing by administering two self-report questionnaires to school-age children between the ages of 7 and 18. Results of the study indicated that although there were no significant differences between speech intelligibility and feelings of loneliness for students in the group inclusion setting (this could be attributed to the fact that they had other means for communication, including signs and speech), there were significant correlates for children who were enrolled in individual included programs. The findings of this study further imply that because difficulties arise due to the level of speech intelligibility, this in itself may create barriers to establishing and maintaining peer interactions, thereby leading to such feelings as loneliness. These findings support previous studies (Weisel, Most, & Efron, 2005) that indicate that preschool children who are deaf and hard of hearing encountered more success while interacting with other children with hearing losses than with children who could hear.

Additional studies examining self-esteem and coping strategies have been conducted with students at the postsecondary level. Jambor and Elliott (2005) collected data from college students who are deaf attending California State University, Northridge. The central purpose of their study was to explore factors that might have a direct bearing on the self-esteem of this collegiate group. The factors studied included: mode of communication used at home, type of educational program (residential, day, mainstream/inclusion) the student attended prior to enrolling in college, age of onset of deafness, severity of loss with hearing aid, and group identification.

Jambor and Elliott's (2005) findings revealed that the majority of the participants were born deaf and most had a moderate hearing loss. Of those surveyed, 48% had attended a mainstream school with support services at some point during the course of their educational experience. The majority of those involved in the study used oral communication at home (54%) or oral communication with some sign language (23%); only 19% used sign language as the primary mode of communication. Most of the participants appeared to have developed strong bicultural skills. This is not surprising considering that the majority of their lives had been spent with hearing people, but most were also exposed to the Deaf world while attending mainstream programs with at least a small group of students who were deaf.

Results from this study further indicate that self-esteem was positively related to severity of hearing loss with hearing aid—individuals exhibiting a profound loss typically reflect a higher level of self-esteem than those functioning with a greater degree of residual hearing. Self-esteem was negatively correlated to oral communication at home, revealing that when individuals who are deaf are required to depend on speech reading only in order to receive information, they may feel isolated and eliminated from daily conversations that are commonplace within the home environment. This in itself has negative implications for their self-esteem. Findings further indicated that students who have acquired bicultural skills and can get along in both the Deaf and the hearing worlds tend to have higher self-esteem (Jambor & Elliott, 2005).

SUCCESSFUL ADULTS WHO ARE DEAF: REFLECTIONS ON SELF-CONCEPT AND SELF-ESTEEM

Luckner and Stewart (2003) interviewed 14 successful adults who are deaf in order to identify alterable patterns and ingredients of success for individuals who are deaf, so recommendations from these adults could then be shared with parents and professionals within the field. Those participating in the study were asked 10 interview questions, 5 of which pertained to their family, education, personality, and social life, as well as why they thought they were successful. The other 5 questions focused on recommendations they would make to children who are deaf, parents, teachers, and employers. The last question was open ended in nature, asking participants to contribute anything else they would want to share. Individuals nominated to participate in the study were selected based on the following criteria: has completed a postsecondary training program, earns more than $30,000 annually, is currently employed, has friends and is respected by peers, and exhibits self-confidence (p. 246).

Responses obtained during the interviews indicated that family support and hard work were key attributes for success. Comments such as "I was always included in different activities," "My parents always told me that education is really important," and "My grandfather told me I must be smart, I must read and learn, practice and study" resonated throughout their responses. Half of those responding indicated they had received a high caliber of education; the other half indicated that their "education was lousy" and "I received a very poor education." Regarding how their personality had affected their success, a number of those responding emphasized they were motivated and enjoyed overcoming challenges.

A recurring theme revolved around what they learned from interacting with others, being included in family conversations, and having a friend they could trust and with whom they could talk. Involvement in sports, activities, and organizations for Deaf individuals were also mentioned. In addition, several reported that they had both Deaf and hearing friends, indicating how the ability to communicate with both groups made this possible, while stressing the overall ease with which communication occurred in the Deaf world.

When asked to provide advice for children who are deaf that would lead them on the path to success, four basic recommendations were provided: set goals, develop friendships, become skilled at reading and writing, and learn to advocate for yourself. When asked to give advice to parents, the resounding response was to communicate with them. As one respondent elaborated, "The key is communication. It doesn't matter if it is ASL, SEE, oral. . . . it's important that the child can communicate. . . . not just the mom, but the whole family" (p. 247).

Summary

Identity develops dramatically throughout each individual's lifetime and is influenced by multiple contexts within society. Ethnic heritage, culture, religious foundation, gender, socioeconomic background, and family dynamics all play contributing roles in the shaping of the person's identity. It is critical to recognize that individuals who are deaf can be immersed in their ethnic cultural heritage and embrace their Native American, Asian, Latino/Hispanic, or African American culture while simultaneously immersing themselves in Deaf culture. Furthermore, they may identify with their religious affiliation and revere that part of their social identity while at the same time functioning as leaders in the Deaf community. Storbeck and Magongwa (2006) remind us that these social identities are fluid and that generally one or two of the variables are generally stronger than the others. The interaction that occurs among these variables contributes to the shaping, forming, and plurality of the unique identity embodied in each individual Deaf person.

Deaf individuals may be faced with the challenge of forming an ethnic as well as a Deaf identity. According to Leigh (2009), the degree to which both identities will be internalized will depend on "circumstance, family communication, environmental influence, and positive/negative associations with the hearing difference and the reactions of others" (p 131). Although it is possible for a Deaf person who also holds minority ethnic status to find a comfortable niche with both identities—the Deaf minority group and the ethnic minority group—this often requires a lifetime of interfacing with and exploring the expectations associated with both group memberships.

As future educators and providers of support services, it is imperative that professionals within the field recognize the diverse group of individuals who identify themselves as being Deaf. While some will embrace a Deaf identity, cherish ASL, and the rich culture and heritage that the community has to offer, others will maintain a hearing identity, preferring to communicate and socialize with those who can hear, oblivious to the world of the Deaf. Throughout their careers, professionals will also encounter Deaf individuals who are able to acknowledge the positive attributes of both cultures and can develop a level of comfort while interacting with each group, thus epitomizing a bicultural Deaf identity.

Developing an identity evolves throughout one's lifetime. Influenced by a multiplicity of events, experiences, and individuals, the persona is formed and adapts to the exigencies of the cumulative life experience. Through offering support, respect, and scaffolding for those seeking to define their identities, professionals can be instrumental in fostering growth and development. By providing individuals who are deaf and hard of hearing with the tools they need to explore and fashion their own identities, all can be provided with a resilient foundation that is essential to their ongoing development as they continue on their journey through life.

12

Economics, Postsecondary Opportunities, and Employment Trends

Entering Adulthood

With a stymied economy creating an increasingly competitive job market, those joining the ranks of the 21st-century workforce are being presented with employment opportunities marked by rapid change, technological advancements, far-reaching opportunities, and endless possibilities. Slowly moving from recession to recovery, astute career seekers are honing their skills so they can compete in a world where digitization, virtualization, and automation are as common today as telephones, typewriters, and copy machines were a decade ago. We are in a period of transition, having moved from a nation that once viewed workers as "an unthinking cog in a great machine" to a new model that is based on the worker as a creative contributor (Timm, 2005, p. 55). Those preparing and competing for jobs today are being challenged to develop a "hard skill set" as well as a "soft skill set." As America continues to advance into the new millennium, men and women seeking employment are being challenged to represent themselves as unique, bright, talented individuals as they compete for jobs with their peers who are equally skilled and qualified.

Employment trends across the United States can be viewed through a kaleidoscope of ethnic, cultural, and multigenerational diversity. Impacted by slowing growth, the graying of America, and increasing diversity, the mosaic of the traditional workforce is changing dramatically. Currently comprised of employees representing the Traditionalists/Silent Generation (born between 1930 and 1945), Baby Boomers (born between 1946 and 1964), Generation X (born between approximately 1965 and 1980), and Millennials/Generation Y (born between approximately 1981 to 1999), the workplace affords numerous opportunities for professional growth and development for all these individuals.

Where do most of these people work? What are the employment trends of the future? What skills do young people need today to become gainfully employed? What are the barriers to employment? Are individuals who are deaf and hard of hearing as prepared as their hearing counterparts to compete for the jobs for which they have trained? What, if any, barriers are preventing this population from achieving their vocational aspirations?

LABOR FORCE PROJECTIONS: A LOOK AT WHERE WE ARE AND WHERE WE ARE EXPECTED TO BE IN 2018

According to the U.S. Bureau of Labor Statistics (BLS) data for 2008–2018, the labor force is expected to increase by 12.6 million, reaching nearly 167 million by 2018. It is anticipated that persons in the 55-and-older age group will comprise 12 million of the additional 12.6 million additional workers accounting for approximately 25% of the labor force. Looking ahead, individuals between the ages of 25 and 54 will make up 63.5% of the total labor force, with those ages 16 to 24 estimated to account for approximately 12.7% of the workers, roughly half of that for the older age group (Toosi, 2009).

Although the annual rate of growth for females is expected to slow to 0.9% over this targeted period, it is still a faster growth rate when compared to males, with women representing 46.9% of the workforce by 2018. Furthermore, with the influx of immigrants entering the United States, it is projected that the Hispanic labor force will reach more than 29 million during this same time frame, thus comprising 17.6% of the labor force. It is further projected that Asians will reach more than 9 million workers by 2018, and the African American labor force will surpass 20 million. During this same period it is anticipated that 37.6 million workers will enter the labor force while 25 million will leave. The majority of those individuals leaving the workforce in 2018 will be the Baby Boomers who are leaving due to their age and arriving at the retirement stage of their lives (Toosi, 2009, pp. 31–46).

The retirement of the Baby Boomers will play a significant role in the occupational outlook for this millennium. With increased members of the population aging, the impact on the field of health care is significant with over half of the 20 fastest-growing occupations related to health care. (See Table 12.1 for a list of the employment opportunities with the fastest growth and the education that is required for each of these jobs.) As consumers age, many of these patients will seek home health care as an alternative to costly stays in hospitals, nursing homes, or other residential care facilities. This accounts for the increased demand for home health care aids. Furthermore, as the population becomes more concerned with self-improvement, the demand for self-enrichment teachers and skin care specialists will also increase. In addition to the increase in health care fields, two of the fastest-growing detailed occupations are found in the computer specialist group. These include network systems and data communications analysts. This field is projected to be the second fastest-growing occupation in the U.S. economy (U.S. Bureau of Labor Statistics, n.d.).

Additional information provided by the U.S. Bureau of Labor Statistics (n.d.) indicates that the occupations with the largest percentage of growth include those in the areas of health occupations, education, sales, and food service. Office and administrative support services occupations are expected to account for about one fifth of the job growth, but many of the other jobs listed in Table 12.2 indicate significant increases in numbers of employees, creating new jobs and representing high growth rates. Only 3 of the 20 fastest-growing fields are also projected to be among the 20 top occupations with the largest increases in employment in numerical growth. (See Table 12.2 for the occupations with the largest numerical growth.) Note that the education or training categories and wages reflected in the areas with the largest numbers of new jobs are considerably different when compared with those listed in the fastest-growing employment opportunities. Of these occupations, 12 are in an on-the-job training category, with only 7 of them reflecting the need for any postsecondary education. Further examination of these categories also indicates that 10 of the 20 fields with the largest numbers of new jobs earned less than the national median wage in May 2008 (U.S. Bureau of Labor Statistics, n.d.).

TABLE 12.1 Occupations Representing the Fastest Growth: 2008–2018

Occupations	Percent Change	Number of New Jobs (in thousands)	Wages (May 2008 median)	Education/Training Category
Biomedical engineers	72	11.6	$77,400	Bachelor's degree
Network systems and data communications analysts	53	155.8	71,100	Bachelor's degree
Home health aides	50	460.9	20,460	Short-term on-the-job training
Personal and home care aides	46	375.8	19,180	Short-term on-the-job training
Financial examiners	41	11.1	70,930	Bachelor's degree
Medical scientists, except epidemiologists	40	44.2	72,590	Doctoral degree
Physician assistants	39	29.2	81,230	Master's degree
Skin care specialists	38	14.7	28,730	Postsecondary vocational award
Biochemists and biophysicists	37	8.7	82,840	Doctoral degree
Athletic trainers	37	6.0	39,640	Bachelor's degree
Physical therapist aides	36	16.7	23,760	Short-term on-the-job training
Dental hygienists	36	62.9	66,570	Associate degree
Veterinary technologists and technicians	36	28.5	28,900	Associate degree
Dental assistants	36	105.6	32,380	Moderate-term on-the-job training
Computer software engineers, applications	34	175.1	85,430	Bachelor's degree
Medical assistants	34	163.9	28,300	Moderate-term on-the-job training
Physical therapist assistants	33	21.2	46,140	Associate degree
Veterinarians	33	19.7	79,050	First professional degree
Self-enrichment education teachers	32	81.3	35,720	Work experience in a related occupation
Compliance officers, except agriculture, construction, health and safety, and transportation	31	80.8	48,890	Long-term on-the-job training

Source: U.S. Bureau of Labor Statistics, Occupational Employment Statistics and Division of Occupational Outlook.

The landscape of employment across the United States will continue to experience significant changes as more production processes are automated and use of labor is streamlined. Moreover, although some companies will further reduce the number of employees due to outsourcing their manufacturing to overseas companies, other businesses throughout the United States will experience a decline in industries that have previously focused on the textile, apparel, footwear, and leather industries. This will be primarily caused by the stiff competition generated from foreign manufacturers (Bartsch, 2009). Those occupations with the fastest decline include

TABLE 12.2 Occupations with the Largest Numerical Growth: 2008–2018

Occupations	Number of New Jobs (in thousands)	Percent Change	Wages (May 2008 median)	Education/Training Category
Registered nurses	581.5	22	$62,450	Associate degree
Home health aides	460.9	50	20,460	Short-term on-the-job training
Customer service representatives	399.5	18	29,860	Moderate-term on-the-job training
Combined food preparation and serving workers, including fast food	394.3	15	16,430	Short-term on-the-job training
Personal and home care aides	375.8	46	19,180	Short-term on-the-job training
Retail salespersons	374.7	8	20,510	Short-term on-the-job training
Office clerks, general	358.7	12	25,320	Short-term on-the-job training
Accountants and auditors	279.4	22	59,430	Bachelor's degree
Nursing aides, orderlies, and attendants	276.0	19	23,850	Postsecondary vocational award
Postsecondary teachers	256.9	15	58,830	Doctoral degree
Construction laborers	255.9	20	28,520	Moderate-term on-the-job training
Elementary school teachers, except special education	244.2	16	49,330	Bachelor's degree
Truck drivers, heavy and tractor-trailer	232.9	13	37,270	Short-term on-the-job training
Landscaping and groundskeeping workers	217.1	18	23,150	Short-term on-the-job training
Bookkeeping, accounting, and auditing clerks	212.4	10	32,510	Moderate-term on-the-job training
Executive secretaries and administrative assistants	204.4	13	40,030	Work experience in a related occupation
Management analysts	178.3	24	73,570	Bachelor's or higher degree, plus work experience
Computer software engineers, applications	175.1	34	85,430	Bachelor's degree
Receptionists and information clerks	172.9	15	24,550	Short-term on-the-job training
Carpenters	165.4	13	38,940	Long-term on-the-job training

Source: U.S. Bureau of Labor Statistics, Occupational Employment Statistics and Division of Occupational Outlook.

those in the textile industry (dyeing machine operators; textile winding; twisting, knitting and weaving machine operators), the postal service (including mail sorters, processors, and processing machine operators), order clerks, desktop publishers, and semiconductor processors. The only two occupations with the fastest decline requiring a postsecondary education include the desktop publishers and the semiconductor processors; all the others require on-the-job training (U.S. Bureau of Labor Statistics, n.d.).

With the employment market quickly changing and jobs remaining competitive, those entering the world of work will be required to possess core competencies that are required for the job as well as "soft skills." Soft skills refer to a cluster of personal qualities, work habits, ethics, attitudes, and social graces that characterize someone as a good employee who co-workers find to be a compatible worker. Employees of the 21st century will need to be committed to developing these skills. According to Martin (2003) today's employees must be able to communicate and be collaborative. Most employers are looking for individuals who are creative and willing to take risks, show initiative and accountability, can collaborate and lead, approach life from a variety of interdisciplinary levels, and have a thirst for knowledge (Friedman, 2005; Gibson, Blackwell, Dominicis, & Dermerath, 2002; The Herman Group, 2005).

Employees of the future will need to be creative and possess the art of "thinking outside the box." Furthermore, they will need to be able to do more with less and adapt quickly to or anticipate change (Marshall, 1995). Those who demonstrate that they are intrinsically motivated and tenacious and will uphold the values as well as the ethics of the workplace will be in high demand. Furthermore, according to Hall (2005) leadership skills will be expected from all individuals. Those gainfully employed will need to remain lifelong learners to stay competitive in the current dynamic and ever-changing job market.

How are people who are deaf and hard of hearing faring in today's job market? Are they better prepared to meet the demands of the ever-changing job force than they were 10 or even 20 years ago? What types of expectations do hearing employers have of their employees who are deaf? What are the barriers to successful employment? Does communication play a major role and impact retention in the workplace, or has technology enabled employers and employees to overcome that hurdle?

SUPPORTING INDIVIDUALS WHO ARE DEAF AND HARD OF HEARING SO THEY CAN BECOME GAINFULLY EMPLOYED

According to the U.S. Department of Education (National Center for Education Statistics, 2006), without appropriate support individuals who are deaf or hard of hearing may experience difficulty finding and maintaining employment, leaving them vulnerable to chronic unemployment or locked into jobs where they continuously experience underemployment (Dew, 1999) with no means to become independent (Employment Management Professionals, 2008). Recognizing the need to provide support for training, assistance with job placement, and job coaching, the federal government passed the Vocational Rehabilitation Act in 1954 to support individuals with disabilities. Under this legislation numerous services are offered to individuals who qualify as vocational rehabilitation clients.

The Federal Vocational Rehabilitation (VR) Program is administered by the Commissioner of the Rehabilitation Services Administration (RSA) in the U.S. Department of Health and Human Services. This agency operates in all 50 states and is primarily responsible for preparing disabled youth and adults for gainful employment. The original Vocational Rehabilitation Act, Public Law 88-565, was amended in 1966 and provides both direct and indirect services to people who are deaf and hard of hearing.

The rehabilitation process is threefold in nature. It involves making a diagnosis and evaluation to determine the extent and vocational implications of the disability (or disabilities); it provides training that will enable the person to adjust to and overcome his or her limitations; and it prepares individuals for a specific vocation or cluster of vocations (Luckner, 2002).

To become a VR client, the individual must meet the eligibility requirements. These requirements are based on four criteria:

1. The client must demonstrate, usually through a medical exam, the existence of a physical or mental disability.
2. Based on the disability, it must then be determined, usually by the individual VR counselor, that the disability constitutes a substantial impediment to employment.
3. There must be a certain level of expectation by the VR counselor that the individual can benefit in terms of an employment outcome.
4. VR services are required for the person to prepare for, engage in, or retain gainful employment. (Luckner, 2002)

Once a client is determined to be eligible for services, the client and the counselor work together to prepare a rehabilitation plan. The Individual Plan of Employment (IPE) (previously referred to as the Individual Written Rehabilitation Program [IWRP]) outlines the training, educational objectives, and career goals for the client. It is subject to review on a periodic basis and includes a listing of the types of services that will be purchased for the client. These services include training programs, medical treatment and restoration, hearing aids, interpreting services, and any other products and services that can reasonably be expected to enhance the client's ability to qualify for and obtain employment.

Within the Division of Rehabilitation, general counselors work with individuals with a myriad of disabilities. These include, but are not limited to, serving those who are visually impaired and those who have physical disabilities, providing services to persons who are deaf or hard of hearing, and supporting individuals with intellectual disabilities. These are some of the groups of individuals for which VR provides services.

Frequently, counselors' caseloads are composed of clients who have a wide range of disabilities. Their caseloads are often large, and their clients' backgrounds may be as diverse as the individuals themselves. Although a number of states have a separate class of counselors referred to as Rehabilitation Counselors for the Deaf (RCD) who focus on serving consumers who are deaf, other states are not as fortunate. As a result, counselors find frequently that they are not prepared to deal with the varying disability groups with whom they are confronted.

Individuals who are deaf or hard of hearing seeking VR services represent four very distinct, diverse groups with very different rehabilitation needs. These groups represent those who are Deaf, clients who are hard of hearing, persons who are late deafened, and those who are low-functioning deaf (Luft, Vierstra, Copeland, & Resh, 2009). In addition, counselors serving this population typically encounter individuals representing a wide variety of communication modes, academic abilities, and career or lack of career aspirations. Some communicate fluently in ASL; others may rely on an English-based sign system; and still others converse orally. Demonstrating varied literacy as well as academic competencies, some will be college ready, and others will require a cadre of support services to render them capable of entering the workforce. Furthermore, although a segment of this population will arrive at the VR counselor's door with a clear sense of his or her identity, others may arrive with evolving Deaf identities and need help resolving some of their identity issues while simultaneously needing assistance with setting realistic career and work goals.

Adults who become deaf later in life (late deafened) may struggle with communication and the impact their hearing loss is having on their lifestyle, current career, and future professional aspirations. As a result, they may seek the assistance of the VR counselor for help with communication strategies and hearing devices (Bat-Chava, Deignan, & Martin, 2002, as cited in Luft et al., 2009). Those who comprise the low-functioning population of deaf individuals present an additional set of challenges for the counselor. These individuals typically read at the third-grade level or lower and may have additional disabilities. Finishing school with a certificate of attendance, they may have limited sign language skills, be undereducated, and often have behavior problems (Ewing & Jones, 2003; Luft et al., 2009; Wheeler-Scruggs, 2003). The services provided for this group of clients vary significantly from those designated to support the college-bound population.

The goal of the VR counselor is to provide clients with the training and support needed to obtain and remain gainfully employed. Serving as a vital link between the high school years and the world of work, VR counselors serve an integral part of the multidisciplinary team by assisting students as they transition from secondary education to the world of work.

As they transition, what types of services and support do individuals typically need to successfully enter the workforce? What kinds of difficulties do they encounter that can contribute to sustained underemployment or loss of employment? What are the workplace expectations of Deaf workers and hearing employers? Where do Deaf professionals traditionally apply for work? Are there still barriers to employment opportunities for individuals who are deaf or hard of hearing entering or remaining in the workforce today?

PROVIDING SUPPORT SERVICES: THE ROLE OF VOCATIONAL REHABILITATION

When VR counselors schedule their initial meetings with individuals who are deaf or hard of hearing, one of the first things they must determine is if the person is eligible for services and, if so, does the person have a career goal in mind. Once eligibility is established, the counselor and client mutually agree upon a prescribed plan designed to help the individual meet his or her goal and eventually become gainfully employed. Eligibility for services begins with documentation of the disability. In most states the hearing tests performed by an audiologist are used to help make this determination; however, some states rely on formulas to determine audiometric eligibility, and others look at the functional status of the individual. According to Mascia and Mascia (2008), individuals are classified by their functional communication skills and abilities for vocational purposes. When conducting the initial assessment, counselors pay particular attention to the following: Is hearing the only limitation involved? How does the individual communicate with others? Does the person wear hearing aids or a cochlear implant? Does the person currently utilize other types of assistive technology? And does the individual rely on the services of an interpreter for communication (p. 98)?

Attention is also given to the cause and type of the hearing loss, the person's age at the time of onset, the degree of hearing loss, and the person's overall health. In addition, attention is paid to the individual's educational history, speech/ language/reading/writing status, the communication mode used by the consumer's family and peers, his or her psychological status, the neurological/cognitive status, and the person's motivation/compliance/acceptance of the hearing loss (p. 98). All these factors will play an important role as the counselor explores the types of job opportunities the person is interested in and the types of services and training the person will need. Some of the clients will arrive with a certificate of attendance in hand and no clearly defined vocational goals; others will enter the office having graduated from high school and will request financial support so they can attend the postsecondary or vocational program of their choice; still others will wait to request services until long after they have left school.

What types of services are generally needed by that segment of the population who are deaf and low functioning? What services do those individuals need who are not equipped to enter the postsecondary arena? What type of support do these clients need so they can secure employment and remain gainfully employed?

Support Services for People Who Are Deaf and Low Functioning

When describing individuals who are deaf and low functioning it is always important to be mindful of the fact that, regardless of the group you are describing, when referring to any group as a whole there is always variation among group members. This is particularly true when discussing persons who are characterized as deaf and low functioning. Although there is no specific denotation of this population, there is one particular salient characteristic upon which the majority of rehabilitation professionals agree: It is that all these individuals experience exceptional difficulty with communication, regardless of whether discourse is conveyed through reading, writing, speech, speechreading, signs, or gestures (Long, 1996, as cited in Wheeler-Scruggs, 2002).

A complicating factor is that, in most cases, these individuals cannot read above the fourth-grade level (Cawthon, 2004; LaSasso & Lollis, 2003; Padden & Ramsey, 2000; Watson, 1998). Many are the products of a failed educational system; deprived of a linguistically rich and culture affirming environment, their psychosocial growth and academic success are stymied (DeLana, Gentry, & Andrews, 2007). These students may begin their career in either residential or public schools and initially experience difficulties by the third grade. Some will remain in the public school system and fall further and further behind in language skill, and in academic content knowledge, but may continue to be socially promoted continuing on through the eighth grade, even though they are reading only at the third-grade level. Others eventually transfer to the residential schools when it is time for them to attend high school. Arriving at residential schools with a weak academic base, they may find their options are limited, often restricting their academic choices to a vocational track rather than a precollege program (Simms, Rusher, Andrews, & Coryell, 2008).

Long, Long, and Ouelette (1993) have stressed that these individuals are not typically able to maintain employment without transitional assistance or support; they may exhibit poor problem-solving skills, lack emotional control, can be described as impulsive, have a low tolerance of frustration, and may engage in inappropriate aggressiveness. Furthermore, many of them may be unable to live independently without transitional assistance or support (as cited in Wheeler-Scruggs, 2002, p. 11). These concerns are not new but, rather, recapitulate previous discussions that have been documented in the literature. Furthermore, they illustrate the factors that affect this population when they attempt to obtain and maintain employment over an extended period of time. Recurring themes include the following:

- They lack the personal and interpersonal skills needed for successful interaction with co-workers and supervisors.
- They frequently display poor work behaviors and habits; they do not understand the value of work; and they are unaware of most career fields and occupations.
- Many of them lack the prerequisite language and reading skills required for job placement as well as for successful on-the-job training.
- Several have limited exposure to the experiences that contribute to the development of independent living skills, personal responsibility, and survival skills.
- They may possess poor decision-making skills. (DiFrancesca, 1978; Melton, 1987)

It is critical to keep in mind the wide variability within this group and that these individuals represent a considerable range of functional levels. Some may primarily need assistance filling out job application forms, while others require support with developing independent living skills, obtaining job readiness skills, and acquiring strategies for getting along with co-workers on the job. The ultimate goal always is to provide clients with the necessary skill set to render them employment ready and to instill in them a sense of accomplishment.

Wheeler-Scruggs (2002) conducted interviews with 23 individuals identified as being both deaf and low functioning who were former or current consumers of VR services. She wanted to gather information regarding their ability to live independently and their satisfaction level based on their current employment. Of those surveyed, the majority were functioning very independently. Her findings further indicated that 16 of the 23 had held jobs in the past. They cited reasons for not remaining employed as follows: inadequate earnings, dissatisfaction, being fired or laid off, sickness, and a lack of transportation. One former employee stated she had been fired from two jobs because she failed to notify her supervisor when she was sick. Although she had a phone, she did not realize the importance of calling and felt it was unfair that she was fired.

The majority of those employed had no idea what their job titles were. Of the individuals who were working, 10 were unsure if they had health insurance, and some had no idea if they had ever had a promotion. Although the majority reported that their quality of work relationships was good, several indicated that they relied on writing to communicate with their supervisors and that interpreters were hired only occasionally for communication purposes. The results of this study indicate the need to work closely with consumers before and after they have become employed. Furthermore, these findings illustrate the need to provide direct instruction to consumers who are deaf with respect to information that consumers who can hear learn incidentally. Without this information these particular clients may have gaps in their vocational training as evidenced in their work behavior, ethics, knowledge of benefits, and promotion (Wheeler-Scruggs, 2002).

Persons who are deaf and low functioning represent one constituency within the overall population of individuals who are deaf or hard of hearing and are currently employed. The opposite end of the spectrum is comprised of individuals who have earned one or more college degrees and are gainfully employed in the professional sector. What are the characteristics of this segment of the population? What types of degrees do they have? Where do they work, and how do they feel about their current employment status?

Professionals in the Workforce Who Are Deaf or Hard of Hearing

During the 2006–2007 academic year 25 million students were enrolled in colleges and universities across the United States (Knapp, Kelly-Reid, & Ginder, 2008). Of this student population an estimated 6% to 16% self-reported that they were college students with disabilities (Horn, Berktold, & Bobbitt, 1999; Horn, Peter, Rooney, & Malizio, 2002). Lewis, Farris, and Greene (1999) report that students who are deaf or hard of hearing are represented at 100% of the institutions with enrollments of more than 10,000 students and at 93% of the institutions that educate between 3,000 and 9,999 students. Those electing to go to college are faced with the same challenges as their hearing counterparts. Required to successfully complete coursework, field experiences, and internships, these students are preparing for the competitive job market with aspirations of entering the fields of computer programming, counseling, computer operations, teaching, and business management (Schroedel & Geyer, 2000). Boutin and Wilson (in press) studied data compiled by the Rehabilitation Services Administration (RSA) for the 2004 fiscal year and determined that 9.1% of eligible consumers with a hearing loss had received college and university training.

What type of support did these individuals rely on while obtaining their education? Once they completed their coursework, where did they find employment? Are most of them currently satisfied with their current job placements?

SUPPORT SERVICES: MAKING POSTSECONDARY INSTITUTIONS ACCESSIBLE FOR STUDENTS WHO ARE DEAF AND HARD OF HEARING

Individuals who become clients of VR are eligible to take advantage of any of the 22 services provided by this agency on an as needed basis. Examples of these services include assessment, transportation, interpreter services, and technical assistance services (Boutin, 2009). However, due to the extensive support services provided by public postsecondary institutions, these services are generally not in large demand through VR.

Students who are deaf and hard of hearing who are enrolled in higher education programs primarily request that their postsecondary institutions provide them with the services of sign language interpreters and note takers. Other services that are frequently provided include preferential seating, extended time for written examinations, tutoring, and the use of computer-assisted real-time translation (CART) and computer-aided speech-to-print transcription (C-Print). Arriving in their late teens or early 20s, these students experience the same transitional issues as their hearing peers. Faced with declaring a major and refining their communication as well as their cognitive skills, they learn to become adept at balancing the rigors of their academic courses with the challenges of discovering a newfound sense of independence and increased opportunities for socialization.

Those who arrive at the halls of higher education with a solid academic foundation possess or quickly develop learning strategies and enjoy the luxury of engaging in fluid communication exchanges. They are better equipped to handle the rigors imposed on them throughout their tenure as students. Some will be very successful; others will struggle and eventually leave the system without earning a degree.

According to Marschark, Lange, and Albertini (2002), students who are deaf who are attending college are much less likely to graduate than their peers who can hear. Approximately 35% of deaf students graduate from 2-year programs, compared to about 40% of their hearing peers. Furthermore, about 30% of students who are deaf graduate from 4-year programs compared to about 70% of their hearing peers. This can be partially attributed to the fact that they have had unmet educational needs prior to entering postsecondary institutions (pp. 151–152). Those who do graduate may find they can secure employment in the workforce but later discover they do not seem to have viable access toward upward mobility.

CAREER EXPERIENCES OF COLLEGE-EDUCATED INDIVIDUALS WHO ARE DEAF AND HARD OF HEARING

Individuals select fields of study for a variety of reasons. Some are driven by monetary rewards; others seek careers with an aura of prestige and social status. Some students enter degree programs with altruistic goals, wanting to major in fields in which they can ultimately secure jobs in the social services sector; others prefer courses of study that will provide them with the challenge of engineering, scientific research, or medical technology. Regardless of the field that is selected, the overall goal is generally to prepare for future employment that can provide the individual with feelings of deep personal satisfaction and self-worth.

Careers do not take place in a vacuum. They are shaped and molded as individual employees interact within the work environment. One's values influence the effort and time given to a career and may affect the amount of satisfaction derived from that occupation (Schroedel & Geyer, 2000). During their tenure in the workforce, some employees will be provided with avenues for promotion and will savor the opportunities for advancement while others will be stymied and remain in the same position throughout their career.

Employees who are deaf and hard of hearing enter the workforce with the same aspirations as their hearing colleagues. Seeking opportunities to produce, create, and apply their skills, they search for environments where they can interact with colleagues and experience professional growth. Engaging in a national longitudinal survey of 240 college graduates with hearing loss, Schroedel and Geyer (2000) examined the career achievements of college alumni who are deaf or hard of hearing to determine their educational attainments, the extent they experienced career mobility, their socioeconomic attainments, and the extent to which they were underemployed.

At the time of the study the majority of those participating were well established in their jobs. Forty-one percent had remained with the same employer for 1 to 3 years, 35% had worked for the same employer for 4 to 9 years, and 24% indicated the same place of employment for 10 years or longer. When asked about the quality of their lives, the majority indicated that they were either happy or very happy with their current situation. However, several indicated they were not similarly satisfied with their current income. (See Table 12.3 for a summary of participants' attitudes about the quality of life.)

Although 59% indicated they were performing the same types of job duties that they had been doing for the previous 5 years, 41% reported that they had been given different responsibilities. Composed of a diverse group of employees, they represented 70 different occupations with the majority of them having been employed in more than one type of job. This implies that college graduates have broader access to a variety of career fields, thus reducing the amount of occupational clustering and segregation often attributed to those with limited job and career skills (Schroedel & Geyer, 2000).

Even though only 45% indicated they had received promotions during the previous 4 years, those who had not advanced stated that this was attributed primarily to lack of opportunities or that the position they were in did not lead to promotion. When examining the annual income of the alumni it was apparent that their earnings were strongly influenced by the college degree they had attained. Furthermore, there was a parallel increase in professional positions as advanced

TABLE 12.3 Attitudes About Quality of Life

Happy or Very Happy	Percent of Individuals Expressing Degrees of Satisfaction
City or Town Where One Resides	81%
Social Life	76%
Friends	80%
Family Life	89%
Health	83%
Overall Quality of Life	78%
Earnings Based on Employment	64%

Source: Based on information from Schroedel and Geyer (2000, p. 306).

degrees were earned. Overall findings indicated that the majority of those participating in the study were successful in their careers and were economically self-sufficient. Female alumni reported earnings that were one third less than their male counterparts, and they continued to be clustered in clerical positions, unlike the men who were working in managerial and technical jobs (Schroedel & Geyer).

Additional research reported by Kavin and Brown-Kurz (2008) has explored the career experiences of supervisors who are deaf in education and social service professions. They interviewed 11 professionals who are deaf and hard of hearing in educational and social service professions and focused specifically on career choices, career mobility, and networking. The researchers asked those participating in the interviews to share their views on why they selected the career they did and if they felt their deafness was a hindrance in their career path.

Regarding career choices, 3 of those responding felt their deafness was a hindrance to their career path, 2 felt it served as an asset, and of the remaining 6, 5 felt it was a hindrance and an asset, while 1 was ambivalent. When asked if they felt they were limited to careers that entailed deafness-specific professions, 8 indicated they felt limitations, while 3 did not view their deafness as specifically imposing limitations (Kavin & Brown-Kurz, 2008). All 11 of those interviewed indicated they chose a deafness-related field for the following reasons: ease of communication access, cultural awareness and sensitivity, staying in the comfort zone, and, primarily, because they had a strong professional interest in the field. Communication was a resounding theme that resonated throughout several of their comments.

One individual picked a profession within the field of deafness because she felt she could succeed there. She stated:

> "I feel limited because I chose to be in a job where the environment is deaf-friendly and communication accessible. . . . I do believe that deaf people are able to work anywhere they want and I made a choice to be in a deaf field because of communication, really." (Kavin & Brown-Kurz, 2008, p. 31)

Ten of the 11 respondents commented on their frustrations at not being able to freely and easily join in informal conversational exchanges that typically occur in hallways, at the water cooler, or in the break room. These impromptu meetings frequently spark interactions enabling co-workers to ask questions, share information, or "catch up" on office details that would routinely be shared in an e-mail. One respondent commented:

> "I do not have good speech skills and I really need an interpreter to communicate with hearing people. Oftentimes, when I see a hearing person in the hall, I needed to talk with them right away but I could not do that, so that is a real barrier. I have to wait until I get back to my office and send e-mail or call that person. I often miss a lot of opportunities with hearing staff for any emerging issues or discussions." (Kavin & Brown-Kurz, 2008, p. 37)

Seven of those responding indicated that they chose to work in a field related to deafness because they felt they could make a contribution to the field. They perceived themselves as positive role models and felt very satisfied being able to demonstrate how barriers could be overcome. Committed to the Deaf community, these individuals felt passionate about what they were doing and enjoyed their level of involvement while serving on professional boards and being recognized for their expertise regarding Deaf culture and the needs of the Deaf community.

Conversely three of those responding indicated their frustration working in a career that focused exclusively on deafness. As one so succinctly stated:

> "Sometimes ... as a therapist, I'm a little jealous of the variety that other therapists have. They talk about mental health treatment, about how they are able to do medical. They're able to do mental mindfulness. These kinds of things; different therapy methods. I'm limited because Deaf people see me [as] [hls4]more of an administrator." (Kavin & Brown-Kurz, 2008, pp. 32–33)

Kavin and Brown-Kurz (2008) further explored the area of career mobility. Respondents to this question believed that if they were not deaf their career path would take a different direction. When asked about their current job, one respondent candidly stated:

> "One thing that bothered me was that I felt stuck there. . . . I watched people change jobs often, easily from one department to another. I saw people work at the women's center . . . and then move on to the employment center and then to the counseling center. I stayed in one place, disability services." (Kavin & Brown-Kurz, 2008, p. 32)

Another participant revealed:

> "I've heard people tell me, the reason you are not considered for that position . . . is because they can't figure out how a deaf people [sic] would be able to do that position." (Kavin & Brown-Kurz, 2008, p. 34)

Previous research available on career mobility indicates that those individuals who are deaf who are hired in entry-level positions traditionally experience difficulties with upward mobility. Although employers hire employees who are deaf and make attempts to accommodate them, they frequently do not address the issues of career education and advancement. It is not uncommon to find these individuals in their same entry-level positions after 20 years of working with the same company. Although they have the potential for advancement, the promotion is often given to the hearing individual who, from the employer's perspective, will be easier to train. Christiansen (1982) reports that although workers who are deaf and hard of hearing report a high degree of job satisfaction, they indicate that they have not had many opportunities for advancement and often remain in the same job for extremely long periods of time.

Johnson (1993) surveyed 490 workers who were deaf to determine longevity of employment and levels of promotion. Of the workers who completed the questionnaire, 81% were between the ages of 31 and 60, and 44% had been employed for 1 to 10 years; 45% had been employed for 11 to 30 years; and over half (52%) had been employed in their current job between 11 and 29 years. Furthermore, 20% had held the same job for over 30 years. Of these workers, 55% had a high school or postsecondary vocational technical education, and 27% were college graduates. In addition, 36% indicated that they were very satisfied with their jobs, 46% were somewhat satisfied, and 14% were not satisfied (p. 347). Previous research conducted by Foster (1987, 1992), Schroedel, Mowry, and Anderson (1992), and Welsh (1993) further indicate that deaf people, in general, have less vertical mobility than their hearing co-workers.

In a more recent study, Punch, Hyde, and Power (2007) reveal that barriers to job mobility are universal. Reporting on the experiences of a group of alumni who are deaf and hard of hearing from Griffith University in Australia, they describe the career barriers imposed on them by their work environments, societal attitudes, and the stigma and discrimination associated with hearing loss. Echoing sentiments reflective of the feelings experienced by individuals in the Kavin and Brown-Kurz (2008) study, their comments regarding communication and networking have resounding similarities. Typical responses included the following:

> I did not anticipate the disadvantage of missing out on gossip, networking opportunities, casual information sharing.
>
> It has always been difficult socializing in groups during lunchtime breaks in the staff room.
>
> Difficulty with fellow staff is always an issue.
>
> Hard to understand at staff socials. Hence difficult to make meaningful friendships in work environment without super-human efforts. (Punch, Hyde, & Power, 2007, p. 512)

Kavin and Brown-Kurz (2008) highlighted comments from some of the respondents indicating the strategies they used to compensate for information that was missed due to informal conversations and networking opportunities. Four of the respondents indicated they scheduled debriefing sessions with their colleagues; others singled out talkative colleagues to solicit information. Deaf individuals who worked in offices with one or two signing colleagues frequently relied on those individuals to provide them with staff and office updates. This body of research supports earlier findings by Foster (1992) that difficulties experienced with informal networking and social interactions can be detrimental to career advancement and obtaining long-range career goals. In essence, these factors can and do contribute to the underemployment experienced by a segment of workers who are deaf or hard of hearing.

A LOOK AT UNDEREMPLOYMENT FOUND WITH RESPECT TO INDIVIDUALS WHO ARE DEAF OR HARD OF HEARING

Underemployment traditionally has been defined as occurring any time individuals are employed in positions that are incompatible with their intelligence, skills, and education. It results in employees filling positions for the sake of "having a job" and usually results in "dead-end" employment. Characteristics of underemployment include failure to place employees in positions affording them the opportunity to draw upon their talents and abilities, reluctance to promote skilled employees into the upper managerial levels, and failure to compensate workers for the quality of work they perform.

Historically, people who are deaf have lagged behind their hearing counterparts in most major measures of work achievement. Studies have shown that these individuals are heavily overrepresented in less prestigious blue-collar occupations and typically earn substantially less than hearing workers. For a historical overview see Schein and Delk (1974), Walter, MacLeod-Gallinger, and Stuckless (1987), Weinrich (1972), and Welsh and Walter (1988).

Due to severely limited achievements, many adults exhibiting various degrees of hearing loss are often compelled to perform manual labor rather than technical work. Statistics compiled from the 1980s onward indicate that nearly 90% of workers who are deaf are employed in jobs requiring manual labor as opposed to less than 50% of their hearing counterparts. Only 17% of employees who are deaf have white-collar jobs as compared with 46% of hearing people (Rosen, 1986).

Siegel (2000) reported statistics compiled by the Northern California Center on Deafness indicating that between 60% and 80% of the individuals who are deaf are underemployed. He attributes this high percentage of underemployment to a mismatch between the skills possessed by the majority of workers who are deaf or hard of hearing and the current demands of the job market. To obtain and secure jobs today in the professional and service sector, employees must have skills in technology or in allied health care. These skills are not possessed by the majority of adults with varying degrees of hearing loss, including those recently graduating from mainstreamed programs. Students wanting to compete in the modern job market must develop a sound academic foundation that will allow them to access and successfully complete vocational and postsecondary programs.

If individuals who are deaf and hard of hearing want to rise above the ranks of the blue-collar worker, it is imperative that they develop a technical or professional skill set so they can compete successfully for the reduced number of jobs that are and will be available. Furthermore, they must also master those nontechnical skills, abilities, and traits referred to as soft skills. Future employees will need to rely on both hard and soft skills to function in today's competitive job market. Without both sets of skills, otherwise very capable and bright future employees will remain among the ranks of the underemployed.

Today's graduates must develop a solid academic foundation prior to exiting their high school programs if they want to be granted admission into vocational, technical, and postsecondary programs. Without this foundation in place, newly admitted postsecondary students will quickly experience frustration and failure and exit the system prior to mastering the necessary skills required to become gainfully employed. Equipped with only minimal skills, these bright, capable individuals will lose their competitive edge and be forced to join the ranks of the unemployed or the underemployed.

EMPLOYMENT TRENDS AND EMPLOYER EXPECTATIONS

It is well established in the literature that youth who are deaf and hard of hearing entering the workforce during the 21st century will be faced with challenges unknown to previous generations of workers. The overall characteristics of the employee spectrum in the United States will be altered as immigrants enter the country. Increased numbers of workers will be fluent in two if not more languages, and English will become their second or third language as they seek to communicate with their co-workers. The cultures they represent will be as unique as the individual countries from which they come. Each of these employees will provide an added dimension to the ever-changing workforce.

Throughout this era the workplace will be characterized by an increase in the number of older workers employed outside the home as a significant number of Baby Boomers remain actively employed. Living longer and remaining in good health, many of them will continue to be very capable of working, feel they still have a contribution to make, and stay actively employed in the workforce on either a full- or part-time basis until their early seventies.

The composition of new employment opportunities will undergo a dramatic change that will likewise be mirrored by the transformation of the future workforce. All potential future employees, including those who are deaf and hard of hearing, will be required to prepare for these positions in the same way as they prepare to enter the workforce. Expected to have an excellent command of reading, writing, and mathematics skills, the employee of the future will be required not only to think outside the box but also to design a new "box" digitally and virtually that is capable of traversing cyberspace. Furthermore, employees will be expected to communicate comfortably with supervisors, co-workers, other office staff, and consumers.

Future employees will be required to meet the expectations of their employers. Employers will be searching for workers who possess the required educational qualifications and vocational skills, including the ability to use the latest technology available at the workplace. Furthermore, they will be seeking employees who possess those personal attributes that include dependability and motivation. Johnson (1993) identifies four characteristics or vocational behaviors that ensure employment retention or consideration for promotion: meeting production expectations, working cooperatively, responding to supervision, and relating interpersonally to co-workers. In addition, the relationship between the Deaf worker and his or her supervisor and co-workers will become an essential and critical requisite needed to sustain employment.

Schierhorn, Endres, and Schierhorn (2001) emphasize that Deaf workers and other potential workers will need to become team players, honing their skills so they can participate in group discussions and become effective team members. Those who arrive on the job with strong interpersonal or social skills will find they have a significant advantage over those who exhibit poor personal and social skills. Prior research has indicated that many Deaf workers lack social and interpersonal skills (Passmore, 1983). Furthermore, their inability to draw from paralinguistic cues, such as intonation, pitch, and frequency, may make it difficult to unravel the implicit meaning couched in the external verbiage. In addition, the absence of vocal stressors that provide the conduit for humor, satire, requests, and commands can make the nuances of these interactions more difficult to detect, thus creating confusion for Deaf individuals (Goss, 2003).

One's ability to successfully interact on a one-to-one basis and engage in group discussions requires two distinct abilities: the ability to comprehend what others are saying and the ability to express oneself clearly through spoken language communication. Spoken communication is built on a foundation of vocabulary, syntax, and one's ability to structure phrases and sentences clearly, thereby expressing ideas, feelings, and experiences efficiently and successfully. When expressing ideas vocally, speech intelligibility (SI) becomes a critical factor in the communication process.

It is well documented in the literature that hearing loss can contribute to voice and speech characteristics that can affect speech intelligibility (Ling, 2002; Monsen, 1983). Research conducted by Most (2007) found that the SI of students who are deaf and hard of hearing in general education classes was directly related to their level of loneliness (as cited in Most, Weisel, & Gali-Cinamon, 2008). Earlier studies conducted by Most and her colleagues (1999) revealed the attitudes toward children with poor SI were significantly less positive than those who exhibited good SI. As the speech intelligibility in children who are deaf and hard of hearing improved, their hearing peers' attitudes regarding their cognitive abilities and their personality features also improved. In essence, children with varying degrees of hearing loss can encounter early and ongoing stigmatizing experiences with their hearing peers that impact their emotional and social development. Those who are readily understood feel comfortable with their ability to express themselves; those who are frequently misunderstood may shy away from interacting with their hearing peers.

Another body of literature has examined the occupational competence (OC) of people who are deaf and hard of hearing with respect to their communication abilities. Several studies (see Most, Weisel, & Gali-Cinamon, 2008, for a description of this body of research) have indicated that parents and teachers of students who are deaf or hard of hearing would limit the scope of possible occupations for this population, relegating them to technical jobs, rather than those requiring communication. In these instances the tendency was to ignore the individual's personal attributes and focus instead on the person's degree of hearing loss (Punch, Hyde, f& Creed, 2004, as cited in Most, Weisel, & Gali-Cinamon). Most, Weisel, and Gali-Cinamon have also studied the relationships between SI and OC. Having administered self-report questionnaires to 36 young adults, their findings indicated that these individuals felt that occupations requiring less communication were more appropriate than those demanding more communication. However, their responses further revealed that SI was not related to OC.

Summary

Gainful employment continues to elude many people who are deaf and hard of hearing. Employment opportunities for these workers hinge on two factors: the individual deaf person's abilities, skills, educational attainments, and soft skills; and the attitudes of the employers engaged in the hiring process. Each factor impacts significantly on the employability and upward mobility of individuals who are deaf.

Research has indicated that annually many students who are deaf graduate from high school unprepared to enter either postsecondary settings or vocational training programs. Many also lack the necessary skills mandatory for entry-level positions in high-tech corporations. Far too many are resigned to the fact that they must accept those jobs involving manual labor or enter the ranks of the unemployed. Although some are fortunate and can continue their education, many more face the grim prospects of unemployment and underemployment.

Studies indicate that those entering the workforce will be challenged with positions that change daily due to automation and advanced technology. This will force them to update their technical knowledge and personal skills in order to remain competitive. Those who are uncomfortable with career change and have no desire to acquire new skills will be left on the fringes of the labor market. To obtain higher levels of employment, appropriate intervention strategies must be incorporated. These strategies need to be designed with the education of this population in mind. It is imperative that they incorporate activities that will enhance feelings of self-confidence. Incentives need to be included that encourage the individual to strive toward upward levels of advancement. Teachers of the deaf, parents, and significant others must change their perceptions regarding the abilities of deaf individuals. These students should be challenged and encouraged to explore the wider range of vocational options available to them.

There are signs of a widening gap between the postsecondary-trained professional deaf individual and the unskilled worker. Unless dramatic changes are made in training programs and rehabilitation efforts, the gap will continue to widen (Rosen, 1986). In addition, an influx of functionally illiterate persons who are deaf and who are welfare dependent or rely on public assistance (e.g., Social Security) will continue. Students need to begin receiving their career education classes in the elementary school years and continue receiving this type of instruction throughout high school. Course material containing information pertaining to the diverse world of work should be shared, and employment availability needs to be stressed. Stereotypic job placements need to be dissolved and replaced with positive attitudes. It is critical that emphasis be placed on job behaviors and socialization as well as on technical skills.

In essence, students must be taught how to learn if they are going to compete in the labor market. Fundamental changes must take place to ensure that the young population of deaf individuals will be prepared to enter the competitive job market rather than remain among the ranks of the unskilled workforce. As the future economic growth in the United States centers around higher levels of education, deaf individuals must receive training to meet this challenge, thus affording them the opportunity to compete equally with their hearing peers.

13

Individuals Who Are Deaf with Additional Disabilities

Prevalence and Characteristics

Children with additional disabilities comprise a unique segment of the population comprised of individuals who are deaf and hard of hearing. Because of the varied etiologies of deafness, these additional conditions may accompany hearing loss and have a significant impact on the child's development. Furthermore, these additional disabilities may impose physical limitations or hamper cognitive/intellectual functioning. Because the extent and nature of particular disabling conditions vary tremendously, each child who is deaf and hard of hearing and has been identified as needing special services must receive individual consideration.

Numerous studies describe the incidence of additional disabilities among this population. A survey conducted by the Gallaudet Research Institute (2008) of more than 36,000 school-age children who are deaf and hard of hearing reports that 39% of the students have been identified as having multiple disabilities. Table 13.1 includes information pertaining to the prevalence within each category.

Miller (2006) indicates that approximately 70% of the school-age population comprised of students who are deaf and hard of hearing. These include disabilities that involve expressive and receptive communication skills, applying reasoning skills, and maintaining attention. Miller further postulates that the assessment protocols currently in use today to identify students with both additional and functional disabilities do not reflect accurate numbers. Because several of the test batteries do not include assessments that evaluate verbal abilities, the potential exists to miss children who have language disabilities. Children can perform exceptionally well on a performance IQ test and score well within the normal limits. However, if evaluated for their proficiency in their preferred mode of communication—sign language, Cued Speech, signed supported speech, or spoken language—it is possible to discover significant deficiencies within the communication skills area (p. 162). Therefore, these statistics may in fact represent depressed numbers.

Additional disabilities are traditionally classified under two general headings: those involving a physical condition and those affecting the cognitive/intellectual functioning of the individual. Physical conditions include visual impairment, deaf-blindness, orthopedic impairment (including cerebral palsy), brain damage, epilepsy, and heart disorders. Those included in the cognitive domain include intellectual disability (previously referred to as mental retardation),

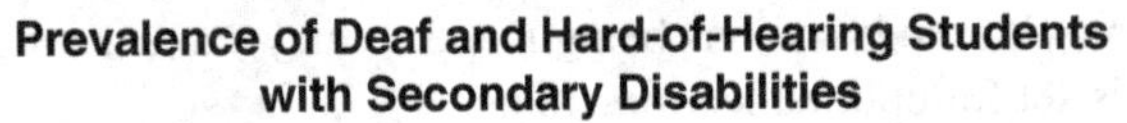

TABLE 13.1 Prevalence of Students Who Are Deaf and Hard of Hearing with Secondary Disabilities

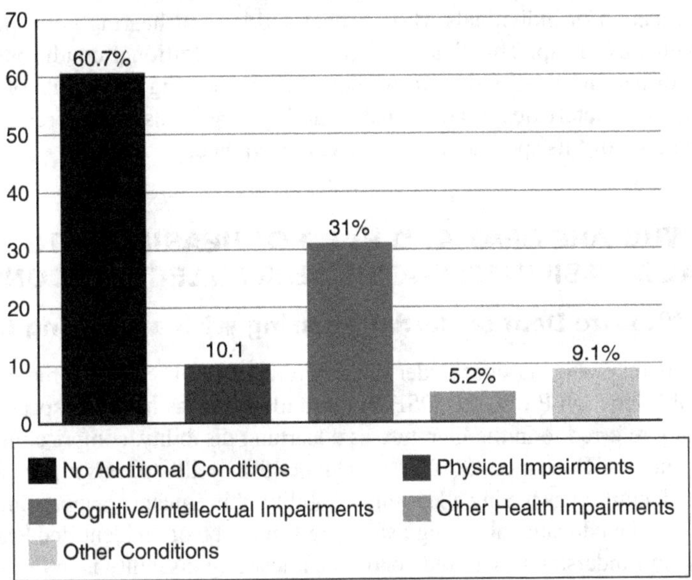

emotional/behavioral problems, autism spectrum disorders (ASD), attention-deficit disorders (ADD/ADHD), and specific learning disabilities.

Individuals who are deaf who have special needs may experience one or more disabling physical conditions in addition to deafness. It is also possible for an individual to have more than one cognitive/intellectual disability in conjunction with a hearing loss. Various combinations of both physical and cognitively/intellectually limiting conditions can occur simultaneously in an individual.

Closer examination of this information reveals the following:

- Special learning disorders and emotional/behavioral problems are the only conditions that are reported alone the majority of the time.
- Students exhibiting legal blindness, brain damage, epilepsy, and orthopedic disorders are reported as having other disabilities in over two thirds of the cases.
- Students diagnosed as learning disabled are more likely to have emotional/behavioral problems than those for whom there is no evidence of learning disabilities.
- Those students with epilepsy and brain damage also tend to have increased incidence of learning disabilities.
- Legal blindness, brain damage, epilepsy, and orthopedic disorders are found more frequently in tandem with mental retardation than in isolation. (Andrews, Leigh, & Weiner, 2004)

Numerous factors can contribute to additional disabling conditions. Diseases and infections, including viruses (rubella, cytomegalovirus, herpes simplex, and HIV) occurring during the prenatal period, genetic factors, conditions present at birth, premature births, early childhood diseases, and trauma can all have a significant impact on the child's development.

In the event any of these diseases or infections occur, children can develop one or more disabling condition. These additional disabilities can play a vital role in the child's overall physical social, and psychological development. Frequently, the child will require a specialized educational placement with modifications being made so they can access the curriculum. When this occurs the stage is set for optimal learning to occur.

The classification of individuals who are deaf and hard of hearing with special needs denotes a heterogeneous group. The characteristics of these additional conditions, concomitant with the degree of hearing loss, will be instrumental in delineating the profile of the individual. By examining the characteristics of additional disabling conditions as they relate to deafness, a greater understanding of this specific population can be gained.

CHILDREN WHO ARE DEAF AND HARD OF HEARING WITH ADDITIONAL DISABILITIES: COGNITIVE/INTELLECTUAL CONDITIONS

Individuals Who Are Deaf or Hard of Hearing with a Learning Disability

Of all the students receiving services under the umbrella of the U.S. Department of Education's Office of Special Education Programs (OSEP), those identified as having a specific learning impairment, typically referred to in the literature as a learning disability, comprise the largest group. The U.S. Department of Education (2007) reports that 45% of all students reported to have a disability have been identified as having a learning disability; this equates to approximately 5% of all students enrolled in the educational setting exhibiting some type of an identified learning problem.

Frequently misunderstood as a mild condition, a learning disability is in fact serious, severe, chronic, and pervasive, and it requires intensive intervention (Bender, 2004; Pierangelo & Giuliani, 2006, as cited in Bryant, Smith, & Bryant, 2008). Children with learning disabilities are a heterogeneous group who display a wide range of strengths and abilities; they approach learning in a variety of ways and respond to interventions inconsistently. Due to their varied abilities and approaches to learning, no single treatment, explanation, or accommodation is uniformly effective. This in itself provides challenges to professionals (Smith & Tyler, 2010). When describing this population, the literature invariably emphasizes first and foremost that those with learning disabilities are primarily characterized as unexpected underachievers who are resistant to treatment (Vaughn & Fuchs, 2003). Unlike other groups of students with disabilities, the low academic achievement of these students is not expected or predicted based on their innate abilities or intelligence. All these students experience difficulties in one or more of the following areas: academic achievement, including reading, written language, or math; cognitive skill deficits, including memory problems, attentional problems, and metacognitive deficits; and social and motivational problems (McLeskey, Rosenberg, & Westling, 2010; Smith & Tyler; Turnbull, Turnbull, & Wehmeyer, 2010). (See Table 13.2 for an overview of the characteristics of learning disabilities.)

One of the most significant challenges for students with learning disabilities frequently lies within the area of reading, and these difficulties are one of the primary reasons students are referred for special education services (Fuchs, Fuchs, Mathes, Lipsey, & Roberts, 2002). Referred to in the educational literature as a reading disorder, and in the medical literature as dyslexia, on occasion the terms are used interchangeably; it is important to note, however, that the term *reading disorder* indicates reading difficulties associated with decoding words, comprehending text, and possessing appropriate speech and fluency whereas dyslexia indicates a more severe reading disorder associated with a neurological dysfunction (McNamara, 2007; Young & Beitchman, 2007).

Often children who experience reading difficulties also encounter problems with written expression. Frequently they struggle with spelling, handwriting, sentence structure, word

TABLE 13.2 Characteristics of Learning Disabilities

Academic	Social	Behavioral Style
Unexpected underachievement	Immature	Inattentive
Resistant to treatment	Socially unacceptable	Distractible
Difficult to teach	Misinterprets social and nonverbal cues	Hyperactive
Inability to solve problems	Makes poor decisions	Impulsive
Uneven academic abilities	Victimized	Poorly coordinated
Inactive learning style	Unable to predict social consequences	Disorganized
Poor basic language skills	Unable to follow social conventions (manners)	Unmotivated
Poor basic reading and decoding skills	Rejected	Dependent
Inefficient information processing abilities	Naïve	
Inability to generalize	Shy, withdrawn, insecure	Dependent

usage, and overall composition. It may be difficult for them to get started with a writing assignment due to feeling overwhelmed with the task put before them. Furthermore, they may struggle as they attempt to convey their ideas, resulting in written assignments that may fall short of the length or organizational requirement (Young & Beitchman, 2007).

Students who experience difficulties within the area of mathematics may struggle with procedural, semantic memory, and visuo-spatial problems. Struggling to understand math concepts and the steps required to solve complex problems, they often lack the ability to remember basic math facts. Although a math disability can occur in isolation, between one half to slightly more than two thirds of children with math disabilities have also been diagnosed as having a reading disability (Barbaresi, Katusic, Colligan, Weaver, & Jacobsen, 2005, as cited in Turnbull et al., 2010).

Two other major characteristics of students with learning disabilities merit discussion: those associated with cognitive skill deficits and those associated with social and motivational problems that impact school performance. Within the area of cognitive skill development, students may experience memory or attentional problems, or metacognitive deficits. However, one should note that these characteristics cannot be attributed to all the students who have learning disabilities. Some members of this population struggle with working memory and experience difficulty remembering sight words or basic math facts; others lack the ability to employ strategies to solve complex problems. Moreover, approximately 25% to 40% of them also have ADHD (Lerner & Kline, 2006). Further evidence suggests that many students with learning disabilities struggle when the situation requires them to monitor their thinking processes. This becomes particularly problematic when reflecting on the needed steps that are required to solve complex math problems (Mercer & Pullen, 2008).

An estimated one third of the students with learning disabilities also have social-skill deficits (Lerner & Kline, 2006). These students lack the skills needed to build social relationships; they may exhibit aggressive actions or nonverbal behaviors and engage in more attention-seeking or disruptive behaviors. Furthermore, when they interact with others they may appear less sensitive, lack tact, and struggle when they try to interact with others (Bryan, Burstein, & Ergul, 2004).

The Individuals with Disabilities Education Act (IDEA) defines the category of learning disabilities as a disorder that includes one or more of the basic psychological processes described here. Referred to as the inclusionary standard, it identifies the conditions that are included within this disability group. The definition further contains an exclusionary standard. Within this standard, conditions that are not included in the category of learning disabilities are described. These include learning problems that exist due to loss of vision or hearing or result from motor disabilities or mental retardation. Further stipulations delineating what is excluded include emotional disturbance or those reflected by the environment, culture, or economic disadvantage.

What impact does the exclusionary standard have on students who are deaf and hard of hearing? How can professionals determine whether the achievement difficulties experienced by this population are due to a processing problem that is characteristic of a learning disability or due to a perceptional problem that can be associated with hearing loss (Soukup & Feinstein, 2007)? What criteria are used to identify students who are deaf and hard of hearing who also have learning disabilities?

A plethora of research documents the effects hearing loss has on language acquisition and academic progress, both factors that impact levels of academic achievement. Furthermore, several causes of deafness are also primary causes of neurological dysfunction. These include prematurity, meningitis, prenatal rubella, certain genetic syndromes, and maternal use of teratogenic medications (Mauk & Mauk, 1993; Morgan & Vernon, 1994, as cited in Soukup & Feinstein, 2007). Confronted with students displaying characteristics that mirror learning disabilities in hearing children, professionals are frequently challenged to determine if the problems their struggling students are facing are attributed solely to their deafness or if their deafness is compounded by a learning disability. It is important to keep in mind that some students who are deaf and hard of hearing who do not have learning disabilities also struggle academically due to the ramifications of deafness. Therefore, when asked to identify those who are struggling due to a learning disability, rather than their deafness, the task can become an arduous one that at times seems both daunting and overwhelming.

According to Soukup and Feinstein (2007), hearing loss is usually not accompanied by attention deficits, visual-perceptual problems, severe inability to learn vocabulary and English-language structures, consistent distractive behaviors, or emotional factors. Therefore, evidence of one or more of these conditions can indicate that the child should be referred for evaluation to determine if a learning disability does in fact exist. Stewart and Kluwin (2001) posit that one way parents and professionals can identify a student who is deaf or hard of hearing with a concomitant learning disability is to compare his or her functioning ability to other students who are deaf or hard of hearing. Characteristics that are atypical of a student who is deaf with a normal nonverbal IQ and a severe hearing loss include low concentration, passive activity level, weak integration processes, weak visual perception, very poor communication skills, weak mother–child relationships, low motivation, and higher incidence of medical problems (Van Vuuren, 1995). These characteristics signify a problem that may not be attributed to hearing loss but, rather, to a processing problem resulting from the brain's inability to organize sensory input in a standard fashion (Stewart & Kluwin, 2001, p. 305).

Within the field of deaf education the consensus is that, without a doubt, children who are deaf are adversely affected by learning disabilities; also, although it can be extremely challenging to make an accurate diagnosis, every attempt must be made to do so. It is significant to note that deafness per se is not a learning disability. Although experiential deprivation of students who are deaf is often exacerbated by hearing loss and can appear to replicate the behavior and learning characteristics of students who can hear with learning disabilities, it is critical to that distinguish those students who are deaf and do have a learning disability from those who do not despite the fact that this is an involved and complex and multidimensional process.

When attempting to complete these evaluations, the practitioner must weigh the impact of poor communication in the home. Furthermore, it is critical that the evaluator pay particular attention to when the diagnosis is made, noting if it takes place after the critical language developmental period has passed. One should also try to determine if the child has failed to thrive because the chosen communication modality has not allowed for optimum development so the child can flourish. When a modality is not a good fit for the child, it can adversely impact the child's cognitive growth and development. In addition, practitioners must be mindful of the fact that parental education, consistent family support, and the quality of early intervention services can all play a critical role impacting the child's development. It is imperative to recognize that all these factors play a significant role in influencing the child's development and can later be manifested in characteristics that mimic those of a child with a learning disability without the child actually having one.

Individuals Who Are Deaf or Hard of Hearing with Emotional or Behavioral Disorders

Emotional or behavioral disorders (E/BD) fall within the high-incidence special education category. Children who display characteristics of this group typically become a concern of parents, family members, school personnel, and other members of the community. Frequently, they display behaviors that are disruptive, aggressive, and verbally abusive. Often these behaviors become pronounced to the extent that the individual engages in violent behaviors that are frequently destructive to oneself or toward other members of this disability group. These behaviors and others may lead to recurring encounters with the criminal justice system (Smith & Lane, 2007; Walker, Ramsey, & Gresham, 2004).

Emotional or behavioral disorders can be difficult to define. However, both IDEA '04 and the National Mental Health and Special Education Coalition agree that individuals exhibiting any characteristic or any group of characteristics among the following can benefit from services designed to support this disability group. The characteristics include those who are unable to build or maintain satisfactory interpersonal relationships with their teachers and peers; those who display inappropriate types of behavior or feelings under normal circumstances; those who have a tendency to develop physical symptoms related to fears associated with personal or school problems; and those who seem to display a general mood of unhappiness or depression (Bryant et al., 2008, p. 73). These defining features occur for extended periods of time and adversely affect the student's educational performance.

Emotional or behavioral disorders are divided into three groups: externalizing, internalizing, and low incidence. Externalizing behaviors include behaviors such as behaving in a defiant manner; exhibiting aggressive behaviors; demonstrating a lack of self-control; and being argumentative, hostile, and threatening physical harm to people or animals. Many students with emotional or behavioral disorders bully and victimize their classmates (Hartung & Scambler, 2006) and engage in physical fighting.

Internalizing behaviors are seen in sharp contrast to externalizing behavior problems; as a result, teachers often experience difficulty in identifying students with these types of problems. Characteristic of students described with internalizing behavior problems include those who are frequently socially withdrawn, experience anxiety disorders, have low self-esteem or a negative self-image, and experience depression. Unlike acting-out problems, depression is often overlooked in school-age children. Termed a *silent disorder,* it may be more prevalent in young boys than young girls. However, this trend changes as students enter the adolescent years. During this time it becomes a more frequent occurrence in girls and can manifest itself in perceptions of a negative body self-image leading to anorexia and bulimia.

Children who experience social withdrawal, play primarily by themselves; they usually have low rates of verbalization; and they may develop feelings of loneliness and depression (Schrepferman, Eby, Snyder, & Stropes, 2006). Furthermore, 8% of those who experience internalizing behavior problems may experience severe anxiety that interferes with their personal, social, and academic development (Kauffman, 2001). Individuals with anxiety disorders can be observed exhibiting excessive worry and fear, and they often display an intense response when separating from their family, friends, or a familiar environment.

Within the low-incidence conditions category are a group of disorders that are rare but very serious when they occur. One of the conditions that frequently appears in the literature is schizophrenia. Although it is a very rare happening when it does occur, it can be very challenging for everyone who has direct contact with the person. Schizophrenia is characterized by bizarre delusions, hallucinations, disconnected thoughts, and significant personal hygiene and organizational problems. Individuals who have schizophrenia find they struggle with class assignments, and frequently they are hospitalized or receive at least part of their education in specialized educational settings. However, one should note that this diagnosis is seldom ascribed to individuals below age 17.

The federal government has reported that slightly less than 1% of all school-age children have emotional or behavioral disorders (OSEP, 2006). However, of those identified with E/BD a national profile of these students revealed that 29% of them were rated low on a self-control social skills measure; slightly less than two thirds of the students had reading scores in the lowest 25% of all students; and 43% were reported to be in the bottom 25% of scores in mathematics. Furthermore, 22% of elementary/middle and 38% of secondary students had been held back one grade level at least once, and two thirds of the students with E/BDs were reported to have expressive and/or receptive language disorders. These disorders remained stable across the entire span of the school years (Wagner, Kutash, Duchnowski, Epstein, & Sumi, 2005). Further statistics regarding this population indicate that about 74% of children identified with emotional or behavioral disorders are male; also, Asian American and Hispanic students tend to be underrepresented in this category and African Americans are overrepresented, indicating that 29% of students identified as having this disability are Black, even though overall they represent only about 14% of the student population (OSEP, 2006).

Although it is difficult to determine the exact causes of students' emotional or behavioral disorders, it is apparent that two of the major causes that contribute to this population are biological and environmental (Gray & Hannan, 2007). The breadth and depth of the different conditions are tremendous, and many may go unidentified to school personnel who are reluctant to attach a stigmatizing label to a child because that diagnosis is viewed negatively by society.

Statistical data concerning the prevalence of emotional or behavioral disorders in the school-age deaf population vary considerably. This is due to identification criteria incorporated by the school as well as formal reporting practices. Furthermore, the causes of emotional disturbances in deaf children are varied. Some can be attributed to the impact of deafness on human development, the way those in the environment respond to deafness, and the manner in which deaf individuals react to their environment. Other cases can be attributed to immaturity and poor home environments.

Theoretically, another significant component may be responsible for this disabling condition. It involves an interactional effect of both the loss of hearing and of other central nervous system lesions associated with the condition causing deafness. Impulse disorders, psychosis, general behavioral disorders, and aphasoid disorders can also be accounted for, in part, due to pathology located within the central nervous system (Vernon & Rothstein, 1967). Additional research conducted by Rainer and Altshuler (1966) has suggested that some deaf mentally ill individuals exhibit symptoms that are similar to characteristics found in brain injured people. In addition, research conducted by Chess and Fernandez (1980) has also documented physiological findings. In studies of children with rubella-related deafness, a high incidence of emotional and behavioral difficulties was noted. This further supports studies cited in the Annual Survey whereby conditions such as rubella, birth trauma, and complications during pregnancy were cited in conjunction with emotional/behavioral problems (Schildroth & Karchmer, 1986, p. 76).

Physiological causes, strained familial and peer relationships, social difficulties, educational environment, and communication factors can all contribute to emotional and behavioral difficulties. Once a dysfunction of this nature has been identified, professional treatment must be secured. However, as with other areas of deafness, due to a scarcity of mental health professionals trained to work with this population and the special needs of this group, needs are not always met.

Individuals Who Are Deaf or Hard of Hearing with an Intellectual Disability

During the past 50 years the term *intellectual disability* has replaced an older and often more familiar term, *mental retardation,* the term still used by IDEA to describe a "significantly subaverage general intellectual functioning, existing concurrently with deficits in adaptive behavior and manifested during the developmental period, that adversely affects a child's educational performance" (Turnbull et al., 2010). National organizations, such as the American Association on Intellectual and Developmental Disabilities (AAIDD), adopted the new term in 2006 and are no longer referred to as the American Association on Mental Retardation. Other organizations that advocate for this group of students have also adopted the newer term, preferring to eliminate a term that has so often stigmatized many people with this disability.

The term *intellectual disability* encompasses the same population of individuals who were diagnosed previously with mental retardation. This diagnostic descriptor has remained consistent with respect to the number of individuals; the level, type, and duration of the disability; and the specialized need for support services for this population. The term *intellectual disability* has been described as being:

> "characterized by significant limitations both in intellectual functioning and in adaptive behavior as expressed in conceptual, social, and practical adaptive skills. This disability originates before age 18." (Schalock et al., 2007, p. 118)

Individuals with intellectual disabilities are generally identified during their school years, and although it is difficult to obtain an accurate prevalence rate, statistics indicate that more males than females are diagnosed, and socioeconomic level (poverty) is a contributing factor to this disability (Emerson, 2007; Harris, 2006). Based on data provided by the Centers for Disease Control (CDC, 2005b), intellectual disabilities are identified in 12 of every 1,000 children. Additional data provided by the CDC indicate that 7.4 of every 1,000 children are of European descent, and 19.7% of every 1,000 children are of African American descent.

Intellectual disabilities are characterized in two major ways: limitations in intellectual functioning and limitations in adaptive behavior. Intellectual functioning is traditionally assessed by administering intelligence tests such as the Wechsler Intelligence Scale for Children or the Stanford-Binet. Those who score approximately 2 standard deviations below the mean, designated as an IQ of 70, are considered to have an intellectual disability. Of the population that is tested, 95% falls between 2 standard deviations above and 2 standard deviations below the mean. Furthermore, approximately 85% of the students with intellectual disabilities have IQs ranging from 50–55 to 70 (Turnbull et al., 2010, p. 243). According to the American Association on Mental Retardation (AAMR, 2002), individuals who have intellectual disabilities are described by adhering to the following classification system:

	Intelligence Quotient Range
Mild intellectual disability	50–55 to approximately 70
Moderate intellectual disability	35–40 to 50–55
Severe intellectual disability	20–25 to 30–40
Profound intellectual disability	below 20–25

When identifying individuals with intellectual disabilities, the current philosophy is to examine functional abilities as well as performance on intelligence measures. Adaptive behavior is not as easy to measure as intelligence. Test instruments designed to measure this function are not readily available. One measure that is frequently included in the test battery is the Vineland Social Maturity Scale. This instrument renders a single score and reflects a level of general social competence. The test is designed to sample various aspects of social ability, such as self-sufficiency, self-direction, communication, and social participation. This instrument also reflects the child's need for direction, assistance, and supervision by others. Although this scale tests a variety of behaviors and contains a section for young children as well as older children and adults, it does not yield the same type of levels found in intelligence testing.

Once evidence is found of significantly lower intelligence and limitations in adaptive behavior, the child can be considered to be eligible to receive special education services. Adaptive behavior consists of three domains: conceptual skills, social skills, and practical skills that have been learned by people in order to function in their everyday lives (Luckasson et al., 2002). Conceptual skills include both receptive and expressive language, literacy (reading and writing), money concepts, and self-direction. Social skills encompass responsibility, self-esteem, gullibility, and the ability to follow rules; and within the area of practical skills are included activities of daily living, occupational skills, and the ability to maintain a safe environment.

Adaptive behavior is examined within the constructs of culture, environment, and age (Borthwick-Duffy, 2007). When a student scores at least 2 standard deviations below the mean on one or more scores reflecting conceptual, social, and practical skills, or demonstrates an overall score on a standardized measure that includes conceptual, social, and practical skills, the student is described as having significant limitations in adaptive behavior (Turnbull et al., 2010, p. 245). These individuals typically experience difficulties knowing how to perform a skill. They struggle with not knowing when to implement a skill that has been previously learned, and they fail to possess the motivational factors that are required to use a skill to complete a task.

There are several contributing factors that can cause an intellectual disability. Within the literature these causes are generally organized in two ways: first, according to time of onset, and second, type or reason for the disability. Time of onset includes three time periods: prenatal, those causes that occur before birth; perinatal, causes that occur during the birth process; and postnatal, causes that happen after birth or during childhood. Prenatal causes include genetic or heredity, toxins that are ingested during pregnancy, disease, and neural tube defects. Genetic causes include conditions such as fragile X syndrome and Down syndrome, as well as phenylketonuria (PKU); toxins include alcohol, tobacco, and drug exposure used by the mother during pregnancy. Perinatal causes occur during the birth process and include prematurity, oxygen deprivation, umbilical cord accidents, or head trauma. Postnatal causes are often attributed to the environment. Toxins such as lead poisoning, traumatic brain injury and infections, as well as child abuse and neglect can result in lifelong disabilities (Smith & Tyler, 2010).

It is recognized in the literature that child abuse and neglect can be directly related to poverty. It has also been established that poverty has a higher correlation with intellectual disabilities than with any of the other disabilities (National Research Council, 2002). According to Emerson (2007) and Fujiura and Parish (2007), poverty during childhood not only creates risks for higher intellectual disability but also contributes to lower educational attainment, poorer physical and mental health, and increased mortality. Emerson, Graham, and Hatton (2006) report that families who represent the bottom 20% of the socioeconomic status are four times more likely to have a child with an intellectual disability when compared with those who comprise the top 20% of the socioeconomic status.

Hassanzadeh (2007) reports that when the school-age population is examined, students who are deaf and hard of hearing are approximately three times as likely to exhibit a secondary disability (30.2%) as their hearing counterparts. This is attributed in part to the varying causes of hearing loss. It is well documented in the literature that several causes of deafness, including maternal rubella (2%), prematurity (5%) cytomegalovirus (1%), and meningitis (9%) are also associated with neurological effects. These etiologies may also contribute to learning disabilities, emotional or behavioral disabilities, or intellectual disabilities. Individuals who are deaf or hard of hearing and who have also been identified as having an intellectual disability represent a unique group of people who have two specific types of needs: those associated with hearing loss, as well as those faced by individuals with an intellectual disability. These needs, when exhibited concomitantly, present a unique set of demands and challenges for family members as well as the professionals who will later provide services for them.

Individuals Who Are Deaf or Hard of Hearing with Autism Spectrum Disorders

Although the federal government still refers to autism as a single disorder to describe different conditions or syndromes that share "autistic-like" symptoms and characteristics (see IDEA, 2006), the term *autism spectrum disorders* (ASD) is becoming more prevalent in the literature. Embracing a broad spectrum of disorders, the term describes five related conditions that include autistic disorder or autism, childhood disintegrative disorder (CDD), Asperger syndrome, Rett syndrome, and pervasive developmental disorder–not otherwise specified (PDD-NOS) (Bryant et al., 2008). The characteristics and spectrum of behaviors that fall under the umbrella of ASD are broad and variable with some exhibiting more severe manifestations of the disability than others.

Even though each child who is affected by autism is unique, exhibiting symptoms that vary in severity and intensity, generally all display a particular set of common characteristics. These include interactive difficulties represented by absence or insufficient smiling, laughing, and making or maintaining eye contact; limited communication abilities; insisting on routines (with disruptions to daily schedules creating major difficulties for them); repetitious play; struggles with creative and make-believe play; and challenges when attempting to relate to their peers (Szymanski & Brice, 2008). Further discussion pertaining to these characteristics is presented here within the confines of the specific diagnoses identified under the umbrella of this spectrum of disorders.

Autism Disorder or Autism is defined in the American Psychiatric Association's (2000) text revision of the *Diagnostic and Statistical Manual of Mental Disorders* (DSM-IV-TR) as a developmental disability that significantly affects verbal and nonverbal communication, and social interaction, with evidence of restricted repetitive and stereotyped patterns of behavior. These behaviors include but are not limited to hand wringing, hand or finger flapping, and complex whole body movements (DSM-IV-TR, p. 75). Onset occurs prior to age 3 and adversely affects the child's educational performance. Furthermore, the child may exhibit abnormal function in any one of the following areas: failure to develop language skills required for social communication, difficulties participating in social interactions, or engaging in symbolic or imaginative play.

Childhood disintegrative disorder (CDD) is another of the conditions that comprise the ASD array. CDD shares similar characteristics with autism, including restricted, repetitive, and stereotyped behavior and interests; impaired communication; and impairments in social interaction; however, unlike children with autism, children with CDD develop normally until they are 5 or 6 years old, when developmental regression begins. Initially possessing language and social skills, as the regression progresses they lose the former skills and fail to develop new ones (Bryant et al., 2008, p. 96).

Asperger syndrome is eponymously named for Dr. Hans Asperger, the individual who first described and classified the behavior characteristics associated with the syndrome. The majority of children diagnosed with Asperger syndrome have normal intelligence; however, they exhibit problems with social skills and display restricted or unusual behaviors or interests. Although they develop language on par with their peers, their comprehension of the language remains on a literal level, making it difficult for them to understand jokes, form conceptual categories, or interpret nonverbal language. Furthermore, the social use of the language can be extremely challenging, limiting their ability to comprehend other people's feelings (Safran, 2001, as cited in Bryant et al., 2008, p. 96).

Rhett syndrome, also referred to as Rhett disorder, is a genetic condition and is more common in girls. Unlike autism, early childhood development appears normal, but then it stops. Characterized by hand wringing, symptoms also include social and communication deficits and lack of muscle control, with most children having mental retardation that is severe.

Pervasive developmental disorder–not otherwise specified (PDD-NOS) is a severe and pervasive disorder. Although the other conditions or disorders along the ASD continuum are characterized by deficits that occur in one or two of the three areas, individuals with PDD-NOS have problems in all three areas: communication, social skills, and unusual behaviors, including a restricted range of interests (Bryant et al., p. 96).

Autism spectrum disorders permeate globally, affecting males four times as often as females (Grinker, 2008; Yeargin-Allsopp et al., 2003). Recent estimates provided by the Autism Information Center (2010) indicate that on an average the number of children who are identified with ASD is 1 in every 110 children. Furthermore, the Centers for Disease Control and Prevention are continuing their research to determine how many children in the United States have been diagnosed with an ASD. What is the prevalence of ASD within the deaf population? What are some of the warning signs that may provide indicators that a child who is deaf also has autism? Do children who are both deaf and have autism display the same characteristics as those who can hear?

Based on statistics cited in the Annual Survey of Deaf and Hard-of-Hearing Children and Youth, conducted by the Gallaudet Research Institute (2008), one can surmise that 1 deaf child in 76 is receiving services for both a hearing loss and autism. This figure represents approximately twice what is currently believed to be the national prevalence rate throughout the United States (Szymanski & Brice, 2008). Based on research conducted by Chess, Fernandez, and Korn (1972), Jure, Rapin, and Tuchman (1991), and Vernon (1969), causes of autism in children who are deaf is attributed to congenital rubella, cytomegalovirus, herpes, chicken pox, toxoplasmosis, syphilis, mumps, hemophilic influenza, bacterial meningitis, profound immaturity, and hypoxia (Vernon & Rhodes, 2009). In the seminal study conducted by Rapin et al., the findings further indicated that, in concert with the hearing population, more boys than girls were diagnosed as being both deaf and having autism (30 of the 46 children were boys, and only 16 were girls). Contrary to hearing children whose autistic tendencies are identified by age 3, the median age for making a similar diagnosis for children who are deaf did not occur until age 4, with the median age of when identification typically occurs being by age 2 (Jure et al., 1991; Mandell, Novak, & Zubritsky, 2005).

Researchers and educators ascertain that one of the reasons the diagnosis occurs later with children who are deaf is based on the difficulty they encounter when distinguishing characteristics of deafness from characteristics of autism. Possible warning signs or signals that children who are deaf may also have autism include resisting being held or cuddled, failing to respond to their name after attention has been gained, and failing to visually track objects in a room or follow the eye gaze of the caregiver. Additional warning signs include making limited use of eye contact, experiencing difficulty imitating facial expressions, and struggling to understand other people's needs and feelings. Children who are deaf with autism may experience difficulty understanding sign language. They do not engage in age-appropriate play with their peers, their play may be rigid and unimaginative, and they can have difficulty interacting with other students who are deaf or hard of hearing, even when sign communication is used. Furthermore, they may show delays in learning sign language and resist changes in routines even when changes are clearly delineated (Szymanski & Brice, 2008, p. 12).

Although a paucity of research has focused on deafness and autism, young scholars of late are beginning to examine the complexities of this multiple disability. With this heightened awareness of the characteristics, causes, and concerns, parents as well as educators are looking to the future with the hope of discovering more answers so the needs of this unique population can be met.

Individuals Who Are Deaf or Hard of Hearing with Attention-Deficit/Hyperactivity Disorder

The American Psychiatric Association (APA) definition of an attention-deficit/hyperactivity disorder (ADHD) is "a persistent pattern of inattention and/or hyperactivity-impulsivity that is more frequent and severe than is typically observed in individuals at a comparable level of development" (APA, 2000, p. 85). Grouped by IDEA within the category of "other health impairments," it is difficult to identify how many children actually fall into this category. This is partially due to the fact that because ADHD is not designated as a separate category, states do not report the number of these students separately to the federal government. Furthermore, not all students with ADHD are eligible for special education services because it does not adversely affect their academic achievement. In addition, students already identified as having another disability are generally reported and served under that category.

Students within this category can be predominantly inattentive (AD), predominantly hyperactive-impulsive (HD), or both inattentive and hyperactive-impulsive (ADHD). (See APA, 2000; Bryant et al., 2008; Smith & Tyler, 2010; Turnbull et al., 2010 for a complete description of the characteristics.) Approximately 3 to 8% of the general population is identified as having ADHD (APA, 2000; Barkley, 2006; Biederman, 2005; Costello Mustillo, Erkanli, Keeler, & Angold, 2003; Smith et al., 2007) with the prevalence rate for preschoolers at 4.2% (Egger,

Kondo, & Angold, 2006). The majority of school districts report that approximately 3 in every 100 students are identified as having ADHD, with between 2 million and 4.5 million students affected nationwide (Gureasko-Moore, DuPaul, & Power, 2005). Therefore, within general education settings teachers can expect to serve 1 to 3 students with ADHD in their classrooms each year (McLeskey et al., 2010). Throughout the early school years approximately twice as many boys as girls are identified as having ADHD; however, as they progress through the educational system the ratio increases, with approximately three or more boys to every girl exhibiting these characteristics (Reiff, 2004; Smith et al., 2006).

Typically, students with the inattentive type of ADHD are identified later than those who are hyperactive, with a higher ratio of the students displaying these characteristic being girls rather than boys (Glanzman & Blum, 2007). They are not as disruptive as those who are hyperactive; thus, their needs may go unnoticed. These students frequently experience difficulties organizing tasks and completing assignments; they are easily distracted and often forgetful.

Children with ADHD face many challenges throughout their lives. Many of them are at risk for failing in school, becoming involved with substance abuse, dropping out of school, and having a high rate of conflict with their families with regard to homework and household chores (Salend & Rohena, 2003). In addition, their hyperactivity and poor social skills can negatively influence peer relationships, resulting in strained, if not altogether nonexistent friendships, leaving them feeling lonely and isolated.

• Based on the 2007–2008 Regional and National Summary published by the Gallaudet Research Institute (2008), 1,795 of the 36,710 students who are identified as deaf or hard of hearing also have ADHD. This number represents 5.6% of deaf individuals who have secondary disabilities. Although a plethora of research is being conducted with hearing children who exhibit characteristics of ADHD, there is a paucity of information regarding students who are deaf who have been identified as having this secondary disability. One can only surmise that the characteristics exhibited by students who are inattentive and/or hyperactive can be masked due to the child's deafness.

Children who are deaf may make frequent mistakes in schoolwork, experience difficulty organizing tasks and activities, and fail to follow through on instructions or complete homework. All these are characteristics of an attention-deficit disorder. However, they can also be characteristics of communication breakdowns that can occur if information is not conveyed in a manner the child can comprehend. Making an accurate diagnosis can become a formidable task for the practitioner in charge of administering the assessment battery.

Professionals in the field are acutely aware of the need to conduct research and gain additional insights into this unique population. Recognizing the needs of these students and enrolling them in programs designed to enhance their learning provides educators with potential tools, thus minimizing disruptions while promoting student success. In addition, by providing parents and significant caregivers with strategies and interventions to encourage socialization and academic learning, the child is given the opportunity to develop to his or her fullest potential.

CHILDREN WHO ARE DEAF AND HARD OF HEARING WITH ADDITIONAL DISABILITIES: PHYSICAL CONDITIONS

Legal Blindness and Uncorrected Visual Problems

Individuals with visual problems can experience difficulty with two important aspects of their vision: acuity and peripheral vision. Visual acuity is described as how well an individual can see at various distances. Normal visual acuity is defined as a person's ability to see an object 20 feet away. Therefore, a person with normal vision is 20/20. A person with 20/60 vision can see at 20 feet what a person with normal vision would be able see at 60 feet away. The other aspect of vision entails the width of a person's field of vision, referred to as peripheral vision. One uses peripheral vision to see things in the environment that are outside the direct line of vision, thus allowing one to move freely within the confines of their surroundings.

IDEA 2004 defines a *visual impairment,* including blindness, as "an impairment in vision that, even with correction, adversely affects a child's educational performance. The term includes both partial sight and blindness" (U.S. Department of Education, 2006, p. 1265). Two different definitions are used to describe visual impairment: the legal definition and the one used to describe how those with visual impairments function on a daily basis and learn about the world and their surroundings. Typically a person's visual disabilities are designated within two subgroups: those with low vision and those who are blind. The term *low vision* is used to describe individuals who can read print, generally with the assistance of optical aids, and who rely primarily on their vision for learning. Those identified with low vision may or may not be legally blind.

The term *blindness* encompasses those who are functionally blind as well as persons who are totally blind. The term *functionally blind* is used to identify individuals who typically use Braille to access printed materials and for writing purposes but rely on their functional vision for navigating their environment. Individuals who are totally blind are unable to receive meaningful information through the visual channel; instead, they rely on tactile and auditory means to glean information from their surroundings.

It is important to note that blindness can occur at any age and that each individual who experiences a visual impairment will use his or her vision differently. When a visual loss occurs at birth or during infancy the child is referred to as being congenitally blind; when the loss occurs after the age of 2 the individual is said to have adventitious blindness. The age at which visual loss occurs can have a direct bearing on the learning process. Those who lose their sight later in childhood have the advantage of storing information in their visual memory and can draw from this resource later as they embark on tasks that require visualization and the formation of visual concepts.

Keep in mind that children who can see receive a tremendous amount of information with seeming ease through the visual channel. Through observations infants learn how to move, how to identify objects, and how to organize, synthesize, and give meaning to their perceptions of the environment (Liefert, 2003). Vision also allows an individual to experience the world meaningfully and safely from a distance (Turnbull et al., 2010, p. 433). Gathering information and navigating the environment are only two of the important life skills that are at least partially accomplished through the visual channel.

Children and young adults also develop a sense of self-esteem and feelings of self-worth through their social interactions that occur throughout one's lifetime. Students who are visually impaired may feel they are left out of the social loop when their classmates discuss recent movies, video games, or other popular activities that they cannot freely access. Left out of these discussions, they may feel excluded and isolated from a very important part of school culture.

Analogous to several of the other disability groups, those with visual impairments comprise a very heterogeneous group. Including people from every socioeconomic and ethnic background, many of these individuals also have additional disabilities. Some are multiply handicapped, others are gifted, and others are both blind and deaf. Each of these children represent unique individuals who are equipped with a desire to learn, an ability to achieve, and a skill set that will enable growth and development to happen.

Individuals Who Are Deaf-Blind

IDEA 2004 defines deaf-blindness in the following way:

> "Deaf-blindness means concomitant hearing and visual impairments, the combination of which causes such severe communication and other developmental and educational needs that they cannot be accommodated in special education programs solely for children with deafness or children with blindness." (U.S. Department of Education, 2006, p. 1261)

According to Muller (2006) deaf-blindness has one of the lowest incidence rates of all disabilities; still it is one of the most diverse when describing learning profiles. Even though some members of this population have no vision and no hearing, and receive virtually no benefit from either sense, the vast majority has some residual hearing and/or vision. Of those students who are identified as being deaf-blind, approximately 50% have enough residual vision to read enlarged print, see sign language, traverse their environment, attend to some loud noises, comprehend some speech sounds, and recognize friends and family members (Miles, 2008). Furthermore, the majority of these individuals have additional disabilities that can complicate their lives and their ability to garner a quality education.

Deaf-blindness is a serious disability that impacts each individual differently, as well as those who come in daily contact with them. Because the degree and amount of vision and hearing loss are not uniform and occur in various combinations, the effect it will have on each individual will be unique to the person who experiences the dual sensory loss. (Table 13.3 highlights the complexity of disabilities included among students with deaf-blindness.)

Even though most causes of deaf-blindness are unknown, the most common reasons cited today for this condition are prematurity and heredity. Currently more than 50 genetic causes of deaf-blindness have been identified, and of those Usher syndrome (also referred to in some literature as Usher's syndrome) is one of the common causes of this condition (Keats & Lentz, 2008; National Consortium on Deaf-Blindness, 2007). Individuals born with Usher syndrome have congenital deafness, progressive blindness, and intellectual disabilities (Smith & Tyler, 2010). It is interesting to note that while nationally only 3% of the student population with deaf-blindness is due to Usher syndrome, in Louisiana between 15% and 20% of students exhibit this syndrome,

TABLE 13.3 Combinations of Disabilities Among Students with Deaf-Blindness

Vision Loss	Hearing Loss	Additional Disabilities
17% totally blind or light perception only	39% severe to profound hearing loss	66% cognitive disabilities
24% legally blind	13% moderate hearing loss	57% physical disability
21% low vision	14% mild hearing loss	38% complex health care needs
17% cortical vision impairment	6% central auditory processing disorder	9% behavioral challenges
21% other	28% other	30% other

Source: Based on information from Killoran (2007).

TABLE 13.4 Variables Associated with Deaf-Blindness

First Disability	Second Disability	Communication Modes
Congenital sensorineural loss resulting in profound hearing loss	Progressive loss in vision	Function as a deaf person, may utilize a sign system or other modes of communication
Congenital visual impairment rendering the person legally blind	Progressive hearing loss	Function as a blind person, may be skilled in Braille
Profound impairments in both disabilities		Utilize alternative modes of communication
Simultaneous progressive blindness and deafness		Communication strategies are learned in respect to the severity of the primary disability

and 30% of all deaf individuals in three Louisiana parishes (referred to in other parts of the country as counties) have Usher syndrome (Melancon, 2000, as cited in Smith & Tyler, 2010).

Each person who is deaf-blind sustains both a visual impairment and an auditory impairment. However, the degree of severity with which they occur can vary. Certain individuals can rely on some residual hearing; others experience a profound loss with partial sightedness. Some are in a transitional stage, adjusting to a second disability acquired long after the first. The severity of each of these impairments and the specific combination in which they are found will influence the types of instructional and rehabilitative techniques that are incorporated. Individuals who are deaf-blind may be categorized according to the primary disability, the severity of each of the disabilities, and time of the onset.) Table 13.4 illustrates these categories.)

Individuals Who Are Deaf with Cerebral Palsy

The term *cerebral* refers to the brain, and palsy describes a motor disability that is not a disease but, rather, can be defined as a disorder of posture and movement due to a nonprogressive lesion in the brain that occurs in the developing central nervous system. The term *cerebral palsy* was coined by Winthrop Phelps, an orthopedic surgeon and a pioneer in this field (Harryman & Warren, 1985). Further described as a neuromotor impairment that is an incurable and nonprogressive condition caused by brain injury, it usually occurs by 6 years of age. It sometimes limits the individual's ability to control muscle groups or motor functioning in specific areas of the body (Bryant et al., 2008; Pelligrino, 2007). Cerebral palsy is a result of damage primarily due to lack of oxygen to the brain. It can occur prenatally, perinatally, or immediately after the child's birth. It can also be caused by brain damage that results from an accident, brain infection, or child abuse.

Statistics indicate that 2 individuals per 1,000 people in the general population have cerebral palsy, a modest increase in prevalence throughout the past three decades (Winter, Autry, Boyle, & Yeargin-Allsopp, 2002). In addition, information provided by the United Cerebral Palsy Association indicates that approximately 0.03% of all children have cerebral palsy, although some of these cases are mild and those affected do not require any special support services (United Cerebral Palsy Association [UCP], 2001). Each of the five major types of cerebral palsy refers to the person's specific movement patterns. The first two types include spastic, which is characterized by tightness in one or more muscle groups (this type affects 70 to 80%

of the individuals who have cerebral palsy), and dyskinetic, which impacts the whole body and involves impairments in muscle tone that can vary throughout the day and week. The third and fourth types are athetoid, which involves abrupt, involuntary movements of the upper body, primarily the head, neck, face, neck and upper extremities; and ataxic, which affects balance and coordinating creating a feeling of unsteadiness that impacts standing and walking. The fifth type is mixed; it combines two or more movement patterns with no evidence that one type dominates the other (Pelligrino, 2007, as cited in Turnbull et al., 2010, p. 335).

Due to the fact that cerebral palsy is caused by brain damage, when it occurs it is sometimes associated with other disabilities. These include intellectual disabilities, visual disabilities, hearing impairments, speech and language disorders, seizures, growth abnormalities, learning disabilities, emotional or behavioral disorders, and attention-deficit/hyperactivity disorder (ADHD). It is important to note that even though some degree of intellectual and developmental disabilities are concomitant in approximately half these children, others among them are intellectually gifted. It is critical to be mindful of this and not make the false and tragic assumption that cerebral palsy and mental retardation always go together (Bryant et al., 2008; McLeskey et al., 2010). Students who are deaf and students who are hard of hearing who also have cerebral palsy function in a variety of ways. The severity of the palsy, the degree of the neuromuscular involvement, and the site of the lesion will all influence students' ability to progress educationally and independently. Educational placements are based on the multidimensional characteristics of the disorder and the individual's motivation to explore his or her potential.

Other Disabling Conditions

Other disabling conditions noted in the 2007–2008 Regional and National Summary Report of Data from the 2007–2008 Annual Survey of Deaf and Hard of Hearing Children and Youth (Gallaudet Research Institute, 2008) include orthopedic handicaps, epilepsy, and heart disorders. In relation to deafness, statistics reveal that these are low-incidence disabilities. The severity and the way in which they interface with deafness will determine the types of support services necessary for the individual to enter the mainstream of society.

Summary

Approximately one third of the population that is deaf or hard of hearing have additional disabilities. These disabilities are varied and are the result of both physical and cognitive/intellectual dysfunctions. The majority of these students are included in general education classrooms; some attend special education facilities; others become hospitalized. Within certain specialized areas, the support services are adequate; in others minimal progress has been made.

Throughout the past decade research has been conducted that sheds new insights into the domain of the deaf population with special needs. Additional research is needed within this field. Educators' interests must be sparked, and programs must be developed to ensure that the potential that lies within this unique group of individuals is tapped.

14

Preparing Personnel to Serve Individuals Who Are Deaf or Hard of Hearing

Roles and Responsibilities

In an era of high-stakes testing, meeting adequate yearly progress (AYP) goals and complying with the mandates set forth by both the Individuals with Disabilities Education Act (IDEA) and No Child Left Behind (NCLB), the old adage "the squeaky wheel gets the most oil" has again come to the forefront of education. Devoting numerous resources to students and problem areas characterized as high risk and in need of immediate improvement, there continues to be a predominant resounding theme echoed by educators and administrators. The message is straightforward and direct; those serving in an instructional capacity are charged with ensuring that all students are equipped with the essential skills required to pass standardized tests while simultaneously preparing them to compete in the larger academic arena. Monopolizing the literature with strategies, interventions, and programs, those who are achieving academic expectations or exceeding the standards are seldom described in the literature. This is especially true within the field of deaf education, where the emphasis has traditionally focused on academic failures, communication debates, and appropriate academic settings coupled with support services.

However, within this macrocosm is a group of people who are deaf and who are not merely succeeding but are excelling both academically and professionally. Identified as successful Deaf adults, they embody a constellation of individuals who have excelled academically, are comfortable self-advocating, and have mastered the art of communicating between two cultures. They represent an extremely motivated group, with high aspirations and parental support. They describe their educational experiences as being taught by teachers who believed in them and their potential and were interested in them as individuals (Luckner & Stewart, 2003). These overarching insights provide an avenue for examining the competencies and skills possessed by exemplary teachers, professionals who personify the requisite salient characteristics that when implemented will promote success among students who are deaf and hard of hearing.

What are the characteristics of master teachers? Are they the same for all teachers, regardless of student population or academic focus? Within the confines of deaf education, what are the exemplary characteristics of other support personnel who work with these students? What role do they play in advancing student success?

CHARACTERISTICS OF MASTER TEACHERS

The literature on teacher qualities is replete with a copious of articles describing the characteristics of the master teacher, with several articles describing the attributes that contribute to the efficacy of exemplary teachers. Research conducted by Salter (2001) has identified 16 characteristics or behaviors that all great teachers possess. These traits include (a) have prior knowledge of students' talents, prior experience, and needs; (b) create a safe environment where learning is emotional, intellectual, and psychological; (c) have a passion for the material and for teaching; (d) tell students the instructional goals and objectives; (d) have the ability to communicate complex ideas by breaking them down and making them understandable; (e) acknowledge that one does not know everything and that teachers do make mistakes; (f) know themselves so that they can know their students more thoroughly; (g) repeat the important parts during instruction; (h) ask good questions; (i) teach students not only the right answers but also how to think; (j) have good listening skills; (k) know what to listen for from their students; (l) encourage student interaction; (m) understand that every student learns differently and adapt accordingly; and (n) develop a trusting, solid relationship with the students (Salter, 2001, pp. 116–124).

Aylor (2003) postulates that communication is an essential element in the teaching process; it is a critical skill that one must possess to be considered an excellent teacher. Through the Communications Functions Questionnaire (CFQ), Aylor identified eight communication skills: (a) *conversational skill,* the ability to initiate and maintain enjoyable conversations; (b) *referential skill,* the ability to convey information clearly and concisely; (c) *ego-supportive skill,* the ability to make a person feel good about themselves, their goals, and their ideas; (d) *comforting skill,* the ability to help a person in times of emotional distress; (e) *conflict management skill,* the ability to reach mutually satisfying solutions to conflicts; (f) *persuasive skill,* the ability to change a person's attitudes, beliefs, and/or behaviors; (g) *narrative skill,* the ability to entertain through storytelling; and (h) *regulative skill,* the ability to help someone realize their mistakes and correct them.

Relationships

Further research conducted by Aylor (2003) recognizes that effective teachers care about their students' feelings, self-image, goals, and emotional stability. When this occurs, students report more cognitive and affective learning. According to Aylor, the two dimensions of a teacher/student relationship are content and relational. This author notes that teachers should understand that the content and relational dimensions of the relationship with their students are interdependent and that they build on each other. That fact can be used to their advantage in teaching and facilitating interactions in order to maximize learning opportunities.

Assessments

Assessments can be reported and used to benefit all parties involved (teacher, student, and parent), but the teacher must know how to use them in that manner (Anonymous, 2002). The anonymous author states, "Effective teaching of young children begins with thoughtful, appreciative, systematic observation and documentation of each child's unique qualities, strengths, and needs" (p. 15). According to this same author, well-prepared teachers should have specific assessment skills. They include (a) being able to communicate the results to parents, (b) knowing a wide range of assessment tools and approaches to align with educational goals, (c) creating opportunities to observe both formally and informally, especially with infants and toddlers, (d) having the ability to conduct, interpret, and reflect on the assessment, (e) possessing the knowledge of definitions and jargon, (f) having the ability to point out and limit test weaknesses and limitations, and (g) understanding and practicing responsible assessment techniques which are ethically grounded, collaborative, and guided by professional standards.

MASTER TEACHERS IN DEAF EDUCATION

Current educators have also explored the characteristics of the master teacher, with respect to teachers of students who are deaf or hard of hearing. The ability to communicate effectively with students, families, colleagues, and administrators has long been an established characteristic of teacher excellence in general education. Likewise, within the field of deaf education the ability to communicate with all these constituencies has been recognized as a desired trait. Because of the diverse nature of the field, effective communication skills may entail using an aural/oral approach, ASL, one of the English sign systems, Cued Speech, Total Communication, or a bilingual approach.

Throughout the history of the field numerous debates have been based on the merits of using sign language in the classroom. In the past the sign-language skills of the teacher have been considered to be the major factor in determining the effectiveness of communication in the classroom, but recent research says otherwise. According to Smith and Ramsey (2004), Long, Stinson, Kelly, and Liu (1999), and Mayer, Akamatsu, and Stewart (2002), effective communication and instruction are not solely dependent on the teachers' sign skills; rather, the manner in which they use the language as a "linguistic resource in classroom discourse" is critical (Mayer et al. p. 486) to encourage student participation. Not only do the overall sign skills of the teacher bear little weight, but the teacher's hearing status has little effect as well. The results of research conducted by Roberson and Serwatka (2000) show that although students who are deaf associate more effective behaviors with the teacher who is herself deaf, the actual achievement level of students is not affected by the hearing status of the teacher. Steering away from strict attention on the teacher's sign skills, Luckner and Howell (2002) have described the importance of the teacher's interpersonal communication skills. They believe that it is crucial that these professionals have the ability to communicate with the families of the students as well as with their colleagues and with other professionals.

As stated by Mayer et al. (2002), a threshold level of sign proficiency is needed for meaningful dialogue to occur; however, they also state the overall quality and effectiveness of the interaction, rather than the sign proficiency, is a better way to measure cogent teacher communication. Interaction is made and mediated through the use of language, signs, and other tools of communication. Mayer et al. (2002) refer to this type of purposeful, educational interaction as dialogic inquiry. Dialogic inquiry is constructed when the teacher possesses three understandings: (a) "learning is a social, interactive enterprise in which the teacher and the learner interdependently co-construct meaning; (b) this joint-meaning making is mediated through language, through classroom conversations that occur within the context of meaningful, purposeful activity; and (c) the interaction is dependent on the ability of the teacher to work in a contingently responsive manner with the student" (p. 487). The authors further state that teachers who are comfortable in their manner of communication will be more equipped to communicate effectively with their students.

When examining recent research that describes a master teacher of students who are deaf or hard of hearing, sign skills are not the primary focus of the research; however, possessing sign skills is still considered an important characteristic. Being able to sign and use this mode of communication to engage students in classroom interactions provides one of the primary avenues for learning to take place. Research conducted by Long et al. (1999) found a correlation with respect to successful interactions between teachers and their students when the teachers were found to possess higher-level skills in both expressive and receptive sign language. Student rating of communication ease was higher for teachers with higher scores on their Sign Communication Proficiency Interview such as Superior through Intermediate Plus rather than lower scores of Intermediate through Novice.

Researchers, such as Smith and Ramsey (2004), advocate for using ASL as one communication option in the classroom; their research findings indicate there are some benefits when fluent users of ASL deliver the instruction while using this language. When comparing teachers using different modes of sign communication during instruction and storytelling, they found that teachers using ASL elicited more participation from the students through question asking, classifier predicates, role-playing, and the full range of ASL morphology. "Fluent signers can smooth out rough spots and ensure coherence in the discourse" (p. 56). To fully participate and learn as active, engaged learners, students who are deaf and hard of hearing need to feel at ease in communicating with their teacher and other students through comfortable, reciprocal communication. Through this effective communication exchange, teacher/student interactions occur as a bridge to learning (Long et al., 1999).

Classroom Discourse

The ability to establish clear and comfortable communication exchanges, regardless of the mode with which they are conveyed (sign or speech), is only one of the attributes that is characteristic of effective teachers. Another is their ability to engage students in effective classroom discourse. The importance of classroom discourse is seen throughout much of the research. Positive occurrences result from meaningful discourse, such as learning to make meaning and sense of the world through the process of applying higher-level thinking skills (Mayer et al., 2002). A teacher must possess and incorporate a myriad of skills and behaviors while teaching in order to facilitate classroom discourse. Smith and Ramsey (2004) believe that the classroom atmosphere must be flexible and free and, to accomplish this, experienced teachers, exhibit less-controlling behaviors with a relaxed attitude while maintaining control and showing an ability to prevent problems. Smith and her colleagues (2004) discovered a high negative correlation between the amount of control assumed by the teacher and the amount of complex language used by the students. However, students whose language skills are inadequate can pose problems and additional challenges for the teacher who is attempting to maintain this type of classroom atmosphere.

In addition, with respect to communication as it relates to discourse, Smith and her colleagues list several strategies and skills that excellent teachers possess. They (a) encourage further comments while boosting student confidence and extending interaction, (b) develop increased sensitivity to students' perceptions of the quality of communication in class, (c) give greater attention to variations in communication needs of the students, and (d) put greater effort into developing teaching strategies for effective interactive communication (Smith & Ramsey, 2004).

Use of Teaching Strategies

To be considered a master teacher of students who are deaf or hard of hearing, certain teaching behaviors and strategies are encouraged, if not expected, that relate to communication while instructing students. One approach advocated by Akamatsu, Stewart, and Mayer (2004) encourages employing a constructivist teaching approach. This teaching approach utilizes communication that relies on symbols and signs, which allows students to eventually become independent in regulating their own language and behaviors. Instructional conversations can be used in the classroom to "support, guide, and assist the learner in achieving fuller participation and understanding" (Mayer et al., 2002, p. 487). Greenspan (2003) delves deeper and with more specificity by stating the importance of using multiple channels to communicate with the child during instruction, including incorporating extensive visual support. Mayer et al. (2002) describe other exemplary practices in order to facilitate language and communication that include, but are not limited to, (a) taking the learners' best attempt as the starting place, (b) inviting suggestions and opinions, (c) requesting explanations, clarifications, justifications, and amplifications, (d) encouraging learners to take risks and express their own points of view, and (e) shaping instruction into meaningful and purposeful language activity (Mayer et al., 2002, p. 490). They sum up exemplary teacher communicative practice in instruction and discourse stating, "Teachers who are responsive to their students, and engaged in joint meaning-making, are constantly stretching to reach the learner's cognitive and linguistic ground" (Mayer et al., 2002, p. 489).

Research conducted by Roberson, Woosley, Seabrooks, and Williams (2004) focuses on measuring the effectiveness of teachers of students who are deaf or hard of hearing by using two broad categories: *teacher* quality, the characteristics and skills teachers bring to the classroom, and *teaching* quality, how they teach once they are in the classroom. Some of the characteristics and skills that are encompassed by teacher quality are preparation, proper assessment-data collection, knowledge of content, ability to provide evidence of pedagogical knowledge, and demonstration that their instruction actually has an effect on student learning.

The major indicator of excellent teaching quality is the presence of academic responding that has been positively correlated with achievement on standardized tests. Academic responding is defined as "the active and appropriate student behaviors that are made in direct response to an academic task, teacher command, or teacher prompt" (Roberson et al., 2004, p. 406).

In addition, research reported by Mayer et al. (2002) and Greenspan (2003) discusses the effect the teacher-created environment and atmosphere have on student learning. Education is a "collaborative enterprise in which the teacher takes a leadership role" (Mayer et al., 2002, p. 486) in creating and providing an atmosphere where students learn from each other and from the teacher while engaging in joint activities. Therefore, the atmosphere must be trusting, flexible, and controlled by the teacher. The results from the study conducted by Greenspan (2003) found that the teacher must create a nurturing, supportive environment where all children benefit by focusing on being patient and understanding each other.

Teacher Attitudes

A body of research exists pertaining to the attitudes that teachers bring with them into the classroom. It reveals that teachers' attitudes toward students and other teachers during the teaching process play a tremendous role in the effectiveness of their teaching and student outcomes. A study conducted by Luckner and Muir (2001) found that excellent teachers have high expectations for their students and are not afraid to challenge them in situations where they might fail. Their findings revealed that when this occurs students attain more skills in dealing with the hearing world and feel more at ease when interacting with their peers who can hear. Within this same study Luckner and Muir interviewed students who were deaf or hard of hearing and were considered successful; their findings further indicated that these successful students were aware and appreciative of the help, support, and high expectations of their teachers.

Teacher Behaviors and Competencies

Woolsey, Harrison, and Gardner (2004) stated that for students who are deaf or hard of hearing to achieve parallel academic levels comparable to their peers who can hear, they must have contact with teachers whose behaviors will accelerate their learning. Further research conducted by Luckner and Carter (2001) have investigated the behaviors teachers need to possess to effectively teach this student population. The following top 10 behaviors identified pertain to general teaching techniques rather than on focusing on any specific disability area: (a) use techniques for modifying instructional methods and materials for students with a variety of special needs, (b) use approaches to create positive learning environments for individuals with a variety of special needs, (c) teach students to use thinking, problem solving, and other cognitive strategies to meet their individual needs, (d) establish a consistent classroom routine for students, (e) design learning environments that are multisensory and that encourage active participation by learners in a variety of group and individual learning activities, (f) provide opportunities for the learner to develop basic concepts through participation in meaningful and motivating real-life experiences, (g) integrate academic instruction, effective education, and behavior management for individual students and groups of students, (h) develop effective behavior support plans, (i) provide opportunities for the learner to actively explore and experience common objects that learners with vision and hearing learn about incidentally, and (j) help parents and other professionals to understand the impact of various disabilities on learning and experience (Luckner & Carter, p. 14).

Luckner conducted an additional study with Howell (2002) in which they identified other disability-specific skills and knowledge. They stated that the teachers who have specialized in deaf education must be knowledgeable about and skilled with technologies such as hearing aids, cochlear implants, and FM systems. Furthermore, they need to be able to provide troubleshooting and auditory training if needed. Additional skills deemed necessary pertained to the ability to collaborate and effectively work as a multidisciplinary team member while contributing to the design and implementation of the Individualized Education Program (IEP).

Further research conducted by Scheetz and Martin (2008) found that teachers who teach students who are deaf or hard of hearing share a set of mutual qualities exhibited by general education teachers. Responses to electronic questionnaires completed by administrators, experienced teachers (e.g., those with 3 or more years of experience), college and university faculty, and follow-up interviews with representatives from each constituency provided data with respect to what constitutes a master teacher. (Table 14.1 provides a list of the characteristics, skills, and abilities that consistently emerged from the three groups.)

Of the behaviors teachers need to possess to effectively teach this student population (see the preceding list), the first five are directly related to the literature and thus show a consistency with the field of general education; however, the remaining items in the list are unique to deaf education.

Research further indicates that when examining the factors that influence student success, the following factors impact student learning: small class size and school; parent education; background factors such as poverty, language, and family characteristics; and teacher qualifications. The National Center for Education Statistics (1999) concluded that small classes and the school were the least important of the factors, parent education accounted for 25% in terms of being influential, and teacher qualifications, at 40%, were the most important factor in influencing student achievement.

TABLE 14.1 Characteristics of a Master Teacher of Students Who Are Deaf

Characteristics of a Master Teacher of Students Who Are Deaf
Strong communication skills
Ability to modify the learning environment
Application of cognitive strategies
Preparation in content
Maintenance of high expectations; challenging students
Remaining up-to-date and open to new ideas
Helping students become autonomous
Being a collaborator
Being certified in deaf education
Showing enthusiasm
Reflecting on one's practice

Source: Scheetz & Martin (2008).

Teaching is a dynamic and complex process. Those engaged in this professional endeavor must possess subject matter competency and comprehend the purpose of the curriculum; they must have a firm understanding of how students learn and develop and how they acquire and use language. Furthermore, they must possess exceptional classroom management skills, be mindful of diverse learners, excel at engaging students in the learning process, and hold high expectations for all students, recognizing that each one has the potential to achieve academically. Teachers exemplify role models for their students; through their passion for learning and teaching, they can instill in their students an intrinsic motivation for them to do their best. Above all, teachers should foster critical thinking skills in their students and be reflective practitioners, good listeners, and passionate about teaching.

Teachers who have specialized in deaf education must possess the same qualities that have been described as important characteristics for general education teachers. In addition, they must be knowledgeable in ASL and the English sign systems and cognizant of the linguistics of both ASL and English. This unique group of teachers must be familiar with specialized curricula, informal and formal assessment procedures, and how to make appropriate accommodations and adaptations for this population. Furthermore, they should become experts responsible for providing assistive technology supports that allow access to academic content, thereby helping to rectify problems and barriers that lead to underachievement (Luft, 2008).

Teachers instruct students who are deaf or hard of hearing in a variety of settings and frequently across more than one setting. Some teach in residential or day schools for the deaf; others serve in a consultant role; still others serve in both resource rooms and as itinerant teachers, providing both direct instruction and indirect support. Within each of these settings, teachers working with this student population continuously rely on a diverse set of skills, thus allowing them to effectively respond to the various demands and expectations that are placed on them in each environment.

What are the essential skills these teachers need to acquire in order to successfully teach students who are deaf and hard of hearing in each of these settings?

Schools for the Deaf or Separate Schools

Until the mid 1970s the majority of students who were deaf were educated within residential schools for the deaf or special day schools designed to serve this population. Between 1977 and

1997 the number of students who received their education in this setting declined as the majority of them began to receive their education in their local neighborhood schools. Currently, under the Individuals with Disabilities Education Act (IDEA), students served in these special environments must demonstrate academic or other deficiencies of such magnitude that they require full-time placement in a segregated setting with a teacher trained specifically to work with them. Although residential schools are the most restrictive, they provide a milieu for student socialization and an opportunity to teach a group of relatively homogenous students who are deaf in a single classroom. Teachers instruct their students through a mutual mode of communication shared by both the teacher and the students. Furthermore, teachers working within the confines of the residential or day school environment must be highly qualified to teach in their content area, proficient in the mode of communication endorsed by the school, and equipped to deal with the students who arrive at their doorstep after failing to achieve academically in their less restrictive, neighborhood school.

Teachers in this setting identify curriculum learning goals and sequences; select materials, methods, and resources that will be used; and determine the learning strategies that are most appropriate for the individual students enrolled in each of their classes. Sometimes they work independently; other times they may collaborate with an instructor from another grade level as part of an educational team (Johnson, 2004; Luft, 2008; Stinson & Kluwin, 2003).

Teachers in Resource Rooms and Separate Classes

Teachers who are certified in deaf education also work in resource rooms and in separate classes, both of which are located in neighborhood schools where the majority of the students can hear. The primary difference between the two types of rooms is determined by the amount of time students who are deaf are assigned to them. Students attending separate classes spend the majority, or all of, their instructional time with other students who are deaf in one classroom under the auspices of a teacher trained specifically to work with them. In contrast, those attending resource rooms typically spend the majority of their day in the general classroom and go to resource rooms only for selected subjects for a portion of their day (Stinson & Kluwin, 2003).

Within resource rooms, teachers of students who are deaf or hard of hearing provide direct instruction that often consists of remedial instruction, pre-teaching or post-teaching the content that is provided in the general education classroom. They also function as tutors when appropriate. Furthermore, resource room teachers frequently address IEP literacy or learning needs and provide students with strategies to promote overall classroom success (Luckner, 2006; Stinson & Kluwin, 2003). Developing materials specifically designed to supplement learning, their major objective is to adhere to the curriculum goals and sequence prescribed by the general education classroom teacher. Furthermore, they are responsible for addressing the student's identified needs with respect to communication, literacy, content, and remediation as well as any other academic areas. All of this occurs through the use of both direct and indirect instruction (Luft, 2008).

The Co-Teacher or Collaborative Teacher

Co-teaching as described by Cook and Friend (1995) occurs when "two or more professionals deliver substantive instruction to a diverse or blended group of students (p. 2). Within the field of special education this collaboration occurs between general and special educators who work together to meet the needs of a diverse population of students. Within these co-taught classrooms teachers share in the planning, presentation, evaluation, and management of the classroom to provide integrated services for all students regardless of their learning needs (Gately & Gately, 2001). (See Table 14.2 for a description of what co-teaching is and is not.) According to Keefe,

TABLE 14.2 A Look at What Co-Teaching Students Who Are Deaf and Hard of Hearing (D/HH) Is and Is Not

Co-Teaching Students Who Are Deaf and Hard of Hearing Is...	Co-Teaching Students Who Are Deaf and Hard of Hearing Is Not...
Two or more teachers working together as peers, professionals, and collaborators. This can include a general education teacher and a teacher of student who are deaf or hard of hearing (D/HH)	A teacher and a teacher's aid; or a teacher and a paraprofessional; or a general education teacher and a teacher of students who are D/HH with one viewing the other as a paraprofessional
When all students are collectively taught in the same classroom, simultaneously using differentiated instruction and appropriate accommodations for students who are D/HH	When the teacher of students who are D/HH pulls them out of the general education classroom on a regular basis for instruction
When both teachers collaborate and plan lessons together. The general education teacher is the content specialist, while the teacher of students who are D/HH might be a content expert, as well as, an expert on individualizing and adapting the curriculum for this population of students	When the general education teacher plans all of the lessons and the teacher of students who are D/HH walks into the room and inquires what the students will be doing on the particular day
When both teachers provide instruction in the course content, planned lessons, grade homework, and facilitate activities for all students	When the teacher of students who are D/HH sits by this population of students, while the general education teacher delivers the content of the lesson and administers the activities
When teachers make maximum use of having two teachers in the room. They are both actively engaged with the students, and provide instruction through the use of various teaching models	When the teacher of students who are D/HH takes turns with the general education teacher of being responsible for the class so the other teacher can use the time to catch up on paper work
When both teachers jointly assess and evaluate student progress.	When there is a division of labor: the general education teacher grades "his" students and the teacher of students who are D/HH grades "her students
When both teachers maintain open and honest communication, reflect on the progress and process, offering each other feedback and professional suggestions that will enhance the overall teaching situation and classroom learning experience for all students	When the teachers get frustrated with each other and vent in the teacher's lounge, or when one teacher becomes overpowering and mandates what the teacher should do and how she should do it

Moore, and Duff (2004), teachers involved in successful collaborative experiences know their personal strengths and weaknesses, and they are in touch with their own perceptions regarding the co-teaching environment. In addition, they know their teaching partner and the students, and they are familiar with daily classroom routines, methods, and materials utilized for instruction. Furthermore, they can take over teaching for a colleague if called upon to do so.

Pivotal to the success of co-teaching are planning early and allowing time throughout the school year for ongoing collaboration to occur. Teachers need this time to determine what and how they will teach, communicate about specific student needs, and discuss necessary modifications to the curriculum (Dieker, 2001; Murawski, 2002). Co-teaching is a developmental process. When two teachers co-teach together for the first time, they generally progress through three stages. These include the beginning stage, characterized by guarded, careful communication; the compromising stage, exemplified when each teacher engages in give-and-take communication, recognizing that they must "give up" something to "get" something that they want; and the collaborating stage, depicted by open communication and interaction, with mutual admiration for each other (Gately & Gateley, 2001, p. 42).

The co-teaching model is designed to allow students who are deaf or hard of hearing to remain in the general education classroom with both a certified teacher who is specifically trained to work with them and a general education teacher working in concert with each other. Depending on the school district, student population, and specific needs of both the students and the general education teacher, the teacher trained to work with students who are deaf may work with one general education teacher or with several different teachers representing the entire span of the curriculum (Antia & Kreimeyer, 2003). While working in this capacity, the teacher with deaf education certification and the general education faculty collaborate on lesson plans, activities, strategies, and interventions. They all assume a variety of roles and responsibilities that include teaching the full class, engaging students in small group work, providing mini-lessons, and delivering individual instruction (Luft, 2008).

When instruction is delivered collaboratively and effectively, the general education teacher provides content knowledge and is responsible for selecting the standards, objectives, and assessments. In addition, they identify the texts, materials, and resources to deliver the lesson. The teacher who is certified in deaf education contributes specific instructional strategies, adaptations, and accommodations, including technology support deemed appropriate for fostering learning. This provides access for the student or students, thus affording them the opportunity to participate fully within the general education classroom experience (Antia, Stinson, & Gaustad, 2002; Friend & Bursuck, 2006; Murawski & Dieker, 2004, as cited in Luft, 2008). Within these settings, the pace of the class is established by the overall progress of the class (Kluwin, Gonsher, Silver, & Samuels, 1996) with support services provided for students who are deaf or hard of hearing.

Co-teaching can be both demanding and rewarding for both deaf education and general education teachers, especially when they are each actively involved in the process. The success of this model hinges on allocating time for collaborative planning, designating a team leader, establishing mutually defined goals, and spending adequate time together (Kluwin et al., 1996; Kreimeyer, Crooke, Drye, Egbert, & Klein, 2000, as cited in Marschark & Spencer, 2003).

The Itinerant Teacher

Bullard (2003) defines the itinerant teacher, certified in deaf education, as a teacher who generally provides direct services to students who are deaf or hard of hearing and consulting services to classroom teachers and other professionals. Although itinerant teachers usually work with one student individually, they can be found working with groups of students, comprised of those with varying degrees of hearing loss as well as those who can hear. Furthermore, services can be furnished inside or outside the regular classroom; due to the low incidence of this population, itinerant teachers must be prepared to work with students enrolled in all grades and attending several different schools in their catchment area.

Smith (1997) describes the job of an itinerant teacher as being extremely diverse. Requiring the teacher to use her car as a traveling office, Smith captures the role of these teachers in the following way:

> "There is no luxury of classroom storage space, because in most cases we have no single classroom! We take our materials and supplies with us wherever we go. We teach and consult wherever each school's staff can find room for us. Sometimes we get lucky and can work in a real classroom. More often we end up working at a table in the supply room, or just making ourselves and our student comfortable in the hallway. . . . In addition to having little control over where she will work, the itinerant sometimes has little influence over what will be taught, and when. The curriculum and implementing lesson plans are determined by the school and the regular classroom teacher, whereas the itinerant is only a visiting professional." (p. 7)

The role of the itinerant is complex. Required to possess expertise within the field of deaf education, exceptional flexibility, and communication and organizational skills, success is often determined by the teacher's ability to understand what her role is and is not, while recognizing how others perceive that role. General education teachers, parents, and administrators may have inaccurate perceptions or expectations of the itinerant teacher who is certified in deaf education. Frequently, the onus of dispelling these misperceptions falls on the shoulders of the itinerant teacher. The ability to develop strong consulting skills is the most essential skill an itinerant must possess (Bullard, 2003, p. 23).

Kluwin, Morris, and Clifford (2004) capitulate that effective itinerant teachers are ones who "can generate a positive composite image of their role as itinerants and are then able to interact on the basis of that image" (p. 62). While conducting interviews with working itinerants and observing their daily routines, they ascertained that these teachers experienced considerable variation in their school settings and expended a substantial amount of time traveling from school to school (sites visited ranged from 4 to 12, with visits per week totaling between 12 and 19). Teachers described the importance of having resources at each school site and across sites. Kluwin et al. further emphasized the need to have a desire to become an itinerant teacher. Attitude was stressed, commenting that it is critical that one possess a love of teaching this way for it to become rewarding and successful. Anticipating problems before they arise, maintaining contact with key personnel in each school (secretaries, janitors, and administrative assistants were frequently mentioned), and maintaining visibility within each setting was of utmost importance in order to sustain credibility. Other key comments included working to fit in and being viewed as a contributing member of the team. Itinerant teachers need to be able to "weave all of the pieces into a seamless pattern of behavior that permits her to operate within the system, not against it" (p. 71).

Yarger and Luckner (1999) provide a list of suggestions for itinerant teachers. These include obtaining experience in the classroom, remaining flexible and open-minded, recognizing that being a team member entails celebrating successes as well as reevaluating disappointments, responding to students on an individualized basis, and becoming an effective team member. Further attributes that foster success include being knowledgeable of a variety of teaching methodologies and sign systems/languages, being professional both in conduct and writing, maintaining healthy boundaries, developing strong organizational skills, and being gentle with oneself (p. 313).

Teachers certified in deaf education entering the field today find they are faced with mixed-ability groupings of students, representing a wide spectrum of languages, communication modalities, ethnic backgrounds, socioeconomic levels, and varying educational and social experiences. Approximately four out of every five children with a hearing loss receive their education in public school settings, while others obtain their instruction in residential or day schools for the deaf. With newborn screening techniques being used to identify infants with hearing loss, and cochlear implants on the rise, the landscape of deaf education is definitely undergoing a metamorphosis. Teachers joining the ranks with their fellow professionals will need to be equipped to interface with general education teachers while recognizing how to modify instructional practices in all classrooms, thus promoting student learning and ultimately academic success.

EDUCATIONAL INTERPRETERS: CHARACTERISTICS OF EFFECTIVE COMMUNICATION FACILITATORS

With the advent of legislation that prompted the mainstream/inclusion movement, schools were charged with providing equal access to students with disabilities who would receive their instruction in general education classrooms. When describing accessibility for students who are deaf and hard of hearing, these learners frequently require accommodations that may include FM and sound field systems; real-time captioning such as C-Print, Typewell, or CART; and tutors, note takers, sign language interpreters, and transliterators. Of all these services, the field of interpreting and transliterating, generally described in the literature under the umbrella term of *interpreting,* has, without a doubt, received the most attention.

The field of educational interpreting has undergone tremendous change. This is due to the complexities involved in the interpreting process, the vital role the interpreter plays in facilitating communication, and the impact the interpreter's skill set has on students' access to the curriculum. In order for interpreters to work effectively in K–12 settings, they must acquire a distinct and specific set of skills.

What do these skills entail? Is the skill set the same for an elementary school interpreter as for a postsecondary-level interpreter? What is the difference between a signer, an interpreter, and a teacher of students who are deaf or hard of hearing?

The Role of the Educational Interpreter

According to the Standard Practice Paper for Interpreting in Educational Settings (K–12), prepared and disseminated by the Registry of Interpreters for the Deaf (RID, 2010), the role of the educational interpreter is defined as follows:

> "Educational interpreters facilitate communication between deaf students and others, including teachers, service providers, and peers within the educational environment. Many educational environments have a communication policy which should be clearly defined to the interpreter applicant. The educational team may be composed of school personnel and parents and may be more structured in some districts than others. The educational interpreter is a member of the educational team and should be afforded every opportunity to attend meetings where educational guidelines are discussed concerning students who are provided services by that interpreter." (p. 2)

Educational interpreters facilitate communication in a variety of settings, both inside and outside the classroom. Throughout the course of a school year they interpret for traditional lectures and classroom activities; field trips; assemblies; club meetings; counseling sessions; athletic practices and competitions; meetings with counselors, principals, and other administrators; and a variety of other extracurricular events. They may serve one or more students, in one or multiple schools, across a wide discipline of academic subjects. Furthermore, they may need to use ASL with one student while relying on contact signing with another.

What qualifications do educational interpreters need to possess in order to effectively perform their role as communication facilitators?

Interpreters: Skills Needed to Become Effective Facilitators of Communication

First and foremost, those professionals serving in the role of educational interpreters must have an exceptional command of both English and ASL. Recognizing that interpreters are professional communicators, they must have an extensive vocabulary and understanding of the linguistics of both languages and a clear understanding of the communication process. Interpreting is interactive in nature, and those functioning as interpreters must be able to accurately express what they hear in a meaningful, visual, conceptual language so that message equivalence can be achieved. Furthermore, it is critical that they are adroit at comprehending ASL and/or messages expressed through one of the sign systems, that they are capable of vocalize these messages in English while adhering to the nuances, idiomatic phrases, and terminology appropriate for the subject being discussed.

Communication is dynamic and interactive, allowing individuals to send and receive multiple and overlapping messages. Transmitted through words, facial expressions, gestures, and body posture, the overall intent and meaning of the message is conveyed through nonverbal elements. Within the English language, only 6% of the meaning is found in the words, 39% of the meaning is imparted through vocal intonation, and 55% of the message is expressed through the accompanying gestures, body language, and facial expressions that are used by the speaker/signer (Burgoon, 1994; Manusov, 1995; Hall & Hall, 1989, as cited in Humphrey & Alcorn, 2001). It is the interpreters' responsibility to decode these nonverbal elements while conveying the intent of the speaker. However, if and when this does not occur the message will not be expressed in the same way that was intended by the sender. To become effective communication facilitators, interpreters must develop analytical skills and the ability to listen carefully while maintaining an exceptional command of both languages.

According to Taylor (1993), an interpreter must acquire 59 skills to achieve equivalency in meaning between the source and the target language. The skills are organized into eight categories that focus on the following major features: fingerspelling, numbers, vocabulary, classifiers/size and shape specifiers (SASSes), structuring space, grammar, interpreting, composure, and appearance (p. 8). While many of these competencies are specifically related to accurate sign production, others address sign concepts while emphasizing the importance of selecting signs that match the meaning (semantics) between the source and target languages. Additional features address sign space while stressing the importance of establishing spatial relationships accurately and consistently. Errors in spatial referencing often result in confusion over where people or objects are located and who said what to whom as well as the juxtaposition of these objects.

Taylor (1993) further elucidates the fact that interpreters must develop a persona of composure and maintain a professional appearance while serving in this role. Remaining mindful of the fact that interpreters are responsible for conveying the speaker's meaning and intent, and not the reactions or feelings of the interpreter, it is critical that they keep their personal feelings in check and refrain from using gestures or displaying facial expressions that are not part of the speaker's message and that, if added, would skew the meaning (p. 71). Professional appearance denotes that one wears plain colors that contrast with one's skin tone; small, if any jewelry; neutral or light colors, if any, of nail polish; and refrain from any hair styles or makeup that could be viewed as distracting.

All qualified interpreters adhere to a code of professional conduct established jointly by the National Association of the Deaf (NAD) and the Registry of Interpreters for the Deaf, Inc. (RID), two organizations that maintain high standards of professionalism and ethical conduct for interpreters. Referred to as the NAD-RID Code of Professional Conduct (CPC), the following seven tenets, described within the document, are designed to serve as guiding principles for interpreters:

1. Interpreters adhere to standards of confidential communication.
2. Interpreters possess the professional skills and knowledge required for the specific interpreting situation.
3. Interpreters conduct themselves in a manner appropriate to the specific interpreting situation.
4. Interpreters demonstrate respect for consumers.
5. Interpreters demonstrate respect for colleagues, interns, and students of the profession.
6. Interpreters maintain ethical business practices.
7. Interpreters engage in professional development. (The Registry of Interpreters for the Deaf, 2005)

Sign language interpreters are employed in a variety of settings, with 85% of them obtaining full-time employment within the public school setting. How are these interpreters evaluated? How do school districts know these individuals have mastered the prerequisite skills to facilitate communication in the classroom?

Evaluation Systems for Sign Language Interpreters

Historically, at the national level, both the Registry of Interpreters for the Deaf, Inc., and the National Association of the Deaf have administered separate evaluations and certified qualified sign language interpreters. In 2005 these organizations combined resources and developed a national interpreting certification evaluation referred to as the NIC. (See www.rid.org for a complete description of the history of the evaluation system.) Previous evaluations, and the current one administered by NIC, have been designed to evaluate the skill set of those wanting to work as interpreters, using adult role models in a variety of everyday situations (vocational, social, educational). However, none of these evaluations included interpreting in the K–12 setting, using young children rather than adults for the signing role models.

As a result the Educational Interpreter Performance Assessment (EIPA) was developed to evaluate interpreting that would transpire within an actual classroom setting. Utilizing children and youth who are deaf within various classroom settings, the EIPA evaluates more than ASL or one type of sign system or vocabulary; rather, it examines a broad range of skills and ascertains whether an interpreter is actively involved in analyzing the incoming message. "The interpreter should be aware of the speaker's goals and integrate the speaker's use of prosody into their signed or spoken interpretations" (Schick & Williams, 2004, p. 24). It is critical that they be able to convey the "big picture" rather than just producing a stream of unrelated signs or words.

Several states throughout the United States use the EIPA to evaluate their educational interpreters. Currently 13 of the states have established a 3.5 on the 5-point EIPA scale as a minimum requirement to work in public schools. Three states have set a minimum requirement of 4.0, and other states require a much lower standard of a 3.0 (Schick, in preparation, p. 22, as cited in Witter-Merithew & Johnson, 2005). Although the scope of this chapter does not allow for an in-depth discussion of the EIPA, those interested in obtaining additional information are encouraged to go to the following website: www.classroominterpreting.org, which provides an in-depth description of this evaluation system.

Educational interpreters work in a variety of settings. Some interpret for young children in the primary grades; others are employed in elementary and middle schools; still others work in high school settings. With the influx of students who are deaf attending college today, several interpreters are hired by postsecondary institutions, including vocational/technical programs, to serve this population.

What are considered best practices in each of these settings?

BEST PRACTICES WHEN INTERPRETING IN THE PRIMARY GRADES

Interpreters wanting to work with pre–K, kindergarten, or first- and possibly second-grade students must have a firm understanding of child development and the developmental changes that take place during childhood. Children who are deaf or hard of hearing arrive at school exhibiting a wide range of competencies within the English language; although some will have acquired a working vocabulary, others will begin their educational journey with virtually no, or very limited, comprehension of the English language. As a result, the interpreter as well as the teacher of students who are deaf will, for all intents and purposes, function as a language role model for these children. By communicating with the child on a daily basis, recognizing the student's existing language, and introducing new information into this knowledge base, the interpreter is facilitating language development (Seal, 2004).

According to Luetke-Stahlman (1992), working within the confines of the primary grades presents additional challenges for the educational interpreter. In addition to becoming role models for both languages, these professionals frequently assist their young pupils in putting on their coats and escorting them to the bus while engaging them in conversation. Interpreters must further possess the innate ability to convey affect, thus representing the dynamic features of the source language. They must further be able to understand what the child is really saying by comprehending his or her signs and the way the signs are produced. When the interpreter can clearly interpret what the child is signing and convey the affect as well as the content of the message to those who can hear, the stage is set to enhance the child's development of language and promote overall thinking skills.

BEST PRACTICES WHEN INTERPRETING IN THE ELEMENTARY AND MIDDLE SCHOOL SETTING

As children transition from elementary to middle school they become engaged in numerous relationships that involve peers, teachers, school personnel, and educational interpreters. Peer relationships may involve students who are also deaf, students who are hard of hearing, or students who can hear. They may form relationships with teachers, independent of the interpreter or with the assistance of the interpreter. Without a doubt, the hallmark of this developmental stage can be captured in the dynamics involved in each of these relationships and social exchanges.

Interpreters working in this setting need to develop an effective mechanism for interpreting in this social milieu. Determining an effective way to decide how and when to interpret "side conversations" and "in-group exchanges" plays a significant role in enhancing or diminishing the relationship between the student who is deaf and the classroom interpreter. In addition to facilitating or enabling peer relationships, the successful classroom interpreter takes time to attend to the communication style(s) of the teacher or teachers, thus enabling teachers to signal to the student when it is appropriate to interrupt and transition from one activity to the next while continuously keeping the student informed of the emotional climate in the room (Seal, 2004, p. 83–84).

Middle school interpreters, in particular, must become familiar with the slang, jargon, and phrases used by students who can hear. When voicing for a middle school student who is deaf, it is imperative that the word choices, phraseology, and sentence structures that are spoken reflect a typical preteen or teenager. By taking on the student's voice and adhering to the proper register, the interpreter must deliver responses to both peers and teachers that are characteristic of what the student is signing. Any hesitancy, sense of caution or confidence, or indications of cockiness should be conveyed.

Beginning in elementary school and continuing throughout middle school, emphasis is placed on the curriculum with an estimated 75% of classroom time being focused on textbooks (Shepherd & Ragan, 1992, as cited in Seal, 2004). Content vocabulary is often complex and ambiguous, challenging the interpreter to search for appropriate sign choices and structures to convey the intended meaning. Frequently interpreters are required to find technical signs that are representative of course content. Capitalizing on their own broad knowledge base, successful interpreters rely on their own expert knowledge of both ASL and English so they can produce the most effective and meaningful interpretation possible. It is not uncommon for middle school interpreters to be asked to interpret classes that deal with everything from algebra to Shakespeare. Drawing from strategies that stem from speech and sign, interpreters must determine which concepts require expansion, restructuring, spatial referencing, or nonmanual markers. All of this must be determined within seconds so that effective communication can take place in real time.

To do their work effectively as communication facilitators, interpreters must be given textbooks for the classes they will be interpreting and a planning period. Like other professionals, they need time to become familiar with the content, determine what signs will most effectively convey the meaning, and review any materials that have been provided by the teacher (i.e., lesson plans, worksheets, outlines, etc.). Although interpreters do not need to master the same level of comprehension that a student must demonstrate while learning, it is still imminent that they achieve a level of comprehension that is required for them to interpret accurately and with meaning (Seal, 2004, p. 93). Exemplary interpreters make good use of their planning time by reading class materials, conferring with other interpreters—especially when questions arise regarding sign choices—and reflecting on how they can use their discipline to most effectively convey course content.

Interpreters provide a vital link in the educational process. When they excel at their job everyone benefits and the access provided to students can be tremendous. However, in the event interpreters do not possess the necessary skill set to equalize communication, they become either a weak or broken link and can negatively impact the learning process. When student(s) who are deaf are prevented from gaining access to the curriculum, they are often unaware of critical information and content they are missing. If they are denied opportunities to master the foundation needed for future academic endeavors, they often arrive at high school lagging behind their peers even though they are bright young adults.

BEST PRACTICES WHEN INTERPRETING IN HIGH SCHOOL SETTINGS

Whereas interpreters working in middle school settings must become competent in learning how and when to interpret social exchanges, those employed in U.S. high schools must possess the trait of flexibility or quickly acquire it. Students who are deaf or hard of hearing attending mainstreamed and included classes represent a heterogeneous group characterized by variability in social skills, communication, motivation, and academic abilities and enter high school with perceptions of who they are and what they can accomplish. Some arrive at the secondary level with supportive families who encourage them to participate in extracurricular activities and achieve academically. Others arrive with or without a great deal of parental support, bringing with them a history of academic struggles and failures, leaving them feeling very inadequate to compete at the high school level.

Interpreters employed to work at the secondary school level find their services are needed for everything from AP English to auto mechanics. Some spend the majority of their days interpreting vocational classes, which may be extremely hands-on in nature; others find they are immersed in courses that require them to impose their own higher order thinking skills on the material being studied. To render messages faithfully and equivalently, they must rely on perception, memory, semantic chunking, lexical retrieval, message analysis, visualization, and imagery to convey the information contained in the material (Kanda & Colonomos, 1990). Prior to these assignments they are required to examine the material, paying particular attention to phrases and sentences that might require restructuring, semantic chunking, and text analysis.

As high school students develop cognitively and are challenged academically, their ability to engage in the learning process changes tremendously. Interpreters working within these settings must frequently engage in critical thinking during the process of interpreting. Often faced with the challenge of laboratory settings, foreign language classes, and college preparatory coursework, they must be prepared to voice for students who are academically prepared to compete alongside their hearing peers. While preparing for these assignments, interpreters pay particular attention to the vocabulary, academic content, and related themes that might become the topics for discussion. Always striving to equalize communication, they continually look for ways to enhance their skills thus affording students who are deaf and hard of hearing full access to the curriculum.

BEST PRACTICES WHEN INTERPRETING IN POSTSECONDARY SETTINGS

Students enrolled in postsecondary settings represent the same diversity as their hearing counterparts. Some arrive on college campuses highly motivated with solid strategies for learning; others attend classes because they are not ready to find a job and have yet to decide what they want to do. Some apply for admission and later attend because their friends have enrolled and they decide to give it a try. There are those who will be very attentive in class; while others will convey an air of disinterest as they go through the daily routine of attending classes. College students typically rely on a host of support services while completing their academic or vocational degrees. Some rely solely on sign language interpreters; others utilize the services of a C-Print or CART captionist in addition to interpreting services. Requests for services are as diverse as the courses in which students enroll.

Sign language interpreters working at the postsecondary level are expected to demonstrate exemplary expressive and receptive skills. Individuals working in this capacity may discover that they will be voicing for undergraduate as well as graduate students who are engaged in lively classroom discussions and are responsible for classroom presentations. Developing the skills to voice effectively for these students requires mastering a postsecondary-level vocabulary, expanding one's current understanding of course content, and enhancing one's discourse skills. Ensuring that students who are deaf and hard of hearing can engage in typical classroom exchanges with little, if any, attention being drawn to the classroom interpreter provides a strong indicator that accessibility is being achieved.

Interpreting in higher education can be extremely challenging as well as rewarding. Course content coupled with students, some of whom are proverbial language learners, create unique situations that require interpreters to reflect on the most effective way they can convey the speaker's message. Furthermore, the diversity exhibited among students, faculty, course content, and class expectations directly impacts the services provided by the interpreter. The role of the college/university interpreter varies considerably from the role of the interpreter who elects to work with kindergarten or first-grade students. Transitioning from language role models to becoming voices for those who model sophisticated discourse, such interpreters provide access to the curriculum at all levels. By performing their job faithfully and accurately, they provide a conduit for students who are deaf and hard of hearing to traverse the academic system seamlessly while gleaning a wealth of information.

Preparing Counselors to Work with Consumers Who Are Deaf or Hard of Hearing

Counseling services are provided in the schools, VR offices, mental health facilities, doctor's offices, and psychiatric hospitals. Although the nature of individuals' problems may vary and the techniques and methods used by professional service providers may be diverse, the professionals' ultimate goal is to assist the individuals who seek their help to gain a better perspective on life and enhance their overall feelings of mental health.

Within residential school settings students frequent counselors' offices with a variety of problems and concerns. Many of these concerns permeate auditory boundaries and are expressed by students of all ages. Regardless of the nature of the problems, those seeking assistance are generally looking for someone who can help them resolve their problem(s) so they can feel better about their feelings and improve their outlook on life. The majority of counselors working in schools for the deaf are trained to work with this population, are knowledgeable about Deaf culture, have varying degrees of fluency in ASL, and have a desire to work with this population. Overall, they feel comfortable dealing with students and their problems.

However, within the public school domain, the majority of counselors hired to work in the K–12 setting are general practitioners with limited exposure, if any, to that population comprised of individuals who are deaf and hard of hearing. When these students arrive for counseling, those serving in professional roles may feel unqualified when trying to assist them as they work through their problems. Although they may be equipped to deal with students who prefer to communicate through spoken exchanges, paying attention to strategies that will enhance communication (facing the person directly, avoiding having one's back to a light source, expressing comments in a conversational manner, making statements or requests in a brief and succinct manner), they often feel inept when asked to work with students who sign.

In such instances interpreters are frequently asked to facilitate communication during the counseling sessions. This allows the practitioner to focus on the problems being conveyed by the individual, rather than struggling with trying to communicate. However, when counselors work in settings where there is a large student population that is deaf, it is beneficial for all parties involved if the counselor has acquired some background knowledge in Deaf culture and understands the ramifications of one's hearing loss. Recognizing the importance of gaining this body of knowledge can further assist the counselor in addressing the problems put forth by those consumers who are deaf and hard of hearing.

Summary

The tapestry of deaf education has changed dramatically over the past several decades. With the majority of students who were once educated in residential schools or special day schools for the deaf joining their peers in neighborhood schools, the majority of them are receiving most, if not all, of their instruction within the general education classroom. Representing a diverse population of learners and teachers, support personnel are being challenged to modify the curriculum to make it accessible to this unique group of learners.

Today's teachers of students who are deaf wear multiple hats while providing itinerant, consultative, collaborative, and direct instruction to students who are deaf and hard of hearing. Sensitive to their communication and instructional needs, these teachers work diligently to provide students with an academic foundation that will support them as they traverse the educational system. Their foremost goal is to ignite in each child a spark of enthusiasm for learning that will support them on the road to becoming independent, lifelong learners. Recognizing the need to instill in students feelings of self-esteem and a sense of positive self-worth, teachers create activities and learning experiences that will support each child's level of learning.

Educational interpreters provide one of the vital links to student learning. When they do their jobs well, they provide seamless communication between those who can hear and those who cannot. Trained to interpret, transliterate, and voice for consumers who are both hearing and deaf, they have at their disposal a phenomenal command of both English and ASL and can equalize messages that are exchanged both inside and outside the classroom. These communication professionals adhere to a strict code of conduct that mandates confidentiality, impartiality, and respect for all consumers. Functioning as members of the educational team, they share their expertise with other team members, providing pertinent information regarding the communication needs of the students they serve, thus ensuring that all members have equal access to communication.

Certified teachers in deaf education as well as sign language interpreters play a critical role in the education of students who are deaf and hard of hearing. Under the auspices of these exemplary practices, students are provided every opportunity to grow, develop, and become self-sufficient, self-satisfied, and independent individuals. Well-trained professionals touch the lives of all students with whom they come in contact, thus providing students who are deaf and hard of hearing the tools that will enable them to fulfill their personal goals and aspirations.

15

Epilogue

Within industrialized nations change is occurring at a rapid pace and altering the landscape of business, education, and social service agencies. Rising to the occasion to meet the changing demands of society, these entities are redesigning the way they interact with consumers to more adequately meet the needs of today's technologically savvy population. These changes are mirrored in the field of deaf education. With universal newborn hearing screenings becoming part of routine evaluations and cochlear implants on the increase, professionals are evaluating this new generation of individuals who will be served under the umbrella of services for individuals who are deaf and hard of hearing.

What types of services will this new generation require? How will they utilize these services, and what modes of communication will they elect to use? With the added benefits of advanced technology, will more of them be able to access the curriculum and achieve academically at levels that will allow them to pursue degrees in higher education? Will they form identities that embrace the cultural values of the Deaf community, or will they reach adulthood oblivious to the rich cultural and linguistic heritage revered by those who are Deaf? Will they be exposed to the benefits offered by sharing joint membership in both hearing and Deaf communities and, therefore, develop a bilingual/bicultural (Bi-Bi) identity?

Will they leave high school reading at a high school level, feeling they have actively participated in social events with their peers, being given a newfound sense of independence? Or will they grow up wondering who they are, if there are any other individuals like them, and where they belong? As they reflect on these questions, will they develop a sense of connectivity to those around them and the world as a whole, or will they feel like the part of the puzzle that does not quite fit?

Although many aspects of the field of deaf education have changed significantly in the past several years, the concerns shared by parents, professionals, consumers, and practitioners remain as salient and germane today as they were 30 years ago. Those with a vested interest in the field are committed to ensuring that all individuals who are deaf or hard of hearing receive the education they require, thus fostering their optimal growth and development. In addition to providing students with a solid academic foundation, these professionals continue to search for ways to avail their students with a sense of independence while concomitantly supporting them in their quest to discover their identities. Focusing on academic as well as social skills, their consummate goal is to prepare their students, who upon graduation from high school, will be able to enter postsecondary institutions or engage in the workforce with the tools they need to be successful.

How can we ensure this will happen? What do we need to do today to foster success for tomorrow's graduates?

SUMMARY OF CURRENT RELEVANT RESEARCH IN THE FIELD

As the field moves forward, four broad but significant themes that merit further research and in-depth analyses appear repeatedly in the literature. Several of these topics have previously received considerable attention and have stimulated robust debates; others have provided excellent research topics, often producing conflicting results. As the field continues to develop a heightened awareness of the need for evidence-based research, many of these topics will be addressed and will reveal new information while providing fresh insights into the field of deaf education. The four major themes focus on language and communication, literacy, educational settings, and the formation of a cultural identity.

Language and Communication

Within the field of deaf education, one of the topics that has caused considerable consternation and debate pertains to what language and which mode of communication parents, family members, educators, and support personnel should use when conversing with and/or instructing individuals who are deaf. Moores and Martin (2006) remind us of the centuries-old "methods war" that remains evident today and is continually fueled by two dichotomous and often contentious groups of professionals. One group still advocates for the use of oral-only instruction emphasizing speech and speechreading; the other group champions the cause for using ASL for all spoken communication. Included in this latter group are those who support employing a bilingual approach or utilizing one of the other visual/manual systems of communication, such as Signed English, Conceptually Accurate Signed English, and so forth (p. 4). Although the debates continue today regarding the efficacy of each of these communication approaches, research findings pertaining to the various modes of communication indicate that there is no clear evidence that one mode is superior in providing students who are deaf and hard of hearing with equal access to the curriculum.

Spencer and Marschark (2010) have succinctly summarized what the research has revealed with respect to language development and the various communication approaches. Recognizing that some students successfully accomplish age-appropriate language that is considered the norm for all children without additional disabilities, they highlight what we have learned and what we still need to investigate. Typical of what we know about the larger hearing population, it is no surprise that factors such as parental involvement and commitment, socioeconomic status, educational resources, and consistency regarding the communication approach used will all contribute to the success or lack of success experienced by children. Furthermore, research within the field as well as outside of deaf education has verified that when children are exposed to rich language models from birth they will readily acquire the source language. This has been substantiated by fostering communication with sign language for children who are deaf, as well as with spoken language for children who can hear.

The field has generated some excellent research within the areas of early intervention that pertains to the specific use of the various language modalities and communication approaches. Although several positive descriptive reports have been made available, further research is needed to demonstrate which populations benefit from which types of approaches. It is time to adjust the lens of how we view the field from an "either/or" approach to a perspective of "one size doesn't fit all" and different children will benefit from different approaches at different times in their developmental process.

Children under the age of 12 months are receiving cochlear implants and are being provided with early intervention services. How will these children fare as they enter the public school system? What types of services will they need? Research indicates that those with severe to profound losses who have cochlear implants typically function as students who are hard of hearing with mild-to-moderate losses; however, even this amount of loss can create difficulties for the individual. It is well documented in the field that children experiencing even a mild degree of hearing loss can be at greater risk for encountering language delays and difficulties accessing the curriculum.

Although early studies are promising, attesting to the fact that children implanted before 2 years of age are developing early age-appropriate language, will this same level of language development continue throughout high school, allowing them to compete alongside their hearing peers while experiencing the same levels of success? If indeed cochlear implants are producing a new generation of students who are hard of hearing, will future professionals know how to most effectively work with them? Will they be able to access the curriculum through an auditory/verbal approach? Will some of them rely on sign-supported speech? Will others use sign language to bridge from a visual/manual modality while they become auditory learners? Will some of them always rely on ASL, finding that they are more visual than auditory learners? Will we see the same diversity in this population that we have seen among those students who are deaf?

Although the field of deaf education contains a rich and robust body of literature regarding how to provide support services to students who are deaf, the profession will need to continue to explore the types of interventions and services that will promote ultimate success among this group of learners. It is critical that parents and professionals remain open to the variety of strategies and interventions available to them and that they recognize that all communication approaches are viable under the right circumstance. They must be willing to accept the fact that if one approach does not appear to be working for any given child, then a new avenue should be explored. Only then will optimum learning environments be fostered that are child focused rather than driven by the debate over philosophically divergent models for communication.

Literacy

Reading and writing provide the cornerstones for academic achievement; thus, programs that produce students who are fluent in both are considered to be successful. McAnally and Spillers (2004) reiterate that teachers of deaf children probably devote more time and energy to thinking about how to promote reading and writing success than does any other group of professionals. That being said, the research clearly indicates that although 50% of students comprising this population read above a fourth-grade level upon graduating from high school, the remaining 50% are still leaving high school having only attained reading levels comparable to hearing students who are in the fourth grade (p. 152). However, when focusing on any underachieving group of students we must be cautious, as Moores (2006) reminds us, to accurately interpret their test results, recognizing that these scores merely reflect the number of questions the student answered correctly on a standardized test. Although these scores mirror those of their hearing peers, they are not representative of how the student arrived at his or her answers. Being cognizant of the path each individual learner uses to attain the same score requires careful consideration (Moores, p. 46).

One of the greatest challenges confronting teachers today is providing students who are deaf or hard of hearing with the skills and strategies they need to become effective readers and writers. The teachers' ultimate goal is to furnish students with the requisite tools needed so they can read age-appropriate materials and write compositions representative of their respective grade levels. Research to date indicates that many of the activities and techniques used to promote increased literacy with students who can hear can also be used effectively with students who are deaf or hard of hearing. Some of these strategies involve engaging in shared reading, enhancing phonological development, and enhancing vocabulary and reading comprehension.

A plethora of research demonstrates the efficacy of engaging in shared reading with children who can hear. Findings illustrate that shared reading activities promote emergent literacy skills, provide young children with exposure to print, encourage vocabulary development and prediction skills, while inculcating skill set necessary to master the skill set required to comprehend, and utilize sequence of events. We also know that although this type of activity can be initiated easily for many Deaf parents, it can become a very daunting task for hearing parents who have children who are deaf. Many of these parents do not possess sign fluency and are not familiar with how to make connections for the child between the signs and the pictures/words that are contained in the child's story. Therefore, engaging in shared reading can become a formidable, if not an altogether impossible, task.

Evidence suggests that when parents, early intervention specialists, and preschool teachers engage in shared reading with children who can hear, it enhances their vocabulary, phonological awareness, and reading comprehension, thus setting the foundation for students to enter elementary school. Research also indicates that when parents are tutored in how to engage in shared reading with the children who are deaf, it can provide similar benefits. However, additional research must be conducted in the field to determine the extent shared reading impacts the child's language or promotes growth in literacy (Spencer & Marschark, 2010).

Within the area of literacy, further research also needs to be conducted, with the promise of gaining a more refined understanding of how students who are deaf and hard of hearing develop a sense of phonological awareness. With programs that rely on speech reading, computer-assisted systems, visual phonics, and Cued Speech, it is becoming increasingly apparent that a segment of the school-age deaf population relies on a combination of one of these visual cues combined with auditory information to develop their phonological abilities. Additional studies that reveal which students can benefit from which of these systems are critical so student needs can further be matched with appropriate and beneficial learning strategies.

Although it is well established that students who are deaf or hard of hearing benefit from direct instruction and exposure to rich language environments upon which they build and expand their vocabularies, a dearth of information provides guidance to teachers on what methods they should use to assist their students in becoming more syntactically correct writers. The results from existing research are inconclusive, indicating that visual/manual modes of communication, with and without cochlear implants, and included settings seem to impact this student population's ability to write grammatically correct sentences. Further research is needed to determine what methods and approaches, when implemented, will facilitate enduring writing skills that will be evident in writing samples (Spencer & Marschark, 2010).

FUTURE PROJECTIONS AND TRENDS

Although numerous topics require and will receive attention throughout this millennium, two of them in particular merit further discussion. One relates to where students who are deaf or hard of hearing are being educated; the second focuses on what impact these educational settings are having on students' familiarity with Deaf culture and the development of a Deaf identity.

Beginning in 1975 students who were deaf began attending their neighborhood schools, receiving instruction in resource rooms as well as general education classrooms. This trend continues today with approximately 85% of students receiving their education in these settings while

15% still attend special schools specifically designed to meet the needs of the students who are deaf and hard of hearing. Those served in resource rooms or mainstreamed or included classes frequently take advantage of support services. These include sign language interpreters and educational professionals specifically trained to work with students who are deaf or hard of hearing. Special schools consist of residential and day schools that support various communication philosophies. Some instruct students using a visual/manual modality that may include ASL, Cued Speech, or a Bi-Bi approach, others are oral in nature, delivering instruction through an auditory/verbal mode and emphasizing speech and speechreading.

The modes of communication they elect to employ differ as significantly as the populations they serve. Over 50% of the students in special schools represent ethnic minorities, and less than 50% of those in included settings represent a diverse population. Furthermore, students attending special schools represent individuals with more severe degrees of hearing loss than their peers enrolled in neighborhood schools. In addition, a significant percentage of the students attending special schools have additional disabilities impacting their ability to access the general curriculum. Because of these stark differences, it is unrealistic to compare the academic achievement levels or the cultural experiences characteristic of each of these groups. Rather, it is appropriate for future research to examine the impact each of these settings has on producing graduates who are comfortable with their present identities and represent independent, self-sufficient, lifelong learners.

Research suggests that students attending visual/manual and bilingual programs have the advantage of establishing a cultural identity due to the very nature of their environment. With increased opportunities to receive instruction under the auspices of Deaf teachers, they are provided with role models who are typically fluent in ASL and represent a cultural identity affording the students an environment in which they can explore who they are, what Deaf culture entails, and whether they want to declare membership in the community. For students raised in families in which they are the sole individual who is deaf, these communities can foster a sense of identity and solace. These schools vary in size and population and provide instruction, extracurricular activities, and leadership opportunities to a diverse student population.

Students attending neighborhood schools may find they have several peers who are also deaf or hard of hearing, or they may discover that they are the only one who is deaf at the school. Some may experience feelings of isolation; others are fortunate to attend schools that have the population to embrace a co-enrollment model. These placement options have been designed to promote more integration of students who are deaf and hard of hearing into general education classes. In programs in which one fourth to one third of the class is represented by students who have hearing losses, the number of students is sufficient to provide a peer group for socialization. These settings require general education teachers and teachers of the deaf to co-teach and work together as a team. In these situations, classes in sign language are frequently taught to hearing students, providing them with insights into Deaf culture. This model represents the best type of inclusion; however, it is difficult to implement across the United States, especially in rural areas.

With the majority of students who are deaf and hard of hearing receiving their academic instruction in mainstreamed and included settings, will there be an impact on Deaf Culture, and if so, how will it affect the future of this cultural/linguistic minority? Will these alternative educational environments diminish opportunities for students to meet other Deaf individuals, to socialize and develop Deaf identities? Will the demise of residential schools and clubs for the Deaf, in conjunction with the increased reliance on cochlear implants, potentially eradicate Deaf culture? Ogden and Classen (2004) address the issue of Deaf culture by poignantly reminding us that although the clubs and residential schools were historically the main conduits through which Deaf culture was transmitted from one generation to another, these institutions are being replaced with

Deaf sports organizations, both nationally and internationally, that will bring Deaf people together in competitive arenas.

Furthermore, with the advent of computer technology specialized Web sites for the Deaf community have emerged, enabling members to engage in conversations and network with each other. The Deaf community, always early adopters of any new visual technology, continues to take advantage of rapidly developing technology to stay connected and interface with others in the Deaf community or bridge to the hearing world. Utilizing video phones, Web cameras, pagers, and smart phones, they remain in close contact with their friends and significant others (G. Ashton, personal communication, 2010).

Today the long tradition of Deaf gatherings and activities continues on the local, state, national, and international levels. Special events such as ASL film showings, trade shows, alumni reunions, and performances at events such as Deafnation World Expo have drawn more than 23,000 deaf people from 70 countries, including a Miss Deaf International pageant with 40 contestants. While some individuals who are culturally Deaf automatically gravitate toward these events, other individuals who were raised in an oral environment may experience a feeling of "coming home" when they find the Deaf community during their teen, college, or adult years (G. Ashton, personal communication, 2010).

With respect to cochlear implants signaling the end of the Deaf community and the culture the members so revere, Ogden and Classen (2004) point out that although cochlear implants are allowing individuals who are deaf to hear substantially more than they could with hearing aids, the device has not altered the fact that the individuals are still deaf. Rather, they view the implant as allowing Deaf individuals the luxury of hearing enough to communicate with hearing people, without interfering with their opportunities to continue socializing and identifying with members of the Deaf community. By rendering them bilingual-bicultural they have been provided with a gift whereby they can experience the best of both worlds. They query how future generations will use the devices to bridge the two cultures, especially for those deaf individuals who have not been exposed to ASL (p. 66). Ogden and Classen further remind us that Deaf culture is not merely represented by the language but is exhibited through a rich body of literature and art that has earned a place of respect within society.

The field of deaf education is as complex as the population that it serves. As teachers enter the classroom prepared to serve future generations of students who are deaf and hard of hearing, they will be met by a variety of students. Some will be ready to learn and will enter the classroom equipped with various language competencies, varying communication modalities, digital hearing aids, and cochlear implants. Others will arrive with additional disabilities, needing the support of a variety of service providers in the classroom. The educator of today and of the future will be asked to draw upon current methodology, technology, and innovative teaching strategies to help equalize the playing field and ensure that this diverse population has access to the curriculum. It is a challenging and exciting time to be part of a field of committed educators and support personnel. Some research questions have been asked that still need to be answered, and many more will come to the forefront as we continue to both collaborate from inside and form partnerships with colleagues from outside the field.

Students entering the classroom today reflect a composite of individual needs. We must adjust our services to match their individual needs, always cognizant of the fact that one model does not fit all students. It is time to reflect and learn from our previous mistakes, remain open to change, and become receptive to new ideas. The future is bright; never before have we had so many resources for tapping into the potential of our students. By asking the right research questions and gathering the evidence, the field, supported by qualified personnel as well as the student population served within varied school environments, stands to reap the benefits of what these findings have to offer.

LIST OF ORGANIZATIONS

Information and Resources for Parents and Professionals

The following list of agencies and organizations provides information about and services for people who are deaf and hard of hearing. After each organization, a brief description from each of the various Web sites describes what services these organizations provide.

ADARA
www.adara.org

ADARA's mission is to facilitate excellence in human service delivery with individuals who are deaf or hard of hearing. This mission is accomplished by enhancing the professional competencies of the membership, expanding opportunities for networking among ADARA colleagues, and supporting positive public policies for individuals who are deaf or hard of hearing. In achieving the mission, ADARA members are committed to full access for members to all aspects of the organization's business, including board matters, conference planning, presentations and journal publications, recognizing and affirming the ethnic, racial, and cultural diversity of the membership, and fostering an inclusive language community through the use of American Sign Language, signed communication, and other communication strategies used by all members at ADARA events in order to strive for barrier-free communication (Mission, para. 1).

Alexander Graham Bell Association
www.agbell.org

The Alexander Graham Bell Association for the Deaf and Hard of Hearing (AG Bell) helps families, health care providers, and education professionals understand childhood hearing loss and the importance of early diagnosis and intervention (About Us, para. 1). AG Bell currently has chapters in thirty-one states, each serving as an extension of AG Bell as well as a local resource for information and support (About Us, para. 2).

American Society for Deaf Children
www.deafchildren.org

The American Society for Deaf Children supports and educates families of children who are deaf and hard of hearing and advocates for high-quality programs and services (Mission Statement, para. 6).

American Speech-Language-Hearing Association (ASHA)
www.asha.org

The American Speech-Language-Hearing Association is committed to ensuring that all people with speech, language, and hearing disorders receive services to help them communicate effectively (Communication for a Lifetime, para. 1)

Better Hearing Institute
www.betterhearing.org

The Better Hearing Institute (BHI) is a not-for-profit corporation that educates the public about the neglected problem of hearing loss and what can be done about it. Founded in 1973, the organization is working to erase the stigma and end the embarrassment that prevent millions of people from seeking help for hearing loss; to show the negative consequences of untreated hearing loss for millions of Americans; and to promote treatment and demonstrate that this is a national problem that can be solved (Overview of Better Hearing Institute, para. 1).

Captioned Media Program
www.msd.k12.mo.us/rcd/Pages/cmp.htm

The Captioned Media Program (CMP) is a free loan service, much like a local library. The only difference is that the CMP loans captioned videos and DVDs to deaf and hard-of-hearing individuals. The CMP is funded by the U.S. Department of Education for selecting, captioning, and distributing captioned media materials. These materials are open captioned. (No special equipment is needed to use them. Just put an item in a VCR/DVD player and press "Play." The captions are embedded in the video.) Materials are loaned free of charge to deaf and hard-of-hearing persons, their families, teachers, interpreters, and anyone who works with deaf and hard-of-hearing persons. There are no age restrictions. The CMP has videos for kindergarten through adult viewers. These videos include educational titles, self-help videos, and classic movies, as well as special interest (crafts, hobbies, etc.) and theatrical titles (Welcome to the Captioned Media Program, para. 1 & 2).

Center for Hearing and Communication
www.chchearing.org

The Center for Hearing and Communication is a leading hearing center offering state-of-the-art hearing testing, hearing aid fitting, speech therapy, and a full range of services for people of all ages with hearing loss. Offices in New York City and Florida provide services that meet all hearing and communication needs (About Us, para. 1).

Children of Deaf Adults Inc.
www.coda-international.org

Children of Deaf Adults (CODA) is an international organization that focuses on hearing children of deaf adults. Membership is primarily but not exclusively composed of hearing children of deaf parents. CODA addresses bicultural identity through conferences, support groups, and resource development. CODA is an organization established for the purpose of promoting family awareness and individual growth in hearing children of deaf parents. This purpose is accomplished through providing educational opportunities, promoting self-help, organizing advocacy efforts, and acting as a resource for the membership and various communities (About CODA, para. 3 & 4).

Conference of Educational Administrators of Schools and Programs for the Deaf Children of Deaf Adults (CEASD)
ceasd.org

Conference of Educational Administrators of Schools and Programs for the Deaf (CEASD) provides an opportunity for professional educators to work together for the improvement of schools and educational programs for individuals who are deaf or hard of hearing. The organization brings together a rich composite of resources and reaches out to both enhance educational programs and influence educational policy makers (Home, para. 1).

Convention of American Instructors of the Deaf
www.caid.org

The Convention of American Instructors of the Deaf (CAID) continues to follow the tradition begun in 1850 and recognizes the value of bringing together fellow teaching professionals to share experiences and ideas for the purpose of improving learning opportunities for deaf and hard-of-hearing children, adolescents, and young adults (Mission Statement, para. 1).

Council for Exceptional Children
www.cec.sped.org

The Council for Exceptional Children (CEC) is the largest international professional organization dedicated to improving the educational success of individuals with disabilities and/or gifts and talents. CEC advocates for appropriate governmental policies, sets professional standards, provides professional development, advocates for individuals with exceptionalities, and helps professionals obtain conditions and resources necessary for effective professional practice (Overview, para. 1).

Council on Education of the Deaf
www.deafed.net

The Council on Education of the Deaf (CED) is designed to enhance the preparation of new teachers while supporting the ongoing professional development of existing teachers. In addition, the CED advocates to expand the array of learning resources and opportunities available to deaf and hard-of-hearing students and to increase collaborative activities between all those individuals involved in the education of deaf and hard-of-hearing students (Mission Statement, para. 1).

Deaf World Web (The International Center for Disability Resources on the Internet)
www.icdri.org/dhhi/dww.htm

Founded in 1998, The International Center for Disability Resources on the Internet (ICDRI) is a nonprofit center based in the United States and designated as a 501(c)(3) entity. The overarching vision is the equalization of opportunities for persons with disabilities. As an internationally recognized public policy center organized by and for people with disabilities, ICDRI seeks to increase opportunities for people with disabilities by identifying barriers to participation in society and promoting best practices and universal design for the global community (Mission and Values, para. 1 & 2).

Described and Captioned Media Program (DCMP)
www.dcmp.org

The DCMP is an idea that works thanks to funding by the U.S. Department of Education and administration by the National Association of the Deaf. The mission of the U.S. Department of Education is to ensure equal access to education and to promote educational excellence throughout the nation. The U.S. Department funds the DCMP through the Office of Special Education Programs (OSEP) , which is part of the Office of Special Education and Rehabilitative Services (OSERS).

OSERS supports programs that assist in educating children with special needs, provides for the rehabilitation of youth and adults with disabilities, and supports research to improve the lives of individuals with disabilities. OSEP is dedicated to improving results for infants, toddlers, children, and youth ages birth through 21 with disabilities by providing leadership and financial support to assist states and local districts. The *Individuals with Disabilities Education Act* (IDEA) authorizes formula grants to states and discretionary grants to institutions of higher education and other nonprofit organizations to support research, demonstrations, technical assistance and dissemination, technology and personnel development, and parent-training and information centers (General Information, para. 2, 3, & 4).

Gallaudet Research Institute
research.gallaudet.edu/Demographics/factsheet.php

Gallaudet University, federally chartered in 1864, is a bilingual, diverse, multicultural institution of higher education that ensures the intellectual and professional advancement of deaf and hard-of-hearing individuals through American Sign Language and English. Gallaudet maintains a proud tradition of research and scholarly activity and prepares its graduates for career opportunities in a highly competitive, technological, and rapidly changing world (Mission Statement, para. 1).

Hands & Voices
www.handsandvoices.org

Hands & Voices is a nationwide nonprofit organization dedicated to supporting families and their children who are deaf or hard of hearing, as well as the professionals who serve them. It is a parent-driven, parent/professional collaborative group that is unbiased toward communication modes and methods. The diverse membership includes those who are deaf, hard of hearing, and hearing impaired and their families who communicate orally, with signs, cue, and/or combined methods. "We exist to help our children reach their highest potential" (Mission, para. 1).

HandsOn
handson.org/node/933

The mission of Hands On is to provide access to arts and cultural programs for the deaf and hard-of-hearing communities. Hands On offers the information and services needed to ensure active participation of the deaf and hard of hearing in New York's vibrant cultural mainstream.

Hands On was founded in 1982 by four individuals, with a small group of names for a mailing list and a first season that was comprised of six interpreted Off-Broadway performances. In 1994, the organization introduced its cultural calendar of events for the deaf community, the first and only comprehensive listing of its kind.

Today, Hands On produces 20 to 30 interpreted performances annually, with a track record of over 500 shows to date. It maintains an active Web site, which features its monthly Cultural Calendar and a comprehensive Resource Directory, and generates input from deaf people locally and around the world (Mission & History, para. 1, 2, & 3).

House Ear Institute
www.hei.org

The House Ear Institute (HEI) is a nonprofit 501(c)(3) organization dedicated to advancing hearing science through research and education to improve quality of life. Established in 1946 by Howard P. House, M.D., as the Los Angeles Foundation of Otology, and later renamed for its founder, the House Ear Institute has been engaged in the scientific exploration of the auditory system from the ear canal to the cortex of the brain for over sixty years.

Institute scientists investigate hearing loss and ear disease at the cellular and molecular level, as well as the complex neurological interactions between the auditory system and brain. They are also working to improve hearing aids and auditory implants, diagnostics, clinical treatments, and intervention methods. House researchers work with House Clinic physicians to integrate medicine and science through clinical and research trials that may directly benefit patients.

The Institute shares its knowledge with the scientific and medical communities as well as the general public through its education and outreach programs. House Clinic physicians volunteer their time to teach specialty courses in the House Ear Institute's professional education programs, attended by more than 22,000 doctors and research fellows since 1946. Outreach programs for the public serve people with hearing loss and related disorders as well as offer information about general hearing health and hearing conservation (About, para. 1, 2, & 3).

John Tracy Clinic
www.jtc.org

John Tracy Clinic provides, worldwide and without charge, parent-centered services to young children with a hearing loss, offering families hope, guidance, and encouragement (Mission, para. 1).

Laurent Clerc National Deaf Education Center, Info to Go
clerccenter.gallaudet.edu/x17217.xml

The Laurent Clerc National Deaf Education Center at Gallaudet University provides information, training, and technical assistance for parents and professionals to meet the needs of children who are deaf or hard of hearing. Its mission is to improve the quality of education afforded to deaf and hard-of-hearing students from birth to age twenty-one throughout the United States.

The Clerc Center also maintains two demonstration schools, Kendall Demonstration Elementary School and the Model Secondary School for the Deaf (About the Clerc Center, para. 1 & 2).

National Association of the Deaf
www.nad.org

The National Association of the Deaf (NAD) is the nation's premier civil rights organization of, by, and for deaf and hard-of-hearing individuals in the United States of America.

Established in 1880, the NAD was shaped by deaf leaders who believed in the right of the American deaf community to use sign language, to congregate on issues important to them, and to have their interests represented at the national level. These beliefs remain true to this day, with American Sign Language as a core value.

The advocacy scope of the NAD is broad, covering a lifetime and impacting future generations in the areas of early intervention, education, employment, health care, technology, telecommunications, youth leadership, and more—improving the lives of millions of deaf and hard-of-hearing Americans. The NAD also carries out its federal advocacy work through coalition efforts with specialized national deaf and hard-of-hearing organizations as well as coalitions representing national cross-disability organizations.

On the international front, the NAD represents the United States to the World Federation of the Deaf (WFD), an international human rights organization.

Individual and organizational membership makes it possible for the NAD to ensure that the collective interests of the American deaf and hard-of-hearing community are seen and represented among our nation's policy makers and opinion leaders at the federal level.

The NAD is a 501(c)(3) nonprofit organization supported by the generosity of individual and organizational donors, including corporations and foundations (About Us, para. 1, 2, 3, 4, 5, & 6).

National Captioning Institute Incorporated
www.ncicap.org

National Captioning Institute is a nonprofit corporation whose primary purposes are to deliver effective captioning services and encourage, develop, and fund the continuing development of captioning, subtitling, and other media access services for the benefit of people who require additional access to auditory and visual information. As its resources permit and opportunities unfold with the development of new technology, NCI will support services to deaf, hard-of-hearing, and other people who, for whatever reason, wherever situated, and irrespective of their economic conditions, are limited in their ability to participate fully in the world of communications, heard, seen, or written (Mission Statement, para. 1).

The National Information Dissemination Center for Children with Disabilities
www.nichcy.org

The National Information Dissemination Center for Children with Disabilities (NICHCY) is the center that provides information to the nation on disabilities in children and youth; programs and services for infants, children, and youth with disabilities; IDEA, the nation's special education law; No Child Left Behind, the nation's general education law; and research-based information on effective practices for children with disabilities (Who We Are, para. 1).

National Institute on Deafness and Other Communication Disorders
www.nidcd.nih.gov

The National Institute on Deafness and Other Communication Disorders (NIDCD) is one of the institutes that comprise the National Institutes of Health (NIH). NIH is the federal government's focal point for the support of biomedical research. NIH's mission is to uncover new knowledge that will lead to better health for everyone. Simply described, the goal of NIH research is to acquire new knowledge to help prevent, detect, diagnose, and treat disease and disability. NIH is part of the U.S. Department of Health and Human Services.

Established in 1988, NIDCD is mandated to conduct and support biomedical and behavioral research and research training in the normal and disordered processes of hearing, balance, smell, taste, voice, speech, and language. NIDCD also conducts and supports research and research training related to disease prevention and health promotion; addresses special biomedical and behavioral problems associated with people who have communication impairments or disorders; and supports efforts to create devices that substitute for lost and impaired sensory and communication function (Mission Statement, para. 1 & 2).

The National Rehabilitation Information Center
www.naric.com

The National Rehabilitation Information Center (NARIC) began as a small collection of research reports housed in a one-room office at Catholic University. The core mission of the center is to collect and disseminate the results of research funded by the National Institute on Disability and Rehabilitation Research (NIDRR). Over a quarter of a century, that mission has expanded to providing information services and document delivery to the disability and rehabilitation communities across the United States. In 1982, NARIC added information and referral services through a toll-free call center. In 1989, NARIC added an electronic bulletin board, facilitating access for libraries and research institutions. With the advent of the Internet, NARIC moved online in 1992 with a small Web site featuring static pages and directories. NARIC.com became fully interactive in 1995, moving REHABDATA online, followed by the organization's other databases. NARIC delivers its resources into mailboxes around the world with REHABDATA Connection, a monthly service (About Us, para. 2)

National Theatre of the Deaf
www.ntd.org

The mission of the National Theatre of the Deaf is to produce theatrically challenging work of the highest quality, drawing from as wide a range of the world's literature as possible; to perform these original works in a style that links American Sign Language with the spoken word; to seek, train, and employ deaf artists; to offer its work to as culturally diverse and inclusive an audience as possible; to provide community outreach activities that will educate and enlighten the general public, opening their eyes and ears to Deaf culture and building linkages that facilitate involvement in the theatre's methods of work (Mission, para. 1).

Office of Special Education and Rehabilitative Services
www2.ed.gov/about/offices/list/osers/index.html

The Office of Special Education and Rehabilitative Services (OSERS) understands the many challenges still facing individuals with disabilities and their families. Therefore, OSERS is committed to improving results and outcomes for people with disabilities of all ages. OSERS supports programs that serve millions of children, youth, and adults with disabilities.

OSERS is comprised of the Office of the Assistant Secretary (OAS) and three program components: the Office of Special Education Programs (OSEP), the National Institute on Disability and Rehabilitation Research (NIDRR), and the Rehabilitation Services Administration (RSA) (About Us, para. 3).

Rainbow Alliance of the Deaf
rad.org

The Rainbow Alliance of the Deaf (RAD) is a 501(c)(3) nonprofit organization established in 1977. The purpose of this alliance is to establish and maintain a society of Deaf GLBT to encourage and promote their educational, economical, and social welfare; to foster fellowship; to defend members' rights; and advance members' interests as Deaf GLBT citizens concerning social justice; to build up an organization in which all worthy members may participate in the discussion of practical problems and solutions related to their social welfare. RAD has over fifteen chapters in the United States and Canada (Purpose, para. 1).

Registry of Interpreters for the Deaf
rid.org

The Registry of Interpreters for the Deaf (RID) is a national membership organization representing the professionals who facilitate communication between people who are deaf or hard of hearing and people who hear. Interpreters serve as professional communicators in a vast array of settings such as churches, schools, courtrooms, hospitals, and theaters, as well as on political grandstands and television (About RID Overview, para. 1).

RID's function is to support its membership by providing the foundation needed to launch and sustain careers while ensuring quality service to the deaf community. RID does this through a four-pronged approach including education, standards, relationships, and resources (About RID Overview, para. 2).

Self-Help for Hard of Hearing People (SHHH)
www.hearinglossweb.com/res/hlorg/shhh/shhh.htm

The Hearing Loss Web is dedicated to people who have hearing loss but are not members of the traditional deaf community. This includes people who consider themselves to be hearing impaired, hard of hearing, late deafened, and oral deaf. The Hearing Loss Web provides information on issues, medical topics, resources, and technology related to hearing loss (Welcome, para. 1).

Telecommunications for the Deaf and Hard of Hearing, Inc.
tdi-online.org

Telecommunications for the Deaf and Hard of Hearing, Inc. (TDI) was established in 1968 to promote further distribution of TTYs in the deaf community and to publish an annual national directory of TTY numbers. Today, it is an active national advocacy organization focusing its energies and resources on addressing equal access issues in telecommunications, media, and information technologies for four constituencies in deafness and hearing loss, specifically people who are deaf, hard of hearing, late deafened, or deaf blind.

TDI is also a founding member of the Coalition of Organizations for Accessible Technology (COAT). COAT is working hard to pass the 21st Century Communications and Video Accessibility Act of 2009 (H.R. 3101) (Home, para. 1, 2, & 3).

USA Deaf Sports Federation
usdeafsports.org

The Akron Club of the Deaf in Ohio sponsored the first national basketball tournament in 1945, at which time it established the American Athletic Union of the Deaf. The organization was later renamed the American Athletic Association of the Deaf and, in 1997, the USA Deaf Sports Federation (USADSF). Its purpose is to foster and regulate uniform rules of competition and provide social outlets for deaf members and their friends; serve as a parent organization of national sports organizations; conduct annual athletic competitions; and assist in the participation of U.S. teams in international competition.

The federation has published a quarterly newspaper, *AAAD Bulletin*, since 1948 and established the Hall of Fame in 1952. Beginning in 1955, Athletes of the Year have been selected on an annual basis. The *Deaf Sports Review* magazine is also published by the organization.

Recognized as the only national athletic association to coordinate the participation of American deaf and hard-of-hearing individuals in international competitions, USADSF is affiliated with the International Committee of Sports for the Deaf (ICSD, formerly known as Comité International des Sports des Sourds—CISS) and has hosted the Summer Deaflympics in 1965 (Washington, DC) and 1985 (Los Angeles) and the Winter Deaflympics in 1975 (Lake Placid, NY) and 2007 (Salt Lake City) (History, para. 1, 2, & 3).

World Federation of the Deaf
wfdeaf.org

Established in Rome, Italy, in 1951, the World Federation of the Deaf (WFD) is an international, nongovernmental central organization of national associations of Deaf people, with a current membership of associations in 130 countries worldwide. Associate members, international members, and individual members also make up WFD's membership base.

WFD's philosophy is one of equality, human rights, and respect for all people, regardless of race, nationality, religion, gender, sexual preference, age, and all other differences. WFD supports and promotes in its work the many United Nations conventions on human rights, with a focus on deaf people who use sign language, and their friends and family. WFD works with the aim of solidarity and unity to make the world a better place.

WFD has consultative status in the United Nations (UN) system, including the Economic and Social Council (ECOSOC); the UN Educational, Scientific and Cultural Organization (UNESCO); the International Labour Organization (ILO); and the World Health Organization (WHO). WFD also cooperates closely with the UN High Commissioner for Human Rights and has representatives on the Panel of Experts on the UN Standard Rules for the Equalization of Opportunities for Persons with Disabilities. WFD is a member of the International Disability Alliance (IDA) (Mission and Objectives, para. 1, 2, & 3).

REFERENCES

Adams, M. J. (1990). *Beginning to read: Thinking and learning about print.* Cambridge, MA: MIT Press.

Akamatsu, C. T., Musselman, C., & Zwiebel, A. (2000). Nature vs. nurture in the development of cognition in deaf people. In P. Spencer, C. Erting, & M. Marschark (Eds.), *Development in context: The deaf children in the family and at school* (pp. 255–274). Mahwah, NJ: Erlbaum.

Akamatsu, C. T., Stewart, D., & Becker, B. J. (2000). Documenting English syntactic development in face-to-face signed communication. *American Annals of the Deaf, 145,* 452–463.

Akamatsu, C. T., Stewart, D. A., & Mayer, C. (2002). It is time to look beyond teachers' signing behavior. *Sign Language Studies*, *2*(3), 230–254.

Akamatsu, E. T., Stewart, D., & Mayer, C. (2004). Is it time to look beyond teacher's signing behavior? In D. Power & G. Leigh (Eds.), *Educating deaf students: Global perspectives* (pp. 40–54). Washington, DC: Gallaudet University Press.

Akers, J., Jones, R., & Coyl, D. (1998). Adolescent friendship pairs: Similarities in identity status development, behaviors, attitudes, and interests. *Journal of Adolescent Research, 13,* 178–201.

Albertini, J. A., & Schley, S. (2005). Writing characteristics, instruction, and assessment. In M. Marschark & P. E. Spencer, *Oxford handbook of deaf studies* (pp. 123–131). New York: Oxford University Press.

Al-Hilawani, Y. (2000). A new approach to evaluating metacognition in hearing average-achieving, hearing underachieving, and deaf/hard-of-hearing elementary school students. *British Journal of Special Education, 27*(I), 41–47.

Al-Hilawani, Y. (2001, March). Examining metacognition in hearing and deaf/hard of hearing students: A comparative study. *American Annals of the Deaf, 146*(1), 45–50.

Allen, T. (1986). Patterns of academic achievement among hearing impaired students: 1974 and 1973. In A. Schildroth & M. Karchmer (Eds.), *Deaf children in America* (pp. 161–206). San Diego, CA: Little Brown.

Allport, G. W. (1965). *Pattern and growth in personality.* New York: Holt, Rinehart & Winston.

Allum, J. H., Greisiger, R., Straubhaar, S., & Carpenter, M. G. (2000). Auditory perception and speech identification in children with cochlear implants tested with the EARS protocol. *British Journal of Audiology, 34,* 293–303.

American Association on Mental Retardation (AAMR). (2002). Mental retardation: Definition, classification, and systems of support (10th ed.) Washington, DC: Author. (*Note:* In 2007 the AAMR changed its name to the American Association on Intellectual and Developmental Disabilities, or AAIDD.)

American Psychiatric Association (APA). (2000). *Diagnostic and statistical manual of mental disorders* (4th ed.), Text Revision (DSM-IV-TR). Washington, DC: Author.

American Speech-Language-Hearing Association (ASHA). (2005). *Technical report: (Central) auditory processing disorders—Working group on auditory processing disorders.* Rockville, MD: ASHA.

American Speech-Language-Hearing Association (ASHA). (2009). Hearing Screening. Retrieved September 16, 2009, from www.asha.org/public/hearing/Hearing-Screening

Anderson, N. B., & Shames, G. H. (2006). *Human communication disorders: An introduction* (7th ed.). Boston: Allyn & Bacon.

Anderson, R., & Freebody, P. (1985). Vocabulary knowledge. In H. Singer & R. Ruddell (Eds.), *Theoretical models and processes of reading* (3rd ed., pp. 343–371). Newark, DE: International Reading Association.

Anderson, R., & Nagy, W. (1993). *The vocabulary conundrum.* Technical Report No. 570. Urbana, IL: Center for the Study of Reading.

Andrews, J., & Mason, J. (1986). How do deaf children learn about prereading? *American Annals of the Deaf, 131,* 210–217.

Andrews, J., Winograd, P., & DeVille, G. (1996). Using sign language summaries during prereading lessons. *Teaching Exceptional Children, 28,* 30–34.

Andrews, J. F., Leigh, I. W., & Weiner, M. T. (2004). *Deaf people: Evolving perspectives from psychology, education, and sociology.* Boston: Pearson.

Andrews, J. F., & Mason, J. M. (1991). Strategy use among deaf and hearing readers. *Exceptional Children, 57,* 536–545.

Angelides, P., & Aravi, C. (2006/2007). A comparative perspective on the experiences of deaf and hard of hearing individuals as students at mainstream and special schools. *American Annals of the Deaf, 15*(5), 476–487.

Anonymous. (2002). Assessment: Partnering with parents. *Scholastic Early Childhood Today, 17*(1), 15–16.

Anthony, D. (1971). *Signing Essential English* (Vols. 1 & 2). Anaheim, CA: Editorial Services Division, Anaheim Union School District.

Antia, S., Reed, S., & Kreimeyer, K. (2005). Written language of deaf and hard of hearing students in public schools. *Journal of Deaf Studies and Deaf Education, 10,* 244–255.

Antia, S., Stinson, M. S., & Gaustad, M. (2002). Developing membership in the education of deaf and hard of hearing students in inclusive settings. *Journal of Deaf Studies and Deaf Education, 1,* 214–229.

Antia, S. D., & Kreimeyer, K. H. (2003). Peer interaction of deaf and hard of hearing children. In M. Marschark & P. E. Spencer (Eds.), *The Oxford handbook of deaf studies, language, and education* (pp. 164–176). New York: Oxford University Press.

Antia, S. D., Kreimeyer, K. H., & Reed, S. (2010). Supporting students in general education classrooms. In M. Marschark & E. Spencer, *The Oxford handbook of deaf studies, language, and education* (Vol. 2, pp. 72–92). New York: Oxford University Press.

Arnold, P., & Mills, M. (2001). Memory for faces, shoes, and objects by deaf and hearing signers and hearing nonsigners. *Journal of Psycholinguistic Research, 30,* 185–195.

Asch, S., & Nerlove, H. (1960). The development of double function terms in children: An exploratory investigation. In B. Kaplan & S. Wapner (Eds.), *Perspectives in psychological theory: Essays in honor of Heinz Werner* (pp. 47–60). New York: International Universities Press.

Atkins, D. V. (1982). *A comparison of older sisters of hearing-impaired and normally hearing children on measures of responsibility and parental attention.* Unpublished doctoral dissertation, University of California, Los Angeles.

Atkins, D. V. (1987). Siblings of the hearing-impaired: Perspectives for parents. *The Volta Review, 89*(5), 32–45.

Atkinson, R. C., & Shiffrin, R. M. (1968). Human memory: A proposed system and its control processes. In W. K. Spence & J. T. Spence (Eds.), *The psychology of learning and motivation (Vol. 2): Advances in learning and theory* (pp. 89–195). New York: Academic Press.

Austin, R. (2006). The role of ICT in bridge building and social inclusion: Theory, policy, and practice issues. *European Journal of Teacher Education, 29*(2), 145–161.

Autism Information Center. (2010). Autism Spectrum Disorders (ASDs): Data & Statistics. Centers for Disease Control and Prevention. Retrieved February 25, 2011, from www.cdc.gov/ncbddd/autism/data.html

Avchen, R. N., Bhasin, T. K., Braun, K. V., & Yeargin-Allsopp, M. (2007). Public health impact: Metropolitan Atlanta developmental disabilities surveillance program. *International Review of Research in Mental Retardation, 33,* 149–190.

Awh, E., & Jonides, J. (2001). Overlapping mechanisms of attention and working memory. *Trends in Cognitive Sciences, 5*(3) 119–126.

Aylor, B. (2003). The impact of sex, gender, and cognitive complexity on the perceived importance of teacher communication skills. *Communication Studies, 54*(4), 496–509.

Azmitia, M., & Hesser, J. (1993). Why siblings are important agents of cognitive development: A comparison of siblings and peers. *Child Development, 64,* 430–444.

Bacon, P. (2009). Deaf Culture: Changes and Challenges. PBS.org. Retrieved January 14, 2011, from pbs.org/wnet/soundandfury/culture/essay.html

Baddeley, A. (2003). Working memory and language: An overview. *Journal of Communication Disorders, 36,* 189–208.

Baddeley, A. D. (1986). *Working memory.* Oxford, England: Oxford University Press.

Baddeley, A. D. (1990). *Human memory: Theory and practice.* Hillsdale, NJ: Erlbaum.

Baddeley, A. D., & Hitch, G. J. (1974). Working memory. In G. H. Bower (Ed.), *The psychology of learning and motivation* (Vol. 8, pp. 47–89). New York: Academic Press.

Bagenholm, A., & Gillberg, C. (1991). Psychosocial effects on sibilings of children with autism and mental retardation: A population-based study. *Journal of Mental Deficiency Research, 35,* 291–307.

Bain, L., Scott, S., & Steinberg, A. G. (2004). Socialization experiences and coping strategies of adults raised using spoken language. *Journal of Deaf Studies and Deaf Education, 9*(1), 120–128.

Bakeman, R., & Adamson, L. (1984). Coordinating attention to people and objects in mother-infant and peer-infant interaction. *Child Development, 55,* 1278–1289.

Baker-Shenk, C., & Cokely, D. (1980). *American sign language: A teacher's resource text on grammar and culture.* Washington, DC: Gallaudet University Press.

Barbaresi, W. J., Katusic, S. K., Colligan, R. C., Weaver, A. L., & Jacobsen, S. J. (2005). Math learning disorder: Incidence in a population-based birth cohort. *Ambulatory Pediatrics, 5,* 281–289.

Barclay, L., & Nghiem, H. T. (2006). Sensorineural hearing loss is common in children with bacterial meningitis. *Archives of Otolaryngoly: Head & Neck Surgery, 132,* 941–945. Retrieved January 15, 2011, from cme.medscape.com/viewarticle/544756

Barkley, R. (2006). Primary symptoms, diagnostic criteria, prevalence, and gender differences. In R. Barkley (Ed.), *Attention-deficit hyperactivity disorder: A handbook for diagnosis and treatment* (3rd ed., pp. 76–121). New York: Guilford.

Bartsch, K. J. (2009, November). Employment outlook: 2008–18; The employment projections for 2008–18. *Monthly Labor Review,* pp. 3–10.

Bat-Chava, Y. (1993). Antecedents of self-esteem in deaf people: A meta-analytic review. *Rehabilitation Psychology, 38,* 221–234.

Bat-Chava, Y. (1994). Group identification and self-esteem of deaf adults. *Personality and Social Psychology Bulletin, 20,* 494–502.

Bat-Chava, Y. (2000). Diversity of deaf identities. *American Annals of the Deaf, 145,* 420–428.

Bat-Chava, Y., & Deignan, E. (2001). Peer relationships of children with cochlear implants. *Journal of Deaf Studies and Deaf Education, 6*(3), 186–199.

Bat-Chava, Y., Deignan, E., & Martin, D. (2002). Rehabilitation counselors' knowledge of hearing loss and assistive technology. *Journal of Rehabilitation, 68,* 33–44.

Bat-Chava, Y., & Martin, D. (2002). Sibling relationships of deaf children: The impact of child and family characteristics. *Rehabilitation Psychology, 47*(1), 73–91.

Bates, E., Marchman, V., Thal, D., Fenson, L., Dale, P., Reznick, S., Reilly, J., & Hartung, J. (1994). Developmental and stylistic variation in the composition of early vocabulary. *Journal of Child Language, 21,* 85–123.

Beattie, R. (2006). The oral methods and spoken language acquisition. In P. Spencer & M. Marschark (Eds.), *Advances in the spoken language development of deaf and hard of hearing children* (pp. 103–135). New York: Oxford University Press.

Becker, G. (1980). *Growing old in silence.* Los Angeles: University of California Press.

Beers, K. (2003). *When kids can't read: What teachers can do.* Portsmouth NH: Heinemann.

Belcastro, F. P. (2004). Rural gifted students who are deaf or hard of hearing: How electronic technology can help. *American Annals of the Deaf, 149*(4), 309–313.

Bellugi, U., & Emmorey, K. (1993). Enhanced spatial abilities in adult signers. *Journal of Psycholinguistic Research, 22,* 153–187.

Bellugi, U., Klima, E. S., & Siple, P. (1975). Remembering in signs. *Cognition, 3,* 93–125.

Bellugi, U., O'Grady, L., Lillo-Martin, D., O'Grady-Hynes, M., Van-Hoek, K., & Corina, D. (1990). Enhancement of spatial cognition in deaf children. In V. Volterra & L. Erting (Eds.), *From gesture to language in hearing and deaf children* (pp. 278–298). New York: Springer-Verlag.

Bender, W. N. (2004). *Learning disabilities: Characteristics, identification, and teaching strategies* (5th ed.). Boston: Allyn & Bacon.

Benderly, B. L. (1980). *Dancing without music.* Garden City, NY: Doubleday.

Bentler, R. A., & Mueller, G. (2009). Hearing aid technology. In J. Katz (Ed.), *Handbook of clinical audiology* (6th ed., pp. 776–793). Philadelphia: Lippincott Williams & Wilkins.

Berchin, J. (1989). Spontaneous comparative behavior and categorization: The links between mediated interaction and reading comprehension. In D. S. Martin (Ed.), *Working Papers of the Second International Symposium on Cognition, Education, and Deafness* (pp. 590–613). Washington, DC: Gallaudet University.

Bernero, R. J., & Bothwell, H. (1966). Relationship of Hearing Impairment to Educational Needs. Illinois Department of Public Health & Office of Superintendent of Public Instruction. Developed by Karen L. Anderson, Ed.S., & Noel D. Matkin, Ph.D. (1991).

Bernstein, D. K., & Tiegerman-Farber, E. (2009). *Language and communication disorders in children* (6th ed.). Boston: Allyn & Bacon.

Bess, F., Dodd-Murphy, J., & Parker, R. (1998). Children with minimal sensorineural hearing loss: Prevalence, educational performance, and functional status. *Ear and Hearing, 19*(5), 339–354.

Bess, F. H., & Humes, L. E. (1995). *Audiology: The fundamentals* (2nd ed.). Philadelphia: Lippincott Williams & Wilkins.

Bettger, J. (1992). *The effects of experience on spatial cognition: Deafness and knowledge of ASL.* Unpublished doctoral dissertation, University of Illinois, Urbana-Champaign.

Bevan, R. C. (1988). *Hearing-impaired children: A guide for concerned parents and professionals.* Springfield, IL: Charles C Thomas.

Biederman, J. (2005). Attention-deficit/hyperactivity disorder: A selective overview. *Biological Psychiatry, 57*(11), 1215–1220.

Blamey, P., Sarant, J., Paatsch, L., Barry, J., Bow, C., & Wales, R. (2001). Relationships among speech perception, production, language, hearing loss, and age in children with impaired hearing. *Journal of Speech, Language and Hearing Research, 44*(2), 264–285.

Blamey, P. J. (2003). Development of spoken language by deaf children. In M. Marschark & P. E. Spencer (Eds.), *Deaf studies, language, and education* (pp. 232–246). Oxford, England: Oxford University Press.

Blatto-Vallee, G., Kelly, R. R., Gaustad, M. G., Porter, J., & Fonzi, J. (2007). Visual-spatial representation in mathematical problem solving by deaf and hearing students. *Journal of Deaf Studies and Deaf Education, 12*(4), 432–448.

Bloom, B. (1984). The 2 Sigma Problem: The Search for Methods of Group Instruction as Effective as One-to-One Tutoring. *Educational Researcher, 13*(6), 4–16.

Bloom, L., & Lahey, M. (1978). *Language development and language disorders.* New York: Wiley.

Bong, M. (1998). Tests of the internal/external frames of reference model with subject-specific academic self-efficacy and frame-specific academic self-concepts. *Journal of Educational Psychology, 90*(1), 102–110.

Borden, B. B. (1996). *The art of interpreting.* Plymouth, MI: Hayden-McNeil Publishing.

Bornstein, H. (1974). Signed English: A manual approach to English language and development. *Journal of Speech and Hearing Disorders, 3,* 330–343.

Bornstein, H., Saulnier, K., & Hamilton, L. (1983). *The comprehensive Signed English dictionary.* Washington, DC: Gallaudet University Press (Clerc Books).

Borthwick-Duffy, S. A. (2007). Adaptive behavior. In J. W. Jacobson, J. A. Mulick, & J. Rojahn (Eds.), *Handbook of intellectual disabilities* (pp. 279–293). New York: Springer Science + Business Media.

Boucher Jones, M. (2001). Response to question 4: Does the auditory-verbal approach differ from the auditory-oral approach and/or traditional aural habilitation? In W. Estabrooks (Ed.), *50 frequently asked questions about auditory-verbal therapy* (pp. 17–19). Toronto, Canada: Learning to Listen Foundation.

Boutin, D. L. (2009). The impact of college training and vocational rehabilitation services on employment for consumers with hearing loss. *Journal of the American Deafness and Rehabilitation Association, 42*(2), 73–89.

Boutin, D. L., & Wilson, K. B. (2009). An analysis of vocational rehabilitation services for consumers with hearing impairments who received college or university training. *Rehabilitation Counseling Bulletin, 52*(3), 156–166.

Boutla, M., Supalla, T., Newport, E., & Bavelier, D. (2004). Short-term memory span: Insights from sign language. *Nature Neuroscience, 7*(9), 997–1002.

Bowe, F. G. (2002). Deaf and hard of hearing Americans' instant messaging and e-mail use: A national survey. *American Annals of the Deaf, 147*(4), 6–10.

Bowen, S. K. (2008). Coenrollment for students who are deaf or hard of hearing: Friendship patterns and social interactions. *American Annals of the Deaf, 153*(3), 285–293.

Boyce, G. C., & Barnett, W. S. (1993). Siblings of persons with mental retardation: A historical perspective and recent findings. In Z. Stoneman & P. W. Berman (Eds.), *The effects of mental retardation, disability, and illness on sibling relationships: Research issues and challenges* (pp. 145–184). Baltimore: Brookes.

Boyd, D., & Bee, H. (2009). *Lifespan development* (5th ed.). Boston: Pearson.

Braden, J. P. (1994). *Deafness, deprivation, and IQ.* New York: Plenum.

Braden, J. P. (1985). The structure of nonverbal intelligence in deaf and hearing subjects. *American Annals of the Deaf, 130,* 496–501.

Breivik, J. (2005). *Deaf identities in the making.* Washington, DC: Gallaudet University Press.

Brody, G., & Stoneman, Z. (1993). Parameters for inclusion in the studies on sibling relationships. In Z. Stoneman & P. W. Berman, (Eds.), *The effects of mental retardation, disability, and illness on sibling relationships: Research issues and challenges* (pp. 275–286). Baltimore: Brookes.

Bryan, T., Burstein, K., & Ergul, C. (2004). The social-emotional side of learning disabilities: A science-based presentation of the state of the art. *Learning Disability Quarterly, 27*(1), 45–51.

Bryant, D. P., Smith, D. D., & Bryant, B. R. (2008). *Teaching students with special needs in inclusive classrooms.* Boston: Allyn & Bacon.

Buehl, K. (2002). Kristin Buehl. In J. Reisler, *Voices of the oral deaf: Fourteen role models speak out.* Jefferson, NC: McFarland & Company.

Bullard, C. (2003). *The itinerant teacher's handbook.* Hillsboro, OR: Butte Publications.

Burch, D. (2005). *Essential language/system competencies for sign language interpreters in pre-college settings.* Alexandria, VA: Journal of Interpretation.

Burgoon, M. (1994). Nonverbal signals. In M. L. Knapp & G. R. Miller (Eds.), *Handbook of interpersonal communication* (pp. 229–285). Beverly Hills, CA: Sage.

Buzzard, D. (2001). Della Buzzard. In R. McKee, *People of the eye: Stories from the deaf world* (pp. 162–167). Wellington, New Zealand: Bridget Williams Books.

Byrne, B. (1984). The general/academic self-concept nomonological network: A review of construct validation research. *Review of Educational Research, 54,* 427–456.

Calkins, L. (1994). *The art of teaching writing.* Portsmouth, NH: Heinemann.

Cappelli, M., Daniels, D., Durieux-Smith, A., McGrath, P., & Neuss, D. (1995). Social development of children with hearing impairments. *The Volta Review, 97,* 197–208.

Carney, A. E., & Moeller, M. P. (1998). Treatment efficacy: Hearing loss in children. *Journal of Speech, Language, Hearing Research, 41,* S61–S84.

Carnine, D. W., Silbert, J., Kame'enui, E. J., Tarver, S. G., & Jungjohann, K. (2006). *Teaching struggling and at-risk readers.* Upper Saddle River, NJ: Pearson.

Carpenter, M., Nagell, K., & Tomasello, M. (1998). Social cognition, joint attention, and communicative competence from 9 to 15 months of age. *Monographs of the Society for Research in Child Development,* Serial No. 255, *63*(4).

Carroll, P. S. (2004). Integrated literacy instruction in the middle grades: Channeling young adolescents' spontaneous overflow of energy. New York: Pearson.

Carver, R. (1990). *Reading rate: A review of research and theory.* San Diego, CA: Academic Press.

Cattani, A., Clibbens, J., & Perfect, T. J. (2007). Visual memory for shapes in deaf signers and nonsigners and in hearing signers and nonsigners: Atypical lateralization and enhancement. *Neuropsychology, 21*(1), 114–121.

Cawthon, S. (2004). Schools for the deaf and the No Child Left Behind Act. *American Annals of the Deaf, 149*(4), 314–323.

Cawthon, S. W. (2008). Accommodations use for statewide standardized assessments: Prevalence and recommendations for students who are deaf or hard of hearing. *Journal of Deaf Studies and Deaf Education, 13*(1), 55–76.

Centers for Disease Control and Prevention. (2005a). DSHPSHWA data summary for reporting year 2003. Retrieved January 17, 2011, from www.cdc.gov/ncbddd/ehdi/2003/Data_Summary_03D.pdf

Centers for Disease Control and Prevention. (2005b). Intellectual disability. Retrieved February 25, 2011, from www.cdc.gov/ncbddd/dd/mr3.htm

Centers for Disease Control and Prevention. (2007). CDC releases new data on autism spectrum disorders (ASDs) from multiple communities in the United States. Retrieved March 9, 2011, from www.cdc.gov/media/pressrel/2007/r070208.htm

Centers for Disease Control and Prevention. (2010). Fetal Alcohol Spectrum Disorders (FASDs). CDC.gov. Retrieved January 15, 2011, from www.cdc.gov/ncbddd/fasd/index.html

Cerney, J. (2007). *Deaf education in America: Voices of children from inclusion settings.* Washington, DC: Gallaudet University Press.

Charlier, B. L., & Leybaert, J. (2000). The rhyming skills of deaf children educated with phonetically augmented speech reading. *The Quarterly Journal of Experimental Psychology, 53,* 349–375.

Chau, M., Thampi, K., & Wight, V. (2010). Basic facts about low-income children, 2009 children under age 6. *Fact Sheet*, National Center for Children in Poverty. Retrieved February 7, 2011, from www.nccp.org/publications/pdf/download_378.pdf

Cheng, G., Xiaoyan, H., & Dajun, Z. (2006). A review of academic self-concept and its relationship with academic achievement. *Psychological Science* (China), *29,* 133–136.

Chermak, G. D., & Musiek, F. E. (1997). *Central auditory processing disorders: New perspectives.* San Diego, CA: Singular Publishing Group.

Chess, S., & Fernandez, P. B. (1980). Neurologic damage and behavior in rubella children. *American Annals of the Deaf, 125,* 998–1001.

Chess, S., Fernandez, P., & Korn, S. J. (1972). *Psychiatric disorders in children with congenital rubella.* New York: Brunner Mazel.

Christiansen, J. B. (1982). The socioeconomic status of the deaf population: A review of the literature. In J. B. Christiansen & J. Egelston-Dodd (Eds.), *Socioeconomic status of the deaf population* (pp. 1–61). Washington, DC: Gallaudet College.

Christiansen, J. B., & I. W. Leigh. (2002). Cochlear implants in children: Ethics and choices. Washington, DC: Gallaudet University Press.

Church, M. W., & Gerkin, K. P. (1988). Hearing disorders in children with fetal alcohol syndrome: Findings from case reports. *Pediatrics, 82*(2), 147–154.

Cicirelli, V. G. (1995). *Sibling relationships across the life span.* New York: Plenum Press.

Clark, S. C. (1995). Advance report of final divorce statistics, 1989 and 1990. *Monthly Vital Statistics Report, 43*(8)(Suppl.).

Cochlear Implant Taskforce of the NAD. (1991). Cochlear implants and children: A position paper of the NAD. *The NAD Broadcaster, 13.*

Conrad, R. (1964). Acoustic confusions in immediate memory. *British Journal of Psychology, 55,* 75–84.

Conrad, R. (1979). *The deaf schoolchild: Language and cognitive function.* London: Harper & Row.

Conrad, R., & Weiskrantz, B. C. (1981). On the cognitive ability of deaf children with deaf parents. *American Annals of the Deaf, 126,* 995–1003.

Cook, L., & Friend, M. (1995). Co-teaching: Guidelines for effective practices. *Focus of Exceptional Children, 28*(3), 1–16.

Corker, M. (1996). *Deaf transitions, images and origins of deaf families, deaf communities and deaf identities.* London: Jessica Kingsley.

Cornell, L. S., & Lyness, K. P. (2004). Therapeutic implications for adolescent deaf identity and self-concept. *Journal of Feminist Family Therapy, 16*(3), 31–49.

Costa, A. L. (2001a). Teaching for, of and about thinking. In Arthur Costa (Ed.), *Developing minds* (3rd ed.) (pp. 354–358). Alexandria, VA: Association for Supervision and Curriculum Development.

Costa, A. L. (2001b). Habits of mind. In Arthur Costa (Ed.), *Developing Minds* (3rd ed., pp. 80–85). Alexandria, VA: Association for Supervision and Curriculum Development.

Costa, A. L., & Kallick, B. (Eds.). (2000). *Discovering and exploring habits of mind.* Alexandria, VA: Association for Supervision and Curriculum Development.

Costello, J., Mustillo, S., Erkanli, A., Keeler, G., & Angold, A. (2003). Prevalence and development of psychiatric disorders in childhood and adolescence. *Archives of General Psychiatry, 60,* 837–844.

Courtin, C. (2000). The impact of sign language on the cognitive development of deaf children: The case of theories of mind. *Journal of Deaf Studies and Deaf Education, 5,* 266–276.

Coyner, L. (1993). Academic success, self-concept, social acceptance, and perceived social acceptance for hearing, hard of hearing, and deaf students in a mainstream setting. *Journal of the American Deafness and Rehabilitation Association, 27,* 13–20.

Craig, H. (1987). Instrumental enrichment: Processes and results with deaf students. *Thinking Skills Newsletter.* Pennsylvania Department of Education.

Crnic, K. A., & Leconte, J. M. (1986). Understanding sibling needs and influences. In R. R. Cummins, J. (1981). The role of primary language development in promoting education success for language minority students. In California State Department of Education (Ed.), *Schooling and language minority students: A theoretical framework.* Los Angeles: California State University, Evaluation, Dissemination and Assessment Center.

Crocker, J., & Quinn, D. M. (2000). Social stigma and self-esteem: The self-protective properties of stigma. *Psychological Review, 96,* 35–53.

Croskery, D. (2001). Douglas Croskery. In R. McKee, *People of the eye: Stories from the deaf world.* Wellington, New Zealand: Bridget Williams Books.

Cummins, J. (1981). The role of primary language development in promoting education success for language minority students. In California State Department of Education (Ed.), *Schooling and language minority students: A theoretical framework.* Los Angeles: California State University, Evaluation, Dissemination and Assessment Center.

Cummins, J. (1984). *Bilingualism and special education: Issues in assessment and pedagogy.* San Diego, CA: College Hill Press.

Davey, B. (1987). Postpassage questions: Task and reader effects on comprehension and metacomprehension processes. *Journal of Reading Behavior, 19,* 261–283.

Davey, B., & King, S. (1990). Acquisition of word meanings from context by deaf readers. *American Annals of the Deaf, 135,* 227–334.

DeBonis, D. A., & Donohue, C. L. (2004). *Survey of audiology fundamentals for audiologists and health professionals.* Boston: Allyn & Bacon.

DeBonis, D. A., & Donohue, C. L. (2008). *Survey of audiology fundamentals for audiologists and health professionals* (2nd ed.). Boston: Allyn & Bacon.

DeLana, M., Gentry, M., & Andrews, J. (2007).The efficacy of ASL/English bilingual education: Considering public schools. *American Annals of the Deaf, 152*(1), 73–87. Retrieved from EBSCOhost.

Della Sala, S., Gray, C., Baddeley, A., Allamano, N., & Wilson, L. (1999). Pattern span: A tool for unwelding visuo-spatial memory. *Neuropsychologia, 37,* 1189–1199.

DeLuca, D., Leigh, I. W., Lindgren, K. A., & Napoli, D. J. (Eds.). (2008). *Access: Multiple avenues for deaf people.* Washington, DC: Gallaudet University Press.

DesJardin, J. L., Eisenberg, L. S., & Hodapp, R. M. (2006). Sound beginnings supporting families of young deaf children with cochlear implants. *Infants & Young children, 19*(3), 179–189.

Desselle, D., & Pearlmutter, L. (1997, January). Navigating two cultures: Deaf children, self-esteem, and parents' communication patterns. *Social Work in Education, 19*(1), 23–30.

Dettman, S. J., Briggs, R. J., Dowell, R. C., & Leigh, J. R. (2007). Communication development in children who receive the cochlear implant younger than 12 months: Risks versus benefits. *Ear and Hearing, 28,* 11S–18S.

deVilliers, P., & Pomerantz, S. (1992). Hearing-impaired students learn new words from written context. *Applied Psycholinguistics, 13,* 409–431.

Dew, D. W. (Ed.). (1999). *Serving individuals who are low-functioning deaf: Report of the Twenty-Fifth Institute on Rehabilitation Issues.* George Washington University, Washington, DC.

Dieker, L. (2001). What are the characteristics of "effective" middle and high school co-taught teams? *Preventing School Failure, 46*(1), 14–25.

Dietz, C. H. (1985). Improving cognitive skills in deaf adolescents using LOGO and Instrumental Enrichment. In D. S. Martin (Ed.), *Cognition, education, and deafness* (pp. 381–385). Washington, DC: Gallaudet University.

DiFrancesca, S. (1978). Developing thinking skills in career education. *The Volta Review, 80,* 351–354.

Dodd, B., McIntosh, B., & Woodhouse, L. (1998). Early lipreading ability and speech and language development of hearing-impaired pre-schoolers. In R. Campbell & B. Dodd (Eds.), *Hearing by the eye II: Advances in the psychology of speechreading and auditory-visual speech* (pp. 229–242). Hove, England: Psychological Press.

Donin, J., Doehring, D., & Brows, F. (1991). Text comprehension and reading achievement in orally educated hearing impaired children. *Discourse Processes, 14,* 307–337.

DuBow, S. (1991). The television decoder circuitry act: TV for all. *Temple Law Review, 64,* 609–618.

Dunn, J. (1985). *Sisters and brothers.* Cambridge, MA: Harvard University Press.

Dunn, J., & Kendrick, C. (1982). *Siblings.* Cambridge, MA: Harvard University Press.

Dunn, J., & McGuire, S. (1992). Sibling and peer relationships in childhood. *Journal of Child Psychology and Psychiatry, 33,* 67–105.

Dyson, L., Edgar, E., & Crnic, K. (1989). Psychological predictors of adjustment by siblings of developmentally disabled children. *American Journal on Mental Retardation, 94*(3), 292–302.

Dyson, L. L. (1996). The experiences of families of children with learning disabilities: Parental stress, family functioning, and sibling self concept. *Journal of Learning Disabilities, 29,* 280–286.

Dyson, L. L. (1998). A support program for siblings of children with disabilities: What siblings learn and what they like. *Psychology in the Schools, 35*(1), 57–65.

Easterbrooks, S., & Baker, S. (2001). Enter the matrix! *Teaching Exceptional Children, 33*(3), 70–77.

Easterbrooks, S., & Stephenson, B. (2006). An examination of twenty literacy, science, and mathematics practices used to educate students who are deaf or hard of hearing. *American Annals of the Deaf, 151*(4), 385–397.

Easterbrooks, S. R., & Baker, S. (2002). *Language learning in children who are deaf and hard of hearing: Multiple pathways.* Boston: Allyn & Bacon.

Easterbrooks, S. R., & Houston, S. G. (2008). The signed reading fluency of students who are deaf/hard of hearing. *Journal of Deaf Studies and Deaf Education, 13*(1), 37–54.

Edwards, J. R. (1979). *Language and disadvantage.* London, England: Edward Arnold.

Egger, H. L., Kondo, D., & Angold, A. (2006). The epidemiology and diagnostic issues in preschool attention-deficit /hyperactivity disorder: A review. *Infants & Young Children, 19*(2), 109–122.

Eleweke, C. J., & Rodda, M. (2000). Factors contributing to parents' selection of a communication mode to use with their deaf children. *American Annals of the Deaf, 145*(4), 375–383.

Emerson, E. (2007). Poverty and people with intellectual disabilities. *Mental Retardation and Developmental Disabilities Research Reviews, 13,* 107–113.

Emerson, E., Graham, H., & Hatton, C. (2006). Household income and health status in children and adolescents: Cross sectional study. *European Journal of Public Health, 16,* 354–360.

Emmorey, K., Kosslyn, S., & Bellugi, U. (1993). Visual imagery and visual-spatial language: Enhanced imagery abilities in deaf and hearing SL signers. *Cognition, 46,* 139–181.

Employment Management Professionals Inc. (2008). Rethinking unemployment workshop information: A non-traditional approach to unemployment issues. Retrieved December 15, 2008, from www.employmentoutcomes.com

Eriks-Brophy, A., Durieux-Smith, A., Olds, J., Fitzpatrick, E., Duquette, C., & Whittingham, J. (2006). Facilitators and barriers to the inclusion of orally educated children and youth with hearing loss in schools promoting partnerships to support inclusion. *The Volta Review, 106*(1), 53–88.

Erting, C., Thurmann-Prezioso, C., & Sonnenstrahl-Benedict, B. (2000). Bilingualism in a Deaf family: Fingerspelling in early childhood. In P. Spencer, C. Erting, & M. Marschark (Eds.), *The deaf child in the family and at school* (pp. 41–54). Hillsdale, NJ: Erlbaum.

Estabrooks, W. (1994). *Auditory-verbal therapy.* Washington, DC: Alexander Graham Bell Association for the Deaf.

Evans, C. J. (2004). Literacy development in deaf students: Case studies in bilingual teaching and learning. *American Annals of the Deaf, 149*(1), 17–27.

Ewing, K. M., & Jones, T. W. (2003). An educational rationale for deaf students with multiple disabilities. *American Annals of the Deaf, 148,* 267–271.

Ewoldt, C., Israelite, N., & Dodds, R. (1992). The ability of deaf students to understand text: A comparison of the perceptions of teachers and students. *American Annals of the Deaf, 137,* 351–361.

Feuerstein, R. (1979). The dynamic assessment of retarded performers: The learning potential assessment, device theory, instruments, techniques. Baltimore: University Park Press.

Feuerstein, R. (1980). *Instrumental Enrichment: An intervention program for cognitive modifiability.* Baltimore: University Park Press.

Fewell, R. R., & Vadasy, P. F. (Eds.), *Families of handicapped children: Needs and supports across the life span* (pp. 75–98). Austin, TX: PRO-ED, Inc.

Finesilver, S. G. (1968). The driving records of deaf drivers. Statement by Sherman G. Finesilver, Denver District Judge, Denver, CO.

Fischer, L. C., & McWhirter, J. J. (2001). The deaf identity development scale: A revision and validation. *Journal of Counseling Psychology, 48,* 355–358.

Fitzgerald, T. (2000). *The educational needs of Deaf and hearing impaired children.* Wellington, New Zealand: Specialist Education Services.

Fitzpatrick, E., Graham, I. D., Durieux-Smith, A., Angus, D., & Coyle, D. (2007). Parents' perspectives on the impact of the early diagnosis of childhood hearing loss. *International Journal of Audiology, 46,* 97–106.

Fleetwood, E., & Metzger, M. (1998). *Cued language structure: An analysis of cued American English based on linguistic principles.* Silver Spring, MD: Calliope Press.

Float, J. (2002). Jeff Float. In J. Reisler, *Voices of the oral deaf: Fourteen role models speak out.* Jefferson, NC: McFarland & Company.

Foehr, U. (2006). Media multitasking among American youth: Prevalence, predictors and pairings. Menlo Park, CA: Henry J. Kaiser Foundation. Retrieved January 20, 2011, from kff.org/entmedia/upload/7592.pdf

Foster, S. (1987). Employment experiences of deaf RIT graduates: An interview study. *Journal of Rehabilitation of the Deaf, 21*(1), 1–15.

Foster, S. (1992). *Working with deaf people: Accessibility and accommodation in the workplace.* Springfield, IL: Charles C Thomas.

Foster, S. (1998). Communication as social engagement: Implications for interactions between deaf and hearing persons. *Social Audiology, 27*(Suppl. 49), 116–124.

Freeman, B., Dieterich, Y. A., & Rak, C. (2002). The struggle for language: perspectives and practices of urban parents with children who are deaf or hard of hearing. *American Annals of the Deaf, 147*(5), 37–44.

Freyman, R., Nerbonne, G., & Cole, H. (1991). Effect of consonant-vowel-ratio modification on amplitude envelope cues for consonant recognition. *Journal of Speech Hearing Research, 34,* 415–426.

Friedman, T. F. (2005, June 2). *The world is flat.* New York: Farrar, Strauss, and Giroux.

Friend, M., & Bursuck, W. D. (2006). *Including students with special needs: A practical guide for classroom teachers* (4th ed.). Boston: Allyn & Bacon.

Fuchs, D., Fuchs, L. S., Mathes, P. G., Lipsey, M. W., & Roberts, P. H. (2002). Is "learning disabilities" just a fancy term for low achievement? A meta-analysis of reading differences between low achievers with and without the label. In R. Bradley, L. Danielson, & D. P. Hallahan (Eds.), *Identification of learning disabilities: Research to practice* (pp. 747–762). Mahwah, NJ: Erlbaum.

Fujiura, G. T., & Parish, S. L. (2007). Emerging policy challenges in intellectual disabilities. *Mental Retardation and Developmental Disabilities Research Reviews, 13*(2), 188–194.

Furth, H. (1964). Research with the deaf: Implications for language and cognition. *Psychological Bulletin, 62*(5), 461–462.

Furth, H. (1966). *Thinking without language.* New York: Free Press.

Furth, H. (1973). *Deafness and learning: A psychological approach.* Belmont, CA: Wadsworth.

Gage, N. L., & Berliner, D. C. (1988). *Educational psychology.* Boston: Houghton Mifflin.

Gallaudet Research Institute. (2006, December). *Regional and national summary report of data from the 2006–2007 annual survey of deaf and hard of hearing children and youth.* Washington, DC: Gallaudet University.

Gallaudet Research Institute. (2008, November). *Regional and national summary report of data from the 2007–2008 annual survey of deaf and hard of hearing children and youth.* Washington, DC: Gallaudet University.

Gallego, M., & Hollingsworth, S. (2000). Introduction: The idea of multiple literacies. In M. Gallego & S. Hollingsworth (Eds.), *What counts as literacy: Challenging the school standard* (pp. 1–23). New York: Teachers College Press.

Gallego, M., & Hollingsworth, S. (Eds.). (2006). *Challenging the school standard.* New York: Teachers College Press.

Gannon, J. R. (1981). *Deaf heritage: A narrative history of deaf America.* Silver Spring, MD: National Association of the Deaf.

Garcia, M. M., Shaw, D. S., Winslow, E. B., & Yaggi, K. E. (2000). Destructive sibling conflict and the development of conduct problems in young boys. *Developmental Psychology, 36,* 44–53.

Gardner, H. (1983). *Frames of mind.* New York: Basic Books, Inc.

Gardner, H. (1985). *The mind's new science: A history of the cognitive revolution.* New York: Basic Books.

Garrison, W., Long, G., & Dowaliby, F. (1997). Working memory capacity and comprehension processes in deaf readers. *Journal of Deaf Studies and Deaf Education, 2,* 78–94.

Gately, S. E., & Gately, F. J. (2001). Understanding coteaching components. *Teaching Exceptional Children, 33*(4), 40–47.

Geers, A., Brenner, C., & Davidson, L. (2003). Factors associated with development of speech perception skills in children implanted by age five. *Ear and Hearing, 24*(Suppl. 24S–35S).

Geers, A., Brenner, C., Nicholas, J., Uchanski, R., Tye-Murray, N., & Tobey, E. (2002). Rehabiitation factors contributing to implant benefit in children. *The Annals of Otology, Rhinology & Laryngology, 111,* 127–130.

Gibson, J. W., Blackwell, C. W., Dominicis, P., & Dermerath, N. (2002, April 1). Telecommuting in the 21st century: Benefits, issues, and a leadership model which will work. *Journal of Leadership & Organizational Studies, 8,* 75.

Ginsburg, C. (2002). Carolyn Ginsburg. In J. Reisler, *Voices of the oral deaf: Fourteen role models speak out.* Jefferson, NC: McFarland & Company.

Glanzman, M. M., & Blum, N. J. (2007). Attention deficits and hyperactivity. In M. L. Batshaw, L. Pellegrino, & N. Roizen (Eds.), *Children with disabilities* (6th ed., pp. 345–365). Baltimore: Brookes.

Glattke, T. J. (1977). Some implications for research. In W. R. Hodgson & P. H. Skinner (Eds.), *Hearing aid assessment and use in audiologic habilitation.* Baltimore: Williams & Wilkins Co.

Gleason, J. B., & Ratner, N. B. (2009). *The development of Lanugage.* Boston: Pearson.

Glickman, N. S. (1993). *Deaf identity development: Construction and validation of a theoretical model.* Unpublished doctoral dissertation, University of Massachusetts.

Goode, R. (1995). Currency status and future of implantable electromagnetic hearing aids: Middle and inner ear electronic implantable devices for partial hearing loss. *Otolaryngologic Clinics of North America, 28*(1), 141–146.

Goss, B. (2003). Hearing from the deaf culture. Intercultural Communication Studies XII-2, New Mexico State University. Retrieved January 21, 2011, from www.uri.edu/iaics/content/2003v12n2/03%20Blaine%20Goss.pdf

Gough, P. (1984). Word recognition. In P. Pearson, R. Barr, M. Kamil, & P. Mosenthal (Eds.), *Handbook of reading research* (Vol. I, pp. 203–211). New York: Longman.

Graves, M. (2006). *The vocabulary book: Learning and instruction.* New York: Teachers College Press.

Graves, M., & Watts-Taffe, S. (2002). The place of word consciousness in research-based vocabulary program. In A. Farstrup & S. J. Samuels (Eds.), *What research has to say about reading instruction* (pp. 140–165). Newark, DE: International Reading Association.

Gray, L., & Hannan, A. J. (2007). Dissecting cause and effect in the pathogenesis of psychiatric disorders: Genes, environment and behaviour. *Current Molecular Medicine, 7*(5), 470–478.

Greenberg, B. L., & Withers, S. (1965). *Better English usage: A guide for the Deaf.* Indianapolis, IN: Bobbs-Merrill.

Greenberg, M. T., Lengua, L. J., & Calderon, R. (1997). The nexus of culture and sensory loss. In S. A. Wolchik & I. N. Sandler (Eds.), *Handbook of children's coping: Linking theory and intervention* (pp. 301–332). New York: Plenum Press.

Greenmum R. M. (1952, September). Stop! That driver's deaf! Safety Education.

Greenspan, S. I. (2003). Working with the hearing impaired child. *Scholastic Early Childhood Today, 17*(7), 20–21.

Gregg, J. L. (2006). Policy-making in the public interest: A contextual analysis of the passage of closed-captioning policy. *Disability & Society, 21,* 537–550.

Gregory, S. (1976). *The deaf child and his family.* New York: Halstead Press. (Republished as *Deaf children and their families.* Cambridge, England: Cambridge University Press, 1995).

Gresham, F., & MacMillan, D. (1997). Social competence and affective characteristics of students with mild disabilities. *Review of Educational Research, 67,* 377–415.

Grieco, E. M., & Trevelyan, E. N. (2010). Place of birth of the foreign-born. American Community Survey Briefs. U.S. Census Bureau. Retrieved February 7, 2011, from www.census.gov/prod/2010pubs/acsbr09-15.pdf

Grinker, R. R. (2008). What in the world is autism: A cross-cultural perspective. *Zero to Three, 28,* 5–10.

Groce, N. (1980). Everyone here spoke sign language. *Natural History, 89*(6), 10–19.

Groce, N. (1985). *Everyone here spoke sign language.* Cambridge, MA: Harvard University Press.

Gureasko-Moore, D., DuPaul, G., & Power, T. (2005). Stimulant treatment for attention-deficit/hyperactivity disorder: Medication monitoring practices of school psychologists. *School Psychology Review, 34*(2), 232–245.

Gustason, G., Pfetzing, D., & Zawolkow, E. (1972). *Signing Exact English.* Rossmoor, CA: Modern Signs Press.

Hadjikakou K., & Nikolaraizi, M. (2007). The impact of personal educational experiences and communication practices on the construction of deaf identity in Cyprus. *American Annals of the Deaf, 152*(4), 398–413.

Hall, B. (2005, February). The top training priorities for 2005. *Training, 42,* 22–28.

Hall, B., Oyer, H., & Haas, W. (2001). *Speech, language, and hearing disorders: A guide for the teacher.* Boston: Allyn & Bacon.

Hall, E. T., & Hall, M. (1989). *Understanding cultural differences: Germans, French and Americans.* Yarmouth, ME: Intercultural Press.

Hamilton, S. (2001). Susan Hamilton. In R. McKey (Ed.), *People of the eye: Stories from the deaf world* (pp. 87–96). Wellington, New Zealand: Bridget Williams Books.

Hammes, D., Novak, M., Rotz, L., Willis, M., & Edmondson, D. (2002). Early identification and cochlear implantation: Critical factors for spoken-language development. *Annals of Otology, Rhinology, and Laryngotogy, 189* (Suppl.), 74–78.

Hanson, V. L. (1982). Short-term recall by deaf signers of American Sign Language: Implications of encoding strategy for order recall. *Journal of Experimental Psychology: Learning, Memory, and Cognition, 8,* 572–583.

Hanson, V. L., Liberman, I. Y., & Shankweiler, D. (1984). Linguistic coding by deaf children in relation to beginning reading success. *Journal of Experimental Child Psychology, 37,* 378–393.

Harper, G. W., Jernewall, N., & Zea, M. C. (2004). Giving voice to emerging science and theory for lesbian, gay, and bisexual people of color. *Cultural Diversity and Ethnic Minority Psychology, 10*(3), 187–199.

Harris, J. C. (2006). *Intellectual disability: Understanding its development, causes, classification, evaluation, and treatment.* Oxford, England: Oxford University Press.

Harris, M., & Beech, J. R. (1998). Implicit phonological awareness and early reading development in pre-lingually deaf children. *Journal of Deaf Studies and Deaf Education, 3,* 205–216.

Harrison, D. R. (1980). Natural oralism: A description. *Journal of British Association Teachers of the Deaf, 4*(4), 8–11.

Harryman, S., & Warren, L. (1985). Physical and occupational therapy models for motor evaluation. In E. Chewor (Ed.), *Hearing impaired children and youth with developmental disabilities*. Washington, DC: Gallaudet College Press.

Harter, S. (1990). Processes underlying adolescent self-concept formation. In R. Montemayor, G. R. Adams, & T. P. Gullotta (Eds.), *From childhood to adolescence: A transitional period?* (pp. 205–239). Newbury Park, CA: Sage.

Harter, S., & Monsour, A. (1992). Developmental analysis of conflict caused by opposing attributes in the adolescent self-portrait. In D. Boyd & H. Bee (Eds.), *Lifespan development* (5th ed., 2009). Boston: Pearson.

Hartung, C. M., & Scambler, D. J. (2006). Dealing with bullying and victimization in schools. *Emotional & Behavioral Disorders in Youth, 6,* 73–96.

Hassanzadeh, A. D. S. (2007). Cochlear implantation in prelingually deaf persons with additional disability. *The Journal of Laryngology & Otology, 121,* 635–638.

Haynes, W. O., & Shulman, B. S. (Eds.). (1998). *Communication development: Foundations, processes, and clinical applications* (pp. 361–386). Baltimore: Williams & Wilkins.

Haywood, H. C., Towery-Woolsey, J., Arbitman-Smith, R., & Aldridge, A. H. (1988). Cognitive education with deaf adolescents: Effects of instrumental enrichment. *Topics in Language Disorders, 8*(4), 23–40.

He, W., Sengupta, M., Velkoff, V. A., & DeBarros, K. A. (2005). 65+ in the United States: 2005 current population reports special studies 23–209. U.S. Census Bureau. Retrieved January 15, 2011, from www.census.gov/prod/2006pubs/p23-209.pdf

Hearing Industries Association (HIA). (1984). *HIA market survey: A summary of findings and business implications for the U.S. hearing aid industry.* Washington, DC: Author.

Heider, F., & Heider, G. (1940). A comparison of sentence structure of deaf and hearing children. *Psychological Monographs, 52,* 42–103.

Heimlich, J. E., & Pittelman, S. D. (1986). *Semantic mapping: Classroom applications.* Newark, DE: International Reading Association, Reading Aids Series.

The Herman Group. (2005, February 9). Secret of effective leadership in 21st century. The Herman Trend Alert. Retrieved January 21, 2011, at www.hermangroup.com/alert/archive_2-9-2005.html

Hermans, D., Knoors, H., Ormel, E., & Verhoeven, L. (2008). Modeling reading vocabulary learning in deaf children in bilingual education programs. *Journal of Deaf Studies, 13*(2), 155–174.

Herrmann, B., Thornton, A., & Joseph, J. (1995). Automated infant hearing screening using the ABR: Development and validation. *American Journal of Audiology, 4,* 6–14.

Heward, W. L. (2003). *Educational children: An introduction to special education* (7th ed.). Upper Saddle River, NJ: Merrill Prentice Hall.

Higgins, P. C. (1980). *Outsiders in a hearing world.* Beverly Hills, CA: Sage Publications.

Hintermair, M. (2006). Parental resources, parental stress, and socioemotional development of deaf and hard of hearing children. *Journal of Deaf Studies and Deaf Education, 11*(4), 493–513.

Hirsh-Pasek, K. (1987). The metalinguistics of fingerspelling: An alternate way to increase reading vocabulary in congenitally deaf readers. *Reading Research Quarterly, 22,* 455–474.

Hocutt, A. M. (1996). Effectiveness of special education: Is placement the critical factor? *The Future of Children: Special Education for Students with Disabilities, 6*(1), 77–102.

Hogg, N., Lomicky, C., & Weiner, S. (2008). Computer-mediated communication and the Gallaudet University community: A preliminary report. *American Annals of the Deaf, 153*(1), 89–96.

Holdaway, D. (1979). *The foundations of literacy.* Portsmouth, NH: Heinemann.

Horn, L., Berktold, J., & Bobbitt, L. (1999). *Students with disabilities in postsecondary education: A profile on preparation, participation, and outcomes* (NCES Publication No. 1999–187). Washington, DC: National Center for Education Statistics, U. S. Department of Education.

Horn, L., Peter, K., Rooney, K., & Malizio, A. G. (2002). *Profile of undergraduates in U.S. postsecondary institutions: 1999–2000* (NCES Publication No. 2002–168). Washington, DC: National Center for Education Statistics, U. S. Department of Education.

Huberty, T. J., & Koller, J. R. (1984). A test of the learning potential hypothesis with hearing and deaf students. *Journal of Educational Research, 78,* 22–28.

Humphrey, J. H., & Alcorn, B. J. (1994). *So you want to be an interpreter: An introduction to sign language interpreting.* Salem, OR: Sign Enhancers.

Humphrey, J. A., & Alcorn, B. J. (2001). *So you want to be an interpreter? An introduction to sign language interpreting* (3rd ed.). Amarillo, TX: H&H Publishers.

Humphries, T. (2005). In C. Padden & T. Humphries (Eds.), *Inside deaf culture.* Cambridge, MA: Harvard University Press.

Individuals with Disabilities Education Act regulations (IDEA), 34 C.F.R 300.8 (2006).

Infoplease. (2007). Pearson Education: U.S. Bureau of the Census, August 2008. Supplement to the Current Population Survey (CPS). Retrieved January 6, 2011, from www.infoplease.com

Israelite, N. K. (1986). Hearing-impaired children and the psychological functioning of their normal-hearing siblings. *The Volta Review, 88*(1), 47–54.

Israelite, N., & Ewoldt, C. (1992). *Bilingual/bicultural education for deaf and hard-of-hearing students: A review of the literature on the effects of native sign language on majority language acquisition.* Toronto, Canada: Queen's Printer for Ontario.

Israelite, N., Ower, J., & Goldstein, G. (2002). Hard-of-hearing adolescents and identity construction: Influences of school experiences, peers, and teachers. *Journal of Deaf Studies and Deaf Education, 7*(2), 134–148.

Jackson, D., Paul, P., & Smith, J. (1997). Prior knowledge and reading comprehension ability of deaf and hard-of-hearing adolescents. *Journal of Deaf Studies and Deaf Education, 2,* 172–184.

Jambor, E., & Elliott, M. (2005). Self-esteem and coping strategies among deaf students. *Journal of Deaf Studies and Deaf Education, 10*(1), 63–80.

James, D. (2002). David James. In J. Reisler, *Voices of the oral deaf: Fourteen role models speak out.* Jefferson, NC: McFarland & Company.

Janger, M. (2002). Michael Janger. In J. Reisler, *Voices of the oral deaf: Fourteen role models speak out.* Jefferson, NC: McFarland & Company.

Jankowski, K. A. (1997). *Deaf empowerment: Emergence, struggle, and rhetoric.* Washington, DC: Gallaudet University Press.

Johnson, C. D. (2009). In J. Katz (Ed.), *Handbook of clinical audiology* (6th ed., pp. 564–583). Philadelphia: Lippincott Williams & Wilkins.

Johnson, H. A. (2004). U.S. Deaf education teacher preparation programs: A look at the present and a vision for the future. *American Annals of the Deaf, 149*(2), 75–91.

Johnson, M. J. (1988, June). *Debugging the human computer: Instrumental enrichment.* Paper presented at the Annual Southeast Regional Summer Conference: New Directions in Resources for Special Needs Hearing Impaired Students, Cave Spring, Georgia. (ERIC Document Reproduction Service No. ED312845)

Johnson, R. (1994). Possible influences on bilingualism in early ASL acquisition. *Teaching English to Deaf and Second Language Students, 10,* 9–17.

Johnson, R. E., Liddell, S. K., & Erting, C. J. (1989). *Unlocking the Curriculum: Principles for Achieving Access in Deaf Education* (Gallaudet Research Institute Working Paper 89–3). Washington, DC: Gallaudet University.

Johnson, V. (1993). Factors impacting the job retention and advancement of workers who are deaf. *The Volta Review, 95,* 341–356.

Jonas, B., & Martin, D. S. (1984). Cognitive improvement of hearing-impaired high school students through instruction in instrumental enrichment. International Symposium on Cognition, Education, and Deafness. Washington, DC: Working Papers, Volumes I & II. (ERIC Document Reproduction Service No. ED 247725)

Josselson, R. (1994). The theory of identity development and the question of intervention: An introduction. In S. L. Archer (Ed.), *Intervention for adolescent identity development* (pp. 12–25). Thousand Oaks, CA: Sage.

Jure, R., Rapin, I., & Tuchman, R. F. (1991). Hearing impaired autistic children. *Developmental Medicine and Child Neurology, 33,* 1062–1072.

Kaminsky, L., & Dewey, D. (2001). Sibling relationships of children with autism. *Journal of Autism and Developmental Disorders, 31,* 399–411.

Kanda, J., & Colonomos, B. (1990). Issues in interpreter education. In C. Baker Shenk (Ed.), *A model curriculum for American Sign Language and teachers of interpreting* (pp. 175–192). Silver Spring, MD: RID Publications.

Karchmer, M. S., & Mitchell, R. E. (2003). Demographic and achievement characteristics of deaf and hard of hearing students. In M. Marschark & P. E. Spencer (Eds.), *The Oxford handbook of deaf studies, language, and education* (pp. 21–37). New York: Oxford University Press.

Katz, J. (Ed.). (2009). *Handbook of clinical audiology* (6th ed.). Philadelphia: Lippincott Williams & Wilkins.

Kauffman, J. M. (1993). How we might achieve the radical reform of special education. *Exceptional Children, 60,* 6–16.

Kauffman, J. M. (2001). *Characteristics of emotional and behavioral disorders of children and youth* (7th ed.). Upper Saddle River, NJ: Merrill/Pearson.

Kavin, D., & Brown-Kurz, K. (2008). The career experiences of deaf supervisors in education and social service professions: Choices, mobility and networking a qualitative study. *Journal of the American Deafness and Rehabilitation Association, 42*(1), 24–47.

Keane, K. J., & Kretschmer, R. E. (1987). Effect of mediated learning intervention on task performance with a deaf population. *Journal of Educational Psychology, 79*(1), 49–53.

Keats, B. J., & Lentz, J. (2008). Usher syndrome Type 1. Gene reviews, NCBI Bookshelf. Retrieved March 3, 2011, from www.ncbi.nlm.nih.gov/books/NBK1265

Keefe, E. B., Moore, V., & Duff, F. (2004). The four "knows" of collaborative teaching. *Teaching Exceptional Children, 36*(5), 36–42.

Keith, R. W. (1996). The audiologic evaluation. In J. L. Northern (Ed.), *Hearing disorders* (3rd. ed., pp. 45–56). Boston: Allyn & Bacon.

Kelly, L. (2003). The importance of processing automaticity and temporary storage capacity to the differences in comprehension between skilled and less skilled college-age deaf readers. *Journal of Deaf Studies and Deaf Education, 8*(3), 230–249.

Kelly, L. P. (1993). Recall of English function words and inflections by skilled and average deaf readers. *American Annals of the Deaf, 138,* 288–296.

Killoran, J. (2007). *The national deaf-blind child count: 1998–2005 in review.* Monmouth, OR: NTAC. Retrieved February 16, 2011, from nationaldb.org/documents/products/population.pdf

Kinsella-Meier, M. A. (1995). Is the audiogram important to consider when determining inclusion? In B. D. Snider (Ed.). *Inclusion? Defining quality education for deaf and hard of hearing students* (pp. 63–77). Washington, DC: Gallaudet University Press.

Kirk, K. I., Miyamoto, R. T., Lento, C. L., Ying, E., O'Neill, T., & Fears, B. (2002). Effects of age at implantation in young children. *The Annals of Otology, Rhinology & Laryingology, 111,* 69–73.

Kirkwood, D. H. (2006). Survey probes the economic realities of the dispensing business. *Hearing Journal, 59*(3), 19–32.

Kluwin, T., & Gaustad, M. (1991). Predicting family communication choices. *American Annals of the Deaf, 136*(1), 28–34.

Kluwin, T., Gonsher, W., Silver, K., & Samuels, J. (1996). Team teaching students with hearing impairments and students with normal hearing together. *Teaching Exceptional Children, 29*(1), 11–15.

Kluwin, T., Moores, D. (1985). The effect of integration on the achievement of hearing impaired adolescents. *Exceptional Children, 52,* 153–160.

Kluwin, T. N. (1999). Coteaching deaf and hearing students: Research on social integration. *American Annals of the Deaf, 144*(4), 339–343.

Kluwin, T. N., Morris, C. S., & Clifford, J. (2004). A rapid ethnography of itinerant teachers of the deaf. *American Annals of the Deaf, 149*(1), 62–72.

Kluwin, T. N., Stinson, M. S., & Colarossi, G. M. (2002). Social processes and outcomes of in-school contact between deaf and hearing peers. *Journal of Deaf Studies and Deaf Education, 7*(3), 200–213.

Knapp, L. G., Kelly-Reid, J. E., & Ginder, S. A. (2008). *Postsecondary institutions in the United States: Fall 2007, degrees and other awards conferred: 2006–07, and 12-month enrollment 2006–07* (NCES Publication No. 2008–359). Washington, DC: National Center for Education Statistics, U. S. Department of Education.

Komesaroff, L. (Ed.). (2007). *Surgical consent bioethics and cochlear implantation.* Washington, DC: Gallaudet University Press.

Kominski, R., & Newburger, E. (1999). Access denied: Changes in computer ownership and use: 1984–1987. Population Division, U.S. Census Bureau. Retrieved January 29, 2011, from www.census.gov/population/socdemo/computer/confpap99.pdf

Kourbetis, V. (1987). Education of the deaf in Greece. First International Conference on Education of the Deaf, Athens, Greece.

Krapf, G. (1985). *The effects of mediated intervention on advance figural analogic problem solving with deaf adolescents: Implications for dynamic assessment.*

Unpublished doctoral dissertation, Temple University, Philadelphia.

Kreider, R. M. (2003). Adopted children and stepchildren: 2000. U.S. Census Bureau. Retrieved January 15, 2011, from www.census.gov/prod/2003pubs/censr-6.pdf

Kreimeyer, K., Crooke, P., Drye, C., Egbert, V., & Klein, B. (2000). Academic benefits of a co-enrollment model of inclusive education for deaf and hard-of hearing children. *Journal of Deaf Studies and Deaf Education, 5*(2), 174–185.

Kusche, C. A., Greenberg, M. T., & Garfield, T. S. (1983). Nonverbal intelligence and verbal achievement in deaf adolescents: An examination of heredity and environment. *American Annals of the Deaf, 128,* 458–466.

Ladd, P. (2003). *Understanding deaf culture: In search of deafhood.* Clevedon, England: Multilingual Matters.

Lamb, M. E., & Sutton-Smith, B. (1982). *Sibling relationships: Their nature and significance across the life span.* Hillsdale, NJ: Erlbaum.

Lane, H., Hoffmeister, R., & Bahan, B. (1996). *A journey into the deaf-world.* San Diego, CA: Dawn Sign Press.

Lang, H. G. (2003). Perspectives on the history of deaf education. In Marschark, M., & Spencer, P. E. (Eds.). (2003). *Deaf studies, language, and education* (pp. 9–19). New York: Oxford University Press.

LaSasso, C., Crain, K., & Leybaert, J. (2003). Rhyme generation in deaf students: The effect of exposure to cued speech. *Journal of Deaf Studies and Deaf Education, 8,* 250–270.

LaSasso, C., & Davey, B. (1987). The relationship between lexical knowledge and reading comprehension for prelingually, profoundly hearing-impaired students. *The Volta Review, 89,* 211–220.

LaSasso, C., & Lollis, J. (2003). Survey of residential and day schools for deaf students in the United States that identify themselves as bilingual-bicultural programs. *Journal of Deaf Studies and Deaf Education, 8*(1), 79–91.

Leigh, I. W. (2009). *A lens on deaf identities.* Oxford, England: Oxford University Press.

Leigh, I. W. (2010) Reflections on identity. In M. Marschark & P. E. Spencer (Eds.), *The Oxford handbook of deaf studies, language, and education* (pp. 195–209). Oxford, England: Oxford University Press.

Leigh, I. W., & Stinson, M. (1991). Social environments, self perceptions, and identity of hearing impaired adolescents. *The Volta Review, 93*(7), 7–22.

Leonard, D. R., Shen, T., Howe, H. L., & Egler, T. (Eds.). (1999). *Trends in the prevalence of birth defects in Illinois and Chicago 1989 to 1997* (Epidemiologic Report Series 99:4). Springfield: Illinois Department of Public Health.

Lerner, J., & Kline, F. (2006). *Learning disabilities and related disorders.* Boston: Houghton Mifflin.

Levitt, A. M., Watchko, J. F., Bennett, F. C., & Folsom, R. C. (1987). Neurodevelopmental outcome following persistent pulmonary hypertension of the neonate. *Journal of Perinatology, 7*(4), 288–91.

Levitt, H. (2007). A historical perspective on digital hearing aids: How digital technology has changed modern hearing aids. *Trends in Amplification, 11*(1), 7–24.

Lewis, L., Farris, E., & Greene, B. (1999). An institutional perspective on students with disabilities in postsecondary education (NCES Publication No. 1999–046). Washington, DC: National Center for Education Statistics, U. S. Department of Education.

Lewis, S. (1996). The reading achievement of a group of severely and profoundly hearing-impaired school leavers educated within a natural aural approach. *Journal of British Association of Teachers of the Deaf, 20*(1), 1–7.

Leybaert, J., & Lechat, J. (2001). Variability in deaf children's spelling. The effect of language experience. *Journal of Educational Psychology, 93,* 554–562.

Liefert, F. (2003). Introduction to visual impairment. In S. A. Goodman & S. H. Wittenstein (Eds.), *Collaborative assessment: Working with students who are blind or visually impaired, including those with additional disabilities* (pp. 1–22). AFB Press: New York.

Ling, D. (2002). *Speech and the hearing-impaired child: Theory and practice* (2nd ed.). Washington, DC: Alexander Graham Bell Association for the Deaf.

Livneh, H., & Antonak, R. F. (1997). *Psychosocial adaptation to chronic illness and disability.* Gaithersburg, MD: Aspen.

Lobato, D., Barbour, L., Hall, L. J., & Miller, C. T. (1987). Psychosocial characteristics of preschool siblings of handicapped and non-handicapped children. *Journal of Abnormal Child Psychology, 15*(3), 329–338.

Logan, G. D. (1978). Attention in character classification tasks: Evidence for the automaticity of component stages. *Journal of Experimental Psychology (Gen.), 107,* 32–63.

Logie, R. H. (1995). *Visuo-spatial working memory.* Hove, England: Erlbaum.

Long, G. (1996). *Assessing workplace communication skills with traditionally underserved persons who are deaf.* DeKalb: Northern Illinois University Research and Training Center on Traditionally Underserved Persons Who Are Deaf.

Long, G., Long, N. M., & Ouelette, S. E. (1993). Service provision issues with traditionally underserved persons who are deaf. In O. M. Welch (Ed.), *Research and practice in deafness: Issues and questions in education, psychology, and vocational service provision* (pp. 107–126). Springfield, IL: Charles C Thomas.

Long, G., Stinson, M., Kelly, R. R., & Liu, Y. (1999). The relationship between teacher sign skills and student evaluations of teacher capability. *American Annals of the Deaf, 144*(5), 354–364.

Luckasson, R., Borthwick-Duffy, S., Buntinx, W. H. E., Coulter, D. L., Craig, F. M., Reeve, A. I., et al. (2002). *Mental retardation: Definition, classification, and systems of supports.* Washington, DC: American Association on Mental Retardation.

Luckner, J. (1991). Skills needed for teaching hearing impaired adolescents: The perception of teachers. *American Annals of the Deaf, 136,* 422–428.

Luckner, J. L. (2006). Providing itinerant services. In D. F. Moores & D. S. Martin (Eds.), *Deaf learners: Developments in curriculum and instruction* (pp. 93–111). Washington, DC: Gallaudet University Press.

Luckner, J. L., & Carter, K. (2001). Essential competencies for teaching students with hearing loss and additional disabilities. *American Annals of the Deaf, 146*(1), 7–15.

Luckner, J. L., & Howell J. (2002). Suggestions for preparing itinerant teachers: A qualitative analysis. *American Annals of the Deaf, 147*(3), 54–61.

Luckner, J. L., & McNeill, J. H. (1994). Performance of a group of deaf and hard-of-hearing students and a comparison group of hearing students on a series of problem-solving tasks. *American Annals of the Deaf, 139,* 371–377.

Luckner, J., & Muir, S. (2001). Successful students who are deaf in general education settings. *American Annals of the Deaf, 146,* 435–446.

Luckner, J. L., & Muir, S. (2002). Suggestions for helping students who are deaf succeed in general education settings. *Communication Disorders Quarterly, 24*(1), 23–30.

Luckner, J. L., & Stewart, J. (2003). Self-assessments and other perceptions of successful adults who are deaf: An initial investigation. *American Annals of the Deaf, 148*(3), 243–250.

Luckner J. L., & Velaski, A. (2004). Healthy families of children who are deaf. *American Annals of the Deaf Volume, 149*(4), 324–335.

Luetke-Stahlman, B. (1992). Hearing-impaired preschoolers in integrated child care. *Perspectives in Education and Deafness, 9,* 8–11.

Luft, P. (2008). Examining educators of the deaf as "highly qualified" teachers: Roles and responsibilities under IDEA and NCLB. *American Annals of the Deaf, 152*(5), 429–440.

Luft, P., Vierstra, C., Copeland, C., & Resh, N. (2009). How staffing patterns impact employment outcomes across diverse D/HH Consumers. *Journal of the American Deafness and Rehabilitation Association,* 2009 Conference Issue Supplement, 210–219.

Luterman, D. M., & Ross, M. (1991). *When your child is deaf: A guide for parents.* Parkton, MD: York Press.

Mackey, E., & La Greca, A. (2007). Adolescents' eating, exercise, and weight control behaviors: Does peer crowd affiliation play a role? *Journal of Pediatric Psychology, 32,* 13–23.

Maller, S. J. (2003). Intellectual assessment of deaf people. In M. Marschark & P. E. Spencer (Eds.), *The Oxford handbook of Deaf studies, language, and education* (pp. 451–460). New York: Oxford University Press.

Mandell, D., Novak, M., & Zubritsky, C. (2005). Factors associated with age of diagnosis among children with autism spectrum disorders. *Pediatrics, 116*(6), 1480–1486.

Maniglia, A. (1989). Implantable hearing devices. *Otolaryngologic Clinics of North America, 22*(1), 36–58.

Mansaram, M., & Lopez, S. J. (2009). Group rehabilitation: Transitioning at-risk youth and adults. *Journal of the American Deafness and Rehabilitation Association,* 2009 Conference Issue Supplement, 220–229.

Manusov, V. (1995). Reacting to changes in nonverbal behaviors: Relational satisfaction and adaptation patterns in romantic dyads. *Human Communication Research, 21,* 456–477.

Markides, A. (1989). Integration: The speech intelligibility, friendship and associations of hearing impaired children in secondary schools. *Journal of the British Association of Teachers of the Deaf,* 13(3), 63–72.

Marschark, M. (1993). *Psychological development of deaf children.* New York: Oxford University Press.

Marschark, M., & Everhart, V. S. (1999). Problem-solving by deaf and hearing students: Twenty questions. *Deafness and Education International, 1*(2), 65–82.

Marschark, M., & Harris, M. (1996). *Raising and educating a deaf child.* New York: Oxford University Press.

Marschark, M., & Hauser, P. C. (Eds.). (2008). Deaf cognition foundations and outcomes. New York: Oxford University Press.

Marschark, M., Lang, H. G., & Albertini, J. A. (2002). *Educating deaf students: From research to practice.* New York: Oxford University Press.

Marschark, M., & Mayer, T. S. (1998). Interactions of language and memory in deaf children and adults. *Scandinavian Journal of Psychology, 39,* 145–148.

Marschark, M., & Spencer, P. E. (Eds.). (2003). *Deaf studies, language, and education.* New York: Oxford University Press.

Marschark, M., & Spencer, P. E. (2010). *The Oxford handbook of deaf studies, language, and education* (Vol. 2). New York: Oxford University Press.

Marschark, M., Young, A., & Lukomski, J. (2002). Perspectives on inclusion. *Journal of deaf studies and deaf Education, 7*(3), 187–188.

Marshall, E. M. (1995, June). The collaborative workplace. *Management Review, 84,* 13–18.

Martin, D., & Bat-Chava, Y. (2003). Negotiating deaf-hearing friendships: Coping strategies of deaf boys and girls in mainstream schools. *Child Care, Health & Development, 29,* 511–521.

Martin, D. C. (Ed.). (2005). The national agenda: Moving forward on achieving educational equality for deaf and hard of hearing students—A forum. Washington, DC: U.S. Department of Education.

Martin, D. S. (1983, April). *Cognitive education for the hearing-impaired adolescent.* Paper presented at the annual conference of the American Educational Research Association, Montreal, Canada. (ERIC Document Reproduction Service No. ED233511)

Martin, D. S. (1984). Cognitive modification for the hearing impaired adolescent: The promise. *Exceptional Children, 51,* 235–242.

Martin, D. S. (1995). *Mediated learning experience and deaf learners.* Paper presented at the meeting of the 18th International Congress on Education of the Deaf, Tel Aviv, Israel. (ERIC Reproduction Service No. ED 390 185)

Martin, D. S., & Jonas, B. S. (1986). Cognitive modifiability in the deaf adolescent. Washington, DC: Gallaudet University. (ERIC Document Reproduction Service No. ED276159)

Martin, D. S., Rohr, C., & Innes, J. (1982, February). *Teaching thinking skills to hearing-impaired adolescents.* Paper presented at the Washington Regional Conference of Educators of the Hearing-Impaired, Kendall Demonstration Elementary School, Washington, DC. (ERIC Document Reproduction Service No. ED221969)

Martin, F. N., & Clark, J. G. (2009). *Introduction to audiology* (10th ed.). Boston: Allyn & Bacon.

Martin, J. (2003, August 2). Rise of the new breed. *Chief Executive,* 24.

Mascia, N., & Mascia, J. (2008). Audiology on the job: the vocational rehabilitation and audiology partnership. *Journal of the American Deafness and Rehabilitation Association, 41*(2), 95–112.

Maslow, A. H. (1954). *Motivation and personality.* New York: Harper.

Mauk, G. W., & Mauk, P. P. (1993). Compounding the challenge: Young deaf children and learning disabilities. *Perspectives in Education and Deafness, 12*(2), 12–17.

Maxwell-McCaw, D. I. (2001). *Acculturation and psychological well-being in deaf and hard of hearing people.* Doctoral dissertation, George Washington University, Washington, DC. *Dissertation Abstracts International, 61*(11-B), 6141.

May, F. B. (1994). *Reading as communication.* New York: Merrill.

Mayer, C., & Akamatsu, C. T. (2003). Bilingualist and literacy. In M. Marschark & P. E. Spencer (Eds.), *The Oxford handbook of deaf studies, language, and education* (pp. 361–370). New York: Oxford University Press.

Mayer, C., Akamatsu, C. T., & Stewart, D. (2002). A model for effective practice: Dialogic inquiry with students who are deaf. *Exceptional Children, 68*(4), 485–502.

McAnally, P., & Spillers, D. (2004). Reading, writing, and technology. In R. K. Rittenhouse (Ed.), *Deaf education at the dawn of the 21st century: Old challenges, new directions* (pp. 151–180). Hillsboro, OR: Butte Publications.

McAnally, P. L., Rose, S., & Quigley, S. P. (2007). *Reading practices with deaf learners* (2nd ed.). Austin, TX: Pro-ed.

McGuinn, P. J. (2006). *No child left behind and the transformation of federal education policy, 1965–2005.* Lawrence: KS: University Press of Kansas.

McGuire, S., Dunn, J., & Plomin, R. (1995). Maternal differential treatment of siblings and children's behavioral problems: A longitudinal study. *Development and Psychopathology, 7,* 515–528.

McHale, S. M., & Pawletko, T. M. (1992). Differential treatment of siblings in two family contexts. *Child Development, 63,* 68–81.

McHale, S. M., Whiteman, S. D., Kim, J., & Crouter, A. C. (2007). Characteristics and correlates of sibling relationships in two-parent African American families. *Journal of Family Psychology, 21*(2), 227–235.

McIntosh, A. (2000). When the deaf and the hearing interact: Communications features, relationships, and disabilities issues. In D. O. Braithwaite & T. Thompson (Eds.), *Handbook of communication and people with disabilities: Research and application* (pp. 353–368). Mahwah, NJ: Erlbaum.

McKee, R. (2001). *People of the eye: Stories from the deaf world.* Wellington, New Zealand: Bridget Williams Books.

McLaughlin, S. (1998). *Introduction to language development.* San Diego, CA: Singular.

McLeskey, J., Rosenberg, M. S., & Westling, D. L. (2010). *Inclusion effective practices for all students.* Boston: Pearson.

McNamara, B. E. (2007). *Learning disabilities: Bridging the gap between research and classroom practice.* Upper Saddle River, NJ: Merrill/Pearson.

Meadow, K. (1980). *Deafness and child development.* Berkeley: University of California Press.

Meadow-Orlans, K. (1980). *Deafness and child development.* Berkeley: University of California Press.

Meadow-Orlans, K., Mertens, D., & Sass-Lehrer, M. (2003). *Parents and their deaf children: The early years.* Washington, DC: Gallaudet University Press.

Meadow-Orlans, K., & Spencer, P. (1996). Maternal sensitivity and the visual attentiveness of children who are deaf. *Early Development and Parenting, 5,* 213–223.

Meadow-Orlans, K. P. (1983). An instrument for assessment of social-emotional adjustment in hearing-impaired preschoolers. *American Annals of the Deaf, 128,* 826–834.

Melancon, F. (2000). A group for students with Usher syndrome in South Louisiana. *Deaf-Blind Perspectives, 8,* 1–3.

Melton, C. (1987). Trends and directions in vocational rehabilitation and their influence upon the education of deaf people. *American Annals of the Deaf, 132,* 315–316.

Meltzoff, A., & Moore, W. (1977). Imitation of facial and manual gestures by human neonates. *Science, 198,* 75–78.

Mercer, C., & Pullen, P. (2008). *Students with learning disabilities* (7th ed.). Upper Saddle River, NJ: Merrill/Pearson.

Mertens, D. M. (1990). A conceptual model of academic achievement: Deaf student outcomes. In D. F. Moores & K. P. Meadow-Orlans (Eds.), *Educational and development aspects of deafness* (pp. 25–72). Washington, DC: Gallaudet University.

Miles, B. (2008, revised). Overview on deaf-blindness. The National Information Clearinghouse on Children Who Are Deaf-Blind, Helen Keller National Center, Hilton/Perkins Program Perkins School for the Blind, Teaching Research Institute. Retrieved February 10, 2011, from www.nationaldb.org/documents/products/Overview.pdf

Miller, G., & Gildea, P. (1987). How children learn words. *Scientific American, 257*(3), 94–99.

Miller, M. (2006). Individual assessment and educational planning: Deaf and hard of hearing students viewed through meaningful contexts. In D. F. Moores & D. S. Martin (Eds.), *Deaf learners: Developments in curriculum and instruction* (pp.161–177). Washington, DC: Gallaudet University Press.

Miller, P. (2002). Communication mode and the processing of printed words: Evidence from readers with prelingually acquired deafness. *Journal of Deaf Studies and Deaf Education, 7,* 312–329.

Miller, P. (2007, Spring). The role of spoken and sign languages in the retention of written words by prelingually deafened native signers. *Journal of Deaf Studies and Deaf Education, 12*(2), 184–208.

Mindel, E. D., & Vernon, M. (1987). *They grow in silence.* Boston: College-Hill Press.

Minor, L. B., Schessel, D. A., & Carey, J. P. (2004). Meniere's disease. Current opinion in neurology. *17*(1), 9–16.

Minuchin, S. (1974). *Families and family therapy.* Cambridge, MA: Harvard University Press.

Mitchell, R. (2005). *Can you tell me how many deaf people there are in the United States?* Washington, DC: Gallaudet Research Institute, Gallaudet University.

Retrieved March 9, 2011, from research.gallaudet.edu/Demographics/deaf-US.php

Mitchell, R., & Karchmer, M. (2004). When parents are deaf versus hard of hearing. *Journal of Deaf Studies and Deaf Education, 9,* 133–152.

Mitchell, R. E. (2004). National profile of deaf and hard of hearing students in special education from weighted survey results. *American Annals of the Deaf, 149*(4), 336–349.

Moeller, M. P. (2000). Early intervention and language development in children who are deaf and hard of hearing. *Pediatrics, 106*(3), 43.

Moeller, M. P., & Schick, B. (2006). Relations between maternal input and theory of mind understanding in deaf children. *Child Development, 77,* 751–766.

Monsen, R. B. (1983). The oral speech intelligibility of hearing-impaired talkers. *Journal of Speech and Hearing Disorders, 48,* 286–296.

Moore, M. S., & Levitan, L. (1993). *For hearing people only.* Rochester, NY: Deaf Life Press.

Moore, M. S., & Levitan, L. (2003). *For hearing people only.* Rochester, NY: Deaf Life Press.

Moores, D. F. (1996). *Educating the deaf.* Boston: Houghton Mifflin.

Moores, D. F. (1999). *Total Communication and Bi-Bi.* [Editorial]. *American Annals for the Deaf, 144*(1), 3.

Moores, D. F. (2001). *Educating the deaf: Psychology, principles, and practices* (5th ed.). Boston: Houghton Mifflin.

Moores, D. F. (2005). The No Child Left Behind and the Individuals with Disabilities Education Acts: The uneven impact of partially funded federal mandates on education of deaf and hard of hearing children. *American Annals of the Deaf, 150*(2), 75–80.

Moores, D. F. (2006). Print literacy: The acquisition of reading and writing skills. In D. F. Moores & D. S. Martin (Eds.), *Deaf learners' developments in curriculum and instruction* (p. 55). Washington, DC: Gallaudet University Press.

Moores, D. F. (2010). The history of language and communication issues in deaf education. In M. Marschark & P. E. Spencer (Eds.), *The Oxford handbook of deaf studies, language, and education* (Vol. 2, pp. 17–30). New York: Oxford University Press.

Moores, D. F., & Martin, D. S. (Eds.). (2006). *Deaf learners: Developments in curriculum and instruction.* Washington, DC: Gallaudet University Press.

Moreno-Torres, I., & Torres, S. (2008). From 1-word to 2-words with cochlear implant and cued speech: A case study. *Clinical Linguistics & Phonetics, 22*(7), 491–508.

Morford, J., & Mayberry, R. (2000). A reexamination of "early exposure" and its implications for language acquisition by eye. In C. Chamberlain, J. Morford, & R. Mayberry (Eds.), *Language acquisition by eye* (pp. 111–127). Mahwah, NJ: Erlbaum.

Morgan, A., & Vernon, M. (1994). A guide to the diagnosis of learning disabilities in deaf and hard of hearing children and adults. *American Annals of the Deaf, 139*(3), 358–369.

Morton, N. (1991). Genetic epidemiology of hearing impairment. *Annals of the New York Academy of Sciences, 630,* 16–31.

Most, T. (2007). Speech intelligibility, loneliness, and sense of coherence among deaf and hard-of-hearing children in individual inclusion and group inclusion. *Journal of Deaf Studies and Deaf Education, 12*(4), 495–503.

Most, T., Weisel, A., & Gali-Cinamon, R. (2008). Is speech intelligibility of deaf and hard of hearing people a barrier for occupational competence? *Journal of the American Deafness and Rehabilitation Association, 42*(1), 7–23.

Most, T., Weisel, A., & Tur-Kaspa, H. (1999). Contact with students with hearing impairment and the evaluation of speech intelligibility and personal qualities. *Journal of Special Education, 33,* 103–111.

Mounty, J. L., & Martin, D. S. (Eds.). (2005). Assessing deaf adults: Critical issues in testing and evaluation. Washington, DC: Gallaudet University Press.

Muller, E. (2006). Deaf-blind child counts: Issues and challenges. In *Forum: Brief policy analysis* (pp. 1–13). Alexandria, VA: National Association of State Directors of Special Education, Project Forum.

Murawski, W. W. (2002). *An analysis of student outcomes in cotaught settings in comparison to other special education service delivery options for students with learning disabilities.* Paper submitted for publication.

Murawski, W. W., & Dieker, L. A. (2004, May/June). Tips and strategies for coteaching at the secondary level. *Teaching Exceptional Children, 36,* 52–58.

Musselman, C. (2000). How do children who can't hear learn to read an alphabetic script? A review of the literature on reading and deafness. *Journal of Deaf Studies and Deaf Education, 5,* 11–31.

Musselman, C., Mootilal, A., & MacKay, S. (1996). The social adjustment of deaf adolescents in segregated, partially integrated, and mainstreamed settings. *Journal of Deaf Studies and Deaf Education, 1*(1), 52–63.

Myklebust, H. (1964). *The psychology of deafness* (2nd ed.). New York: Grune & Stratton.

Myklebust, H., & Brutton, M. (1953). A study of visual perception in deaf children. *Acta Otolaryngologica* (Supplementum), 105.

Nagy, W. E., & Herman, P. A. (1987). Breadth and depth of vocabulary knowledge: Implications for acquisition and instruction. In M. G. McKeown & M. E. Curtis (Eds.), *The nature of vocabulary acquisition* (pp. 19–35). Hillsdale, NJ: Erlbaum.

Najarian, C. G. (2006). Deaf mothers, maternal thinking and intersections of gender and ability. *Scandinavian Journal of Disability Research, 8*(2–3), 99–119.

National Association of the Deaf. (2000). Position statement on cochlear implants (2000). Retrieved January 29, 2011, from www.nad.org/issues/technology/assistive-listening/cochlear-implants

National Center for Education Statistics. (1998). Cited in D. W. Carnine, J. Silbert, E. J. Kame'enui, S. G. Tarver, & K. Jungjohann. (2006). *Teaching struggling and at-risk readers* (p. 4). Upper Saddle River.NJ: Pearson.

National Center for Education Statistics. (2006). Findings from the condition of education 2006: U.S. student and adult performance on international assessments of educational achievement. Retrieved February 23, 2011, from nces.ed.gov/pubsearch/pubsinfo.asp?pubid=2006073

National Center for Education Statistics. (2007). Digest of education statistics. Retrieved March 2, 2011, from nces.ed.gov/programs/digest/d07

National Center for Education Statistics. (2009a). Digest of educational statistics. Retrieved February 14, 2011, from nces.ed.gov/programs/digest/d09/tables/dt09_051.asp

National Center for Education Statistics (2009b). The Nation's Report Card: Reading 2009 (NCES 2010–458). Washington, DC: Institute of Education Sciences, U.S. Department of Education. Retrieved February 23, 2011, from nces.ed.gov/pubsearch/pubsinfo.asp?pubid=2010458

National Center for Hearing Assessment and Management. (2011). Newborn hearing screening. Retrieved March 9, 2011, from www.infanthearing.org/screening/index.html

National Commission on Excellence in Education (April, 1983). A nation at risk: The imperative for educational reform. Retrieved February 11, 2011, from http://www2.ed.gov/pubs/NatAtRisk/index.html

National Consortium on Deaf-Blindness (NCDB). (2007). Primary etiologies of deaf-blindness - Frequency. Retrieved February 16, 2011, from www.nationaldb.org/ISSelectedTopics.php?toicID=990topicCatID=24

National Consortium on Deaf-Blindness (NCDB). (2010). Primary etiologies of deaf-blindness - Frequency. Retrieved February 16, 2011, from www.nationaldb.org/ISSelectedTopics.php?toicID=990topicCatID=24

National Institute of Child Health and Human Development (NICHD). (2000). *Report of the National Reading Panel: Teaching children to read: An evidence-based assessment of the scientific research literature on reading and its implications for reading instruction* (NIH Publication No. 00–4769). Washington, DC: U.S. Government Printing Office.

National Institute of Mental Health (NIMH) (2006). New NIMH research program launches autism trials. Retrieved March 9, 2011, from www.nimh.nih.gov/science-news/2006/new-nimh-research-program-launches-autism-trials.shtml

National Institute on Deafness and Other Communication Disorders (NIDCD). (1990). Deafness: A fact sheet. Publications from the National Information Center on Deafness (085). Washington, DC: Gallaudet University.

National Institute on Deafness and Other Communication Disorders (NIDCD). (2002). Cochlear implants (fact sheet). NIDCD.nih.gov. Retrieved June 18, 2006, from www.nidcd.nih.gov/health/hearing/coch.htm

National Institute on Deafness and Other Communication Disorders (NIDCD). (2006). Cochlear implants (fact sheet). NIDCD.NIH.gov. Retrieved March 15, 2007 from www.nidcd.nih.gov/health/hearing/coch.htm

National Institute on Deafness and Other Communication Disorders (NIDCD). (2010). Cochlear implants (fact sheet). NIDCD.NIH.gov. Retrieved January 10, 2011, at www.nidcd.nih.gov/health/hearing/coch.htm

National Research Council. (2002). *Minority students in special and gifted education.* Washington, DC: National Academy Press.

Naulty, C. M., Weiss, I. P., & Herer, G. R. (1986). Progressive sensorineural hearing loss in survivors of persistent fetal circulation. *Ear & Hearing, 7*(2), 74–77.

Newport, E., & Meier, R. (1985). The acquisition of American Sign Language. In D. Slobin (Ed.), *The crosslinguistic study of language acquisition* (Vol. 1, pp. 881–938). Hillsdale, NJ: Erlbaum.

Nicholas, J., & Geers, A. E. (2006). Effects of early auditory experience on the spoken language of deaf children at 3 years of age. *Ear & Hearing, 27,* 286–298.

Nicholas J. C., & Geers, A. E. (2007). Will they catch up? The role of age at cochlear implantation in the spoken language development of children with severe to profound hearing loss. *Journal of Speech Language and Hearing Research, 50*(4), 1048–1062.

Nieto, S., & Bode, P. (2008). *Affirming diversity: The sociopolitical context of multicultural education* (5th ed.). Boston: Allyn & Bacon.

National Institutes of Health. (1993, March 1–3). Early identification of hearing impairment in infants and young children: National Institutes of Health Development Conference Statement. Retrieved March 3, 2011, from www.ncbi.nlm.nih.gov/books/NBK15109

Nikolopoulos, T. P., O'Donoghue, G.M., & Archbold, S. M. (1999). Age at implantation: its importance in pediatric cochlear implantation. *Laryngoscope, 109*(4), 595–599.

Nippold, M. (1994). Persuasive talk in social contexts. Development, assessment, and intervention. *Topics in Language Disorders, 14*(3), 1–12.

Nippold, M. (1998a). *Later language development: The school-age and adolescent years.* Austin, TX: Pro-Ed.

Nippold, M. (Ed.). (1998b). *Later language development: Ages nine through nineteen.* Boston: Little, Brown & Company.

Nippold, M. (2000). Language development during the adolescent years: Aspects of pragmatics, syntax, and semantics. *Topics in Language Disorders, 20*(2), 15–28.

Nixon, C. L., & Cummings, E. M. (1999). Sibling disability and children's reactivity to conflicts involving family members. *Journal of Family Psychology, 13*(2), 274–285.

No Child Left Behind Act of 2001. (2001). Public Law No. 107-110. 1201-1226, 115 Stat. 425 (2001).

Northern, J. L., & Downs, M. P. (1991). *Hearing in children* (4th ed.). Baltimore: Williams & Wilkins.

Office of Special Education Programs (OSEP). (2006). Students served under IDEA, Part B, by disability category and state. Data Accountability Center, Individuals with Disabilities Education Act (IDEA) Data. Retrieved January 22, 2011, from www.ideadata.org

Ogden, P. W., & Classen, K. M. (2004). *The future of deaf culture.* Hillsboro, OR: Butte Publications.

O'Grady, W. (2005). *How children learn language.* New York: Cambridge University Press.

Oh, S., & Kim, M. (2004). The role of spatial working memory in visual search efficiency. *Psychonomic Bulletin & Review, 11,* 275–281.

Oliva, G. (2004). *Alone in the mainstream.* Washington, DC: Gallaudet University Press.

Osberger, M. J., Zimmerman-Phillips, S., & Koch, D. B. (2002). Cochlear implant candidacy and performance trends in children. The Annals of Otology, Rhinology & Laryngology, *111,* 52–65.

Owens, R. E. (1990). Communication, language, and speech. In G. Shames & E. Wiig (Eds.), *Human communication disorders* (3rd ed., pp. 30–73). Columbus, OH: Merrill Publishing Co.

Owens, R. E. (2000). *Language development: An introduction* (5th ed). Boston: Allyn & Bacon.

Owens, R. E. (2005). *Language development: An introduction* (6th ed.). Boston: Allyn & Bacon.

Padden, C. (1991). The acquisition of fingerspelling by deaf children. In P. Siple & S. Fischer (Eds.), *Theoretical issues in language for research, Volume 2: Psychology* (pp. 191–210.) Chicago: University of Chicago Press.

Padden, C. (1996). From the cultural to the bicultural: The modern deaf community. In I. Parasnis (Ed.), *Cultural and language diversity and the Deaf experience* (pp. 79–98). New York: Cambridge University Press.

Padden, C. A., & Hanson, V. L. (2000). Search for the missing link: The development of skilled reading in deaf children. In K. Emmorey and H. Lane (Eds.), *The signs of language revisited* (pp. 435–448). Mahwah, NJ: Erlbaum.

Padden, C., & Humphries, T. (1989). *Voices in Deaf culture.* Washington, DC: Gallaudet University Press.

Padden, C., & Humphries, T. (2005). *Inside deaf culture.* Cambridge, MA: Harvard University Press.

Padden, C., & Ramsey, C. (2000). American Sign Language and reading ability in deaf children. In C. Chamberlain, J. Morford, & R. Mayberry (Eds.), *Language acquisition by eye* (pp. 165–189). Hillsdale, NJ: Erlbaum.

Pan, B., & Gleason, J. (2008). The study of language loss: Models and hypotheses for an emerging discipline. *Applied Psycholinguistics, 7*(3), 193–206.

Parasnis, I., & Long, G. L. (1979). Relations among spatial skills, communications skills, and field dependence in deaf students. *Directions, 1,* 26–37.

Passmore, D. L. (1983). Employment of deaf people. In D. Watson, G. Anderson, S. Ouellette, N. Ford, P. Marut, & P. Ouellette (Eds.), *Job placement of hearing-impaired persons: Research and practice*. Little Rock, AR: Arkansas Rehabilitation and Training Center.

Patterson, T. (2009). The life of Riley. Unpublished essay.

Paul, P. (1996). Reading vocabulary knowledge and deafness. *Journal of Deaf Studies and Deaf Education, 1*(1), 3–15.

Paul, P. (1998). *Literacy and deafness: The development of reading, writing, and literate thought.* Boston: Allyn & Bacon.

Paul, P. (2001). *Language and deafness* (3rd ed.). San Diego, CA: Singular/Thompson Learning.

Paul, P. (2003). Processes and components of reading. In M. Marschark & P. Spencer (Eds.), *The Oxford handbook of deaf studies, language, and education* (pp. 97–109). New York: Oxford University Press.

Paul, P. (2005). Perspectives on literacy: A rose is a rose, but then again . . . maybe now [Review of Brueggemann, B. (Ed.). (2004). *Literacy and deaf people: Cultural and contextual perspectives*]. *Journal of Deaf Studies and Deaf Education, 10*(2), 222.

Paul, P. (2009). *Language and deafness* (4th ed.). Boston: Jones and Bartlett.

Paul, P. V., & Whitelaw, G. M. (2011). *Hearing and deafness: An introduction for health and education professionals.* Boston: Jones & Bartlett Publishers.

Pierangelo, R., & Giuliani, G. (2006). *Learning disabilities: A practical approach to foundations, assessment, diagnosis, and teaching.* Boston: Allyn & Bacon.

Pelligrino, L. T. (Ed.). (2007). *Handbook of motor skills: Development, impairment, and therapy.* Hauppauge, NY: NOVA Science Publishers.

Perfetti, C. (1985). *Reading ability.* New York: Oxford University Press.

Petitto, L. (1994). Are signed languages "real" languages? Evidence from American Sign Language and Langue des signes quebecoise. *Signpost, 7*(3), 1–10.

Petitto, L. (2000). On the biological foundations of human language. In K. Emmorey & H. Lane (Eds.), *The signs of language revisited: An anthology in honor of Ursula Bellugi and Edward Klima* (pp. 447–471). Mahwah, NJ: Erlbaum.

Pintner, R., Eisenson, J., & Stanton, M. (1941). *The psychology of the physically disabled.* New York: Crofts & Company.

Plante, E., & Beeson, P. (2008). *Communication and communication disorders: A clinical introduction* (3rd ed.). Boston: Allyn & Bacon.

Pollard, R. (1994). Public/mental health services and diagnostic trends regarding individuals who are deaf or hard of hearing. *Rehabilitation Psychology, 39*(3), 147–161.

Pollard, R., & Rendon, M. (1999). Mixed deaf-hearing families: Maximizing benefits and minimizing risks. *Journal of Deaf Studies and Deaf Education, 4,* 156–161.

Powell, T. H., & Ogle, P. A. (1985). *Brothers and sisters: A special part of exceptional families.* Baltimore: Brookes.

Powers, S., Gregory, S., Lynas, W., McCracken, W., Watson, L., Boulton, A., et al. (1999). *A review of good practice in deaf education.* London: Royal National Institute for Deaf People (RNID).

Preisler, G., Tvingstedt, A., & Ahlstrom, M. (2002). A psychosocial follow-up study of deaf preschool children using cochlear implants. *Child Care, Health and Development, 28*(5), 403–418.

Prezbindowski, A., Adamson, L., & Lederberg, A. (1998). Joint attention in deaf and hearing 22 month-old children and their hearing mothers. *Journal of Applied Developmental Psychology, 19,* 377–387.

Prizant, B. M., Meyer, E. C., & Lobato, D. J. (1997). Brothers and sisters of young children with communication disorders. *Seminars in Speech and Language, 18,* 263–282.

Proksch, J., & Bavelier, D. (2002). Changes in the spatial distribution of visual attention after early deafness. *Journal of Cognitive Neuroscience, 14,* 687–701.

Punch, R., Hyde, M., & Creed, P. A. (2004). Issues in the school-to-work transition of hard of hearing adolescents. *American Annals of the Deaf, 149,* 29–38.

Punch, R., Hyde, M., & Power, D. (2007, Fall). Career and workplace experiences of Australian University graduates who are deaf or hard of hearing. *Journal of Deaf Studies and Deaf Education, 12*(4), 504–517.

Quigley, S., McAnally, P., King, C., & Rose, S. (1991). *Reading milestones.* Austin, TX: PRO-ED.

Quigley, S., McAnally, P., King, C., & Rose, S. (2001). *Reading milestones.* Austin, TX: PRO-ED.

Quigley, S., McAnally, P., Rose, S., & Payne, J. (1991). *Reading bridge.* Austin, TX: PRO-ED.

Quigley, S., McAnally, P., Rose, S., & Payne, J. (2003). *Reading bridge.* Austin, TX: PRO-ED.

Quigley, S., & Paul, P. (1984). *Language and deafness.* San Diego: College-Hill Press.

Quigley, S., Wilbur, R., Power, D., Montanelli, D., & Steinkamp, M. (1976). Syntactic structures in the language of deaf children. Urbana: University of Illinois, Institute for Child Behavior and Development. (ERIC Document Reproduction Service No. ED119447)

Race to the Top Fund. (2009). 74 Fed. Reg. 59688 (to be codified 34 C.F.R. Subtitle B, Chapter II).

Raghuraman, R. S. (2008). The emotional well-being of older siblings of children who are deaf or hard of hearing and older siblings of children with typical hearing. *The Volta Review, 108*(1), 5–35.

Rainer, J. D., & Altschuler, K. Z. (1966). *Comprehensive mental health services for the deaf.* New York: New York Psychiatric Institute, Columbia University.

Reed, S. (2003). Beliefs and practices of itinerant teachers of deaf and hard of hearing children concerning literacy development. *American Annals of the Deaf, 148*(4), 333–343.

The Registry of Interpreters for the Deaf (RID). (2005). NAD-RID Code of Professional Conduct. Retrieved February 16, 2011, from rid.org/UserFiles/File/NAD_RID_ETHICS.pdf

Registry of Interpreters for the Deaf (RID). (2010). An overview of K-12 interpreting (Professional Standards Committee, 1997–1999, REV4/00). Alexandria, VA: Author, 1–3.

Reiff, M. (2004). *ADHD: A complete and authoritative guide.* Elk Grove Village, IL: American Academy of Pediatrics.

Reisler, J. (2002). *Voices of the oral deaf: Fourteen role models speak out.* Jefferson, NC: McFarland & Company.

Reynolds, D., & Titus, A. (1991, June). *Bilingual/bicultural education: Constructing a model for change.* Paper presented at the meeting of the Convention of American Instructors of the Deaf, New Orleans, LA.

Rhoades, E. A., Price, F., & Perigoe, C. B. (2004). The changing American family & ethnically diverse children with hearing loss and multiple needs. *The Volta Review, 104*(4), 285–305.

Rhoades, E. A. (2006). Research outcomes of auditory-verbal intervention: Is the approach justified? *Deafness & Education International, 8*(3), 125–143.

Ricketts, T. (2009). Digital hearing aids: Current "state of the art." Accessed January 17, 2011, from www.Asha.org/public/hearing/treatment/digital_aid.htm

Roberson, L., & Serwatka, T. S. (2000). Student perceptions and instructional effectiveness of deaf and hearing teachers. *American Annals of the Deaf, 145*(3), 256–262.

Roberson, L., Woosley, M. L., Seabrooks, J., & Williams, G. (2004). Data-Driven assessment of teacher candidates during their internships in deaf education. *American Annals of the Deaf,* 148(5), 403–412.

Robinson-Riegler, G., & Robinson-Riegler, B. (2008). *Cognitive psychology: Applying the science of the mind.* Boston: Allyn & Bacon.

Rodda, M. (1966). Social adjustment of deaf adolescents. In Proceedings of a Symposium on the Psychological Study of Deafness and Hearing Impairment. Institute of Child Health. London: British Psychological Society.

Roeyers, H., & Mycke, K. (1995). Siblings of a child with autism, with mental retardation and with normal development. *Child Care, Health and Development, 21,* 305–319.

Rogers, C. R. (1961). *On becoming a person.* Boston: Houghton Mifflin.

Rogers, T. (1998). Access to information on computer networks by the Deaf. *Communication Review,* 2(4),497–521.

Romero, A., Baumle, A., Badgett, M., & Gates, G. (2007). Census snapshot. The Williams Institute. Retrieved February 7, 2011, from www2.law.ucla.edu/williamsinstitute/publications/USCensusSnapshot.pdf

Rose, S., McAnally, P., & Quigley, S. (2004). *Language learning practices with deaf children* (3rd ed.). Austin, TX: Pro-Ed.

Rosen, R. (Ed.). (1986). *Life and work in the 21st century: The deaf person of tomorrow.* Proceedings of the 1986 National Association of the Deaf Forum. Silver Spring, MD: National Association of the Deaf.

Rosenberg, M. (1986). Self-concept from middle childhood through adolescence. In J. Suls & A. G. Greenwald (Eds.), *Psychological perspectives on the self* (Vol. 3, pp. 107–136). Hilldale, NJ: Erlbaum.

Rosenstein, J. (1961). Perception, cognition and language in deaf children. *Exceptional Children, 27*(3), 276–284.

Ross, M. (2006). Are binaural hearing aids better? *Hearing Loss, 27*(2), 32–37.

Ross, M., Brackett, D., & Maxon, A. (1991). *Assessment and management of mainstreamed hearing-impaired children.* Austin, TX: Pro-Ed.

Ruble, D. N. (1987). The acquisition of self-knowledge: A self-socialization perspective. In N. Eisenberg (Ed.), *Contemporary topics in developmental psychology* (pp. 243–270). New York: Wiley-Interscience.

Ruddell, R. B., & Unrau, N. J. (Eds.). (2004). Theoretical models and processes of reading (5th ed.). Newark, DE: International Reading Association.

Rumelhart, D. E. (1977). Toward an interactive model of reading. In S. Dornic (Ed.), Attention and Performance IV(Vol. 6, pp. 573–603). New York: Academic Press.

Sadker, D. M., & Zittleman, K. R. (2009). *Teachers, schools, and society: A brief introduction to education* (2nd ed.). Boston: McGraw Hill.

Safran, S. P. (2001). Asperger syndrome: The emerging challenge to special education. *Exceptional Children, 67,* 151–160.

Salend, S. J., & Rohena, E. (2003). Students with attention deficit disorders: An overview. *Intervention in School and Clinic, 38,* 259–266.

Salter, C. (2001). Attention, class!!! 16 ways to be a smarter teacher. *Fast Company, 53,* 114–126.

Santrock, J. (1999). *Life span development.* Boston: McGraw Hill.

Sass-Lehrer, M., & Bodner-Johnson, B. (2003). Early intervention: Current approaches to family-centered programming. In M. Marschark & P. E. Spencer (Eds.), *The Oxford handbook of deaf studies, language, and education* (pp. 65–81). New York: Oxford University Press.

Scarr, S. (1981). *Race, social class, and individual differences in I.Q.* Hillsdale, NJ: Erlbaum.

Schalock, R., Luckasson, R., Shogren, K., Bradley, V., Borthwick-Duffy, S., Buntix, W., et. al. (2007). The renaming of mental retardation: Understanding the change to the term *intellectual disability. Intellectual and Developmental Disabilities, 45,* 116–124.

Schaper, M. W., & Reitsma, P. (1993). The use of speech-based recoding in reading by prelingually deaf children. *American Annals of the Deaf, 138,* 46–54.

Scheetz, N. (1998). *Sign communication for everyday use: A multimedia guide.* Gaithersburg, MD: Aspen Publishers.

Scheetz, N. (2001). *Orientation to deafness.* Boston: Allyn & Bacon.

Scheetz, N. (2004). *Psychosocial aspects of deafness.* Boston: Allyn & Bacon.

Scheetz, N. (2009). *Building ASL interpreting and translation skills.* Boston: Allyn & Bacon.

Scheetz, N., & Martin D. (2008). National study of master teachers in deaf education: Implications for teacher education. *American Annals of the Deaf, 153*(3), 328–343.

Schein, J. (1984). *Speaking the language of sign.* New York: Doubleday.

Schein, J. (1989). *At home among strangers.* Washington, DC: Gallaudet University Press.

Schein, J., & Delk, M. (1974). *The deaf population of the United States.* Silver Spring, MD: National Association of the Deaf.

Schein, J., & Stewart, D. (1995). *Language in motion: Exploring the nature of sign.* Washington, DC: Gallaudet University.

Schessel, D. A. (1999). Meniere's disease. *The Volta Review, 99*(5), 177–193.

Schick, B. (2003). The development of American Sign Language and manually coded English systems. In M. Marschark & P. E. Spencer (Eds.), *The Oxford handbook of deaf studies, language, and education* (pp. 219–231). New York: Oxford University Press.

Schick, B., de Villiers, J., de Villiers, P., & Hoffmeister, R. (2007). Language and theory of mind: A study of deaf children. *Child Development, 78,* 376–396.

Schick, B., & Williams, K. (2004). Evaluating educational interpreters using classroom performance. In B. C. Seal (Ed.). *Best practices in educational interpreting* (2nd ed., pp. 243–251). Boston: Allyn & Bacon.

Schick, B., Marschark, M., & Spencer, P. (2006). *Advances in the sign language development of deaf children.* New York: Oxford University Press.

Schick, B., Williams, K., & Haggai, K. (2005). *Look who's being left behind: Educational interpreters and access to education for deaf and hard-of-hearing students.* New York: Oxford University Press.

Schick, B., Williams, K., & Kupermintz, H. (2005). Look who's being left behind: Educational interpreters and access to education for deaf and hard-of-hearing students. *Journal of Deaf Studies and Deaf Education, 11*(1), 3–20.

Schierhorn, A. B., Endres, F. E., & Schierhorn, C. (2001). Newsroom teams enjoy rapid growth in the 1990s. *Newspaper Research Journal, 22*(3), 2–15.

Schildroth, A. N. (1994). (1992–93, Annual survey). Gallaudet University Center for Assessment and Demographic Studies. Unpublished raw data.

Schildroth, A. N., & Karchmer, M. A. (Eds.). (1986). *Deaf children in America.* San Diego: College-Hill Press.

Schirmer, B. R. (2001). *Psychological, social, and educational dimensions of deafness.* Boston: Allyn & Bacon.

Schirmer, B. R., & McGough, S. M. (2005, Spring). Teaching reading to children who are deaf: Do the conclusions of the national reading panel apply? American Educational Research Association. Retrieved January 19, 2011, from www.jstor.org/stable/3516081

Schirmer, B. R., & Woolsey, M. L. (1997). Effect of teacher questions on the reading comprehension of deaf children. *Journal of Deaf Studies and Deaf Education, 2,* 47–56.

Schlauch, R. S., & Nelson, P. (2009). Puretone evaluation. In J. Katz (Ed.), *Handbook of clinical audiology* (6th ed., pp. 30–49). Philadelphia: Lippincott Williams & Wilkins.

Schleper, D. (1996). *Shared reading, shared success. (Preview, Pre-College Programs, 1–5).* Washington, DC: Gallaudet University.

Schleper, D. R. (1995). Reading to deaf children: Learning from deaf adults. *Perspectives in Education & Deafness, 13*(4), 4–8.

Schley, S., & Albertini, J. (2005). Assessing the writing of deaf college students: Reevaluating a direct assessment of writing. *Journal of Deaf Studies and Deaf Education, 10*(1), 96–105.

Schmidt, J., & Cagran, B. (2008). Self-concept of students in inclusive settings. *International Journal of Special Education, 23*(1), 8–17.

Schrepferman, L. M., Eby, J., Snyder, J., & Stropes, J. (2006). Early affiliation and social engagement with peers: Prospective risk and protective factors for childhood depressive disorders. *Journal of Emotional and Behavioral Disorders, 14,* 50–60.

Schroedel, J. G., & Geyer, P. D. (2000). Long-term career attainments of deaf and hard of hearing college graduates: Results from a 15-year follow-up survey. *American Annals of the Deaf, 145,* 303–314.

Schroedel, J. G., Mowry, R. L., & Anderson, G. B. (1992, November). *Experiences of deaf Americans with accommodations and advancement on the job: A qualitative study.* Paper presented at the International Scientific Colloquium on Functional Limitations and Their Social Consequences: Report and Outlook, Montreal, Quebec.

Schwirian, P. M. (1976). Effects of the presence of a hearing-impaired preschool child in the family on behavior patterns of older, "normal" siblings. *American Annals of the Deaf, 121*(4), 373–380.

Seagoe, M. V. (1970). *The learning process and school practice.* Scranton, PA: Chandler.

Seal, B. C. (2004). *Best practices in educational interpreting* (2nd ed.). Boston: Allyn & Bacon.

Sell, E. J., Gaines, J. A., Gluckman, C., & Williams, E. (1985). Early identification of learning problems in neonatal intensive care graduates. *American Journal of Diseases of Children, 139*(5), 460–463.

Senghas, R. J., & Monaghan, L. (2002). Sign of their times: Deaf communities and the culture of language. *Annual Review of Anthropology, 31,* 69–97.

Shavelson, R. J., Hubner, J. J., & Stanton, G. C. (1976). Self-concept: Validation of construct interpretations. *Review of Educational Research, 46,* 407–441.

Shaver, K. (1988). Genetics and deafness. In F. H. Bess (Ed.), *Hearing impairment in children* (pp. 15–32). Parkton, MD: York Press.

Shepherd, G. D., & Ragan, W. B. (1992). *Modern elementary curriculum* (7th ed.). Fort Worth, TX: Harcourt Brace Jovanovich.

Sheridan, M. (2008). *Deaf adolescents: Inner lives and lifeworld development.* Washington, DC: Gallaudet University Press.

Shiffrin, R. M. (1999). 30 years of memory. In C. Izawa (Ed.), *On human memory: Evolution, progress, and reflection on the 30th anniversary of the Atkinson-Shiffrin model* (pp. 17–34). Mahwah, NJ: Erlbaum.

Siegel, L. (2000). The educational and communication needs of deaf and hard of hearing on fundamental educational change. *American Annals of the Deaf, 145*(2), 64–77.

Siegel, L. (Esq.). (2002). The argument for a constitutional right to communication and language. *Journal of Deaf Studies and Deaf Education, 7*(3), 258–66.

Simms, L., Rusher, M., Andrews, J. F., & Coryell, J. (2008). Apartheid in deaf education: Examining workforce diversity. *American Annals of the Deaf, 153*(4), 384–394.

Simms, L., & Thumann, H. (2007). In search of a new, linguistically and culturally sensitive paradigm in deaf education. *American Annals of the Deaf, 152*(3), 302–311.

Singleton, J., Supalla, S., Litchfield, S., & Schley, S. (1998). From sign to word: Considering modality constraints in ASL/English bilingual education. *Topics in Language Disorders, 18*(4), 16–30.

Sisco, F. H., & Anderson, R. J. (1980). Deaf children's performance on the WISC-R relative to hearing status of parents and child-rearing experiences. *American Annals of the Deaf, 125,* 923–930.

Smaldino, J., Crandell, C., Kreisman, B., John, A., & Kreisman, N. (2009). Room acoustics and auditory rehabilitation technology. In J. Katz (Ed.), *Handbook of Clinical Audiology* (6th ed., pp. 745–775). Philadelphia: Lippincott Williams & Wilkins.

Smith, F. (1978). *Understanding reading* (2nd ed.). New York: Holt, Rinehart, & Winston.

Smith, L. (2001). Lynne Smith. In R. McKey (Ed.), *People of the eye: Stories from the deaf world* (pp. 124–131). Wellington, New Zealand: Bridget Williams Books.

Smith, M. D. (1997). *The art of itinerant teaching for teachers of the deaf and hard of hearing.* Hillsboro, OR: Butte Publications.

Smith, M. M. (1996). Interference with rehearsal in spatial working memory in the absence of eye movements. *Quarterly Journal of Experimental Psychology A, 49,* 940–949.

Smith, B., Barkley, R., & Shapiro, C. (2006). Attention deficit/hyperactivity disorder. In E. Mash & R. Barkley (Eds.), *Treatment of childhood disorders* (3rd ed., pp. 53–122). New York: Guilford Press.

Smith, B., Barkley, R., & Shapiro, C. (2007). Attention deficit/hyperactivity disorder. In E. Mash & R. Barkley (Eds.), *Treatment of childhood disorders* (3rd ed., pp. 65–136). New York: Guilford Press.

Smith, C., Lentz, E. M., & Mikos, K. (1988). *Signing naturally.* San Diego, CA: Dawn Sign Press.

Smith, D. D., & Lane, K. L. (2007). *Introduction to special education: Making a difference* (6th ed.). Boston: Allyn & Bacon.

Smith, D. D., & Tyler, N. C. (2010). *Introduction to special education: Making a difference* (7th ed.). Upper Saddle River, NJ: Merrill.

Smith, D. H., & Ramsey, C. L. (2004). Classroom discourse practices of a deaf teacher using American Sign Language. *Sign Language Studies, 5*(1), 39–62.

Snik, A. F. M., Mylanus, E. A. M., & Cremers, C.W.R.J. (1994). Speech recognition with bone-anchored hearing aid determined objectively and subjectively. *Ear, Nose and Throat Journal, 73,* 115–117.

Snodden, K. (2008). American Sign Language and early intervention. *The Canadian Modern Language Review, 64*(4), 581–604.

Snow, C. E., Burns, M. S., & Griffin, P. (Eds.). (1998). *Preventing reading difficulties in young children.* Washington, DC: National Academy Press.

Snowling, M., & Hulme, C. (Eds.). (2005). *The science of reading: A handbook.* Malden, MA: Blackwell.

Soukup, M., & Feinstein, S. (2007). Identification, assessment, and intervention strategies for deaf and hard of hearing students with learning disabilities. *American Annals of the Deaf, 152*(1), 56–62.

Spencer, P. (2004). Language at 12 and 18 months: Characteristics and accessibility of linguistic models. In K. Meadow-Orlans, P. Spencer, & L. Koester (Eds.), *The world of deaf infants: A longitudinal study* (pp. 147–167). New York: Oxford University Press.

Spencer, P. (2010). Play and theory of mind: Indicators and engines of early cognitive growth. In M. Marschark & P. Spencer (Eds.), *The Oxford handbook of deaf studies, language, and education* (Vol. 2, pp. 407–424). New York: Oxford University Press.

Spencer, P., & Marschark, M. (2006). *Advances in the spoken language development of Deaf and hard-of-hearing children.* New York: Oxford University Press.

Spencer, P., & Marschark, M. (2010). Paradigm shifts, difficult truths, and an increasing knowledge base in deaf education. In M. Marschark & P. Spencer (Eds.). *The Oxford handbook of deaf studies, language, and education* (Vol. 2, pp. 473–479). New York: Oxford University Press.

Spencer, P. E. (2000). Looking without listening: Is audition a prerequisite for normal development of visual attention during infancy? *Journal of Deaf Studies and Deaf Education, 5,* 291–302.

Spencer, P. E. (2004). Individual differences in language performance after cochlear implantation at one to three years of age: Child, family, and linguistic factors. *Journal of Deaf Studies and Deaf Education, 9,* 396–412.

Spinath, F. M., Prince, T. S., Dale, P. S., & Plomin, R. (2004). The genetic and environmental origins of language disability and ability. *Child Development, 75,* 445–454.

Spring, J. (1976). *The sorting machine: National educational policy since 1945.* New York: David McKay, p. 225.

Stahl, S., & Nagy, W. (2006). *Teaching word meanings.* Mahwah, NJ: Erlbaum.

Stanovich, K. (1986). Cognitive process and the reading problems of learning disabled children: Evaluating the problems of specificity. In J. Torgesen & B. Wong (Eds.), *Psychological and educational perspectives on learning disabilities* (pp. 87–131). New York: Academic Press.

Stanovich, L. E. (1980). Toward an interactive-compensatory model of individual differences in the development of reading fluency. *Reading Research Quarterly 16*(1), 32–71.

Sternberg, R. J. (1985). *Beyond IQ: A triarchic theory of human intelligence.* Cambridge, England: Cambridge University Press.

Sterne, A., & Goswami, U. (2003). Phonological awareness of syllables, rhymes, and phonemes in deaf children. *Journal of Child Psychiatry, 41*(5), 609–625.

Stewart, D. A., & Kluwin, T. N. (2001). *Teaching deaf and hard of hearing students: Content, strategies, and curriculum.* Boston: Allyn & Bacon.

Stierman, L. (1994). Birth defects in California: 1983–1990. Sacramento: California Department of Health Services, The California Birth Defects Monitoring Program.

Still, P. (2001). Patty Still. In R. McKey (Ed.), *People of the eye: Stories from the deaf world* (pp. 69–74). Wellington, New Zealand: Bridget Williams Books.

Stinson, M. (2010). Current and future technologies in the education of deaf students. In M. Marschark & P. E. Spencer (Eds.), *The Oxford handbook of deaf studies, language, and education* (Vol. 2, pp. 93–110). New York: Oxford University Press.

Stinson, M., & Antia, S. (1999). Considerations in educating deaf and hard-of-hearing students in inclusive settings. *Journal of Deaf Studies and Deaf Education, 4*(3), 163–175.

Stinson, M., Whitmire, K., & Kluwin, T. (1996). Self-perceptions of social relationships in hearing impaired adolescents. *Journal of Educational Psychology, 88,* 132–143.

Stinson, M. S., & Antia, S. D. (1999). Considerations in educating deaf and hard-of-hearing students in inclusive settings. *Journal of Deaf Studies and Deaf Education, 4,* 163–175.

Stinson, M. S., & Foster, S. (2000). Socialization of deaf children and youths in school. In P. E. Spencer, J. J. Ertine, & Marschark (Eds.), *The deaf child in the family and at school* (pp. 191–209). Mahwah, NJ: Erlbaum.

Stinson, M., & Kluwin, T. (2003). Educational consequences of alternative school placements. In M. Marschark & P. E. Spencer (Eds.), *The Oxford handbook of deaf studies, language, and education* (pp. 52–64). New York: Oxford University Press.

Storbeck, C., & Magongwa, L. (2006). Teaching about deaf culture. In D. F. Moores & D. S. Martin (Eds.), *Deaf learners: Developments in curriculum and instruction* (pp. 113–126). Washington, DC: Gallaudet University Press.

Strassman, B. K. (1992). Deaf adolescents' metacognitive knowledge about school-related reading. *American Annals of the Deaf, 137,* 326–330.

Stredler-Brown, A. (2010). Communication choices and outcomes during the early years: An assessment and evidence-based approach. In M. Marschark & P. E. Spencer, *The Oxford handbook of deaf studies, language, and education* (pp. 292–315). New York: Oxford University Press.

Streissguth, A. P., Clarren, S. K., & Jones, K. L. (1985). Natural history of the fetal alcohol syndrome: A 10-year follow-up of eleven patients. *U. S. National Library of Medicine, 2,* 85–91.

Strong, M. (1995). A review of bilingual/bicultural programs for deaf children in North America. *American Annals of the Deaf, 140,* 84–90.

Strong, M., & Prinz, P. (1997). A study of the relationship between American Sign Language and English literacy. *Journal of Deaf Studies and Deaf Education, 2*(1), 37–46.

Strong, M., & Prinz, P. (2000). Is American Sign Language skill related to English literacy? In C. Chamberlain, J. Morford, & R. Mayberry (Eds.), *Language acquisition by eye* (pp. 131–141). Mahwah, NJ: Erlbaum.

Stuckless, E. R., & Marks, C. H. (1966). Assessment of the written language of deaf students (Report of Cooperative Research Project 2544, U.S. Department of Health, Education, and Welfare). Pittsburgh, PA: University of Pittsburgh.

Sullivan, P., & Schulte, L. (1992). Factor analysis of WISC-R with deaf and hard-of-hearing children. *Psychological Assessment, 4*(4), 537–540.

Sunstrom, R., Van Laer, L., Van Camp, G., & Smith, R. (1999). Autosomal recessive non-syndromic hearing loss. *American Journal of Human Genetics, 89,* 123–129.

Supalla, S. (1994). Equality in educational opportunities: The Deaf version. In J. Erting, R. C. Johnson, D. L. Smith, & B. D. Snider (Eds.), *The Deaf way: Perspectives from the International Conference on Deaf Culture* (pp. 40–43). Washington, DC: Gallaudet University Press.

Supalla, S., Wix, T., & McKee, C. (2001). Print as a primary source of English for deaf learners. In J. Nichol & T. Langendoen (Eds.), *One mind, two languages: Bilingual language processing* (pp. 177–190). Malden, MA: Blackwell.

Swaim, K., & Bracken, B. A. (1997). Self-concepts of adolescent runaways as compared to the self-concepts of a matched sample of non-runaways. *Journal of Clinical Child Psychology, 26,* 397–403.

Szymanski, C., & Brice, P. J. (2008, Spring/Summer). When autism and deafness coexist in children: What we know now. *Odyssey: New Directions in Deaf Education, 9*(1),10–15.

Taylor, M. M. (1993). *Interpretation skills: English to American Sign Language.* Edmonton, Alberta, Canada: Interpreting Consolidated.

Taylor, M. T. (2001). *Interpretation skills: English to American Language.* Edmonton, Alberta, Canada: Interpreting Consolidated.

Thériault, J. (1998). Assessing intimacy with the best friend and the sexual partner during adolescence: The PAIR-M inventory. *The Journal of Psychology, 132*(5), 493–506.

Thompson, D. C., McPhillips, H., Davis, R. L., Lieu, T. A., Homer, C. J., & Helfand, M. (2001). Universal newborn hearing screening: Summary of evidence. *Journal of the American Medical Association, 286,* 2000–2010.

Tillery, K. L. (2009). Central auditory processing evaluation: A test battery approach. In J. Katz (Ed.), *Handbook of clinical audiology* (6th ed.) (pp. 627–641). Philadelphia: Lippincott Williams & Wilkins.

Timm, J. A. (2005, December). Preparing students for the next employment revolution. *Business Education Forum, 60*(2), 55–59.

T-Mobile. (2010). Company Information: The T-Mobile Timeline. T-mobile.com. Retrieved January 14, 2011, from www.t-mobile.com/Company/CompanyInfo.aspx?tp=Abt_Tab_CompanyOverview=tsp=Abt_Sub_History

Tobey, E. A., Geers, A. E., Brenner, C., Altuna, D., & Gabbert, G. (2003). Factors associated with development of speech production skills in children implanted by age five. *Ear and Hearing, 24*(1), 36S–45S.

Toosi, M. (2009, November). Employment outlook: 2008–18, Labor force projections to 2018: Older workers staying more active. *Monthly Labor Review, 132*(11), 30–51.

Traci, M., & Koester, L. S. (2003). Parent-infant interactions a transactional approach to understanding the development of deaf infants. In M. Marschark & P. E. Spencer, (Eds.), *Deaf studies, language, and education* (pp. 190–202). New York: Oxford University Press.

Traxler, C. B. (2000). The Stanford Achievement Test, 9th Edition: National norming and performance standards for deaf and hard-of-hearing students. *Journal of Deaf Studies and Deaf Education, 5*(4), 337–348.

Tronick, E., Als, H., & Brazelton, T. B. (1980). Monadic phases: A structural descriptive analysis of infant-mother face to face interaction. *Merrill-Palmer Quarterly, 21*(1), 3–24.

Trybus, R., & Karchmer, M. (1977). School achievement scores of hearing impaired children: National data on achievement status and growth patterns. *American Annals of the Deaf, 122,* 62–69.

Turnbull, A., Turnbull, R., & Wehmeyer, M. L. (2010). *Exceptional lives: Special education in today's schools* (6th ed.). Upper Saddle River, NJ: Merrill.

Turnbull, R., Turnbull, A., Shank, M., Smith, S., & Leal, D. (2002). *Exceptional lives.* Upper Saddle River, NJ: Merrill.

Tye-Murray, N. (1998). *Foundations of aural rehabilitation.* San Diego, CA: Singular Publishing Group.

Tye-Murray, N. (2009). *Foundations of aural rehabilitation: Children, adults, and their family members* (3rd ed.). Clifton Park, NY: Delmar/Cengage Learning.

U. S. Department of Education. (2006). Assistance to states for the Education of Children with Disabilities Program and the Early Intervention Program for Infants and Toddlers with Disabilities; Final rule. Federal Register, 34. CRF Parts 300 and 301.

U.S. Bureau of Labor Statistics. (n.d.). Occupational outlook handbook, 2010–11 edition: Overview of the 2008–18 projections. Retrieved January 21, 2011, from www.bls.gov/oco/oco2003.htm

U. S. Department of Education. (2006). Assistance to states for the Education of Children with Disabilities Program and the Early Intervention Program for Infants and Toddlers with Disabilities; Final rule. *Federal Register, 34,* CRF Parts 300 and 301.

U. S. Department of Education. (2007). 27th annual report to Congress on the implementation of Individuals with Disabilities Education Act, 2005 (Vol. 1). Washington, DC: Author.

U.S. Public Health Service. (1990). Health objectives for the Nation—Healthy People 2000: National Health Promotion and Disease Prevention Objectives for the Year 2000. Washington, DC: Government Printing Office. Retrieved January 29, 2011, from www.cdc.gov/mmwr/preview/mmwrhtml/00001788.htm

Ulissi, S. M., Brice, P. J., & Gibbins, S. (1989). Use of the Kaufman-Assessment Battery for Children with the hearing impaired. *American Annals of the Deaf, 134,* 283–287.

United Cerebral Palsy Association (UPC). (2001). Cerebral palsy—Facts and figures. Retrieved January 22, 2011, from www.ucp.org/ucp_generaldoc.cfm/1/9/37/37-37/447

Unrau, N. (2008). *Content area reading and writing: Fostering literacies in middle and high school cultures* (2nd ed.). Upper Saddle River, NJ: Pearson.

Urberg, K., Degirmencioglu, S., & Tolson, J. (1998). Adolescent friendship selection and termination: The role of similarity. *Journal of Social & Personal Relationships, 15*(5), 703–710.

Vacca, R. T., & Vacca, J. L. (1996). *Content area reading.* New York: Harper Collins Publishers.

Vacca, R. T., Vacca, J. A., & Mraz, M. (2011). *Content area reading literacy and learning across the curriculum* (10th ed). Boston: Pearson.

Vaccari, C., & Marschark, M. (1997). Communication between parents and deaf children: Implications for social-emotional development. *Journal of Child Psychology and Psychiatry, 38*(7), 793–801.

Valente, M., Meister, M., McCauley, K., & Cass, W. (1994). Selecting and verifying hearing aid fittings for unilateral hearing loss. In Valente, M. (Ed.), *Strategies for selecting and verifying hearing aid fittings* (pp. 228–248). New York: Thieme Medical Publishers.

Valli, C., & Lucas, C. (2000). *Linguistics of American Sign Language.* Washington, DC: Gallaudet University Press.

Van Cleve, J. V., & Crouch, B. (1989). *A place of their own.* Washington, DC: Gallaudet University Press.

Van Eldik, T., Veerman, J. W., Treffers, F. D. A., & Verhulst, F. C. (2000). Probleemgedrag en opvoedingsomgeving van dove kinderen [Problem behavior and parental environment of children who are deaf or hard of hearing]. *Kind en Adolescent, 21,* 232–251.

van Gurp, S. (2001). Self-concept of deaf secondary school students in different educational settings. *Journal of Deaf Studies and Deaf Education, 6*(1), 54–69.

VanKleek, A. (1984). Metalinguistic skills: Cutting across spoken and written language and problem solving abilities. In G. Wallach & K. Butler (Eds), *Language learning disabilities in school age children* (pp. 129–153). Baltimore: Williams and Wilkins.

Van Vuuren, E. (1995). *The deaf pupil with learning disabilities.* (ERIC Document Reproduction Service No. ED392177)

Vaughn, S. R., Bos, C. S., & Schumm, J. S. (2003). *Teaching exceptional, diverse, and at-risk students in the general education classroom* (3rd ed.). Boston: Allyn & Bacon.

Vaughn, S., & Fuchs, L. S. (2003). Redefining learning disabilities as inadequate response to instruction: The promise and potential problems. *Learning Disabilities Research and Practice, 18,* 137–146.

Vento, B. A., & Durrant, J. D. (2009). Assessing bone conduction thresholds in clinical practice. In J. Katz (Ed.), *Handbook of clinical audiology* (6th ed., pp. 50–63). Philadelphia: Lippincott Williams & Wilkins.

Vernon, M. (1967). Relationship of language to the thinking process. *Archives of Genetic Psychiatry, 16*(3), 325–333.

Vernon, M. (1968). Fifty years of research on the intelligence of deaf and hard of hearing children: A review of literature and discussion of implications. *Journal of Rehabilitation of the Deaf, 1,* 1–12.

Vernon, M. (1969). *Multiple-handicapped deaf children: Medical education and psychological considerations.* Reston, VA: Council for Exceptional Children.

Vernon, M. (2005). Fifty years of research on the intelligence of deaf and hard-of-hearing children: A review of literature and discussion of implications. *Journal of Deaf Studies and Deaf Education, 10,* 225–231.

Vernon, M., & Andrews, J. (1990). *The psychology of deafness: Understanding deaf and hard of hearing people.* White Plains, NY: Longman.

Vernon, M., & Rhodes, A. (2009). Deafness and autistic spectrum disorders. *American Annals of the Deaf, 154*(1), 5–14.

Vernon, M., & Rothstein, D. A. (1967). *Deafness: The interdependent variable.* Paper presented at the (5th) Congress of the World Federation of the Deaf, Warsaw, Poland.

Verte, S., Hebbrecht, L., & Roeyers, H. (2006). Psychological adjustment of siblings of children who are deaf or hard of hearing. *The Volta Review, 106*(1), 89–110.

Volterra, V., Iverson, J., & Castrataro, M. (2006). The development of gesture in hearing and deaf children. In B. Shick, M. Marschark, & P. Spencer (Eds.), *Advances in the sign language development of deaf children* (pp. 46–70). New York: Oxford University Press.

Vostanis, P., Hayes, M., DuFeu, M., & Warren, J. (1997). Detection of behavioral and emotional problems in deaf children and adolescents: Comparison of two rating scales. *Child Care, Health and Development, 23,* 233–246.

Wagner, M., Kutash, K., Duchnowski, A. J., Epstein, M. H., & Sumi, W. C. (2005). The children and youth we serve: A national picture of the characteristics of students with emotional disturbances receiving special education. *Journal of Emotional and Behavioral Disorders, 13*(2), 79–96.

Walberg, H. (1984). Improving the productivity of America's Schools. *Educational Leadership, 41*(8), 19–30.

Wald, R., & Knutson, J. (2000). Deaf cultural identity of adolescents with and without cochlear implants. *Annals of Otology, Rhinology & Laryngology, 12*(2)(Suppl. 185), 87–89.

Walden, T. A. (1993). Communicating the meaning of events through social referencing. In D. B. Gray & A. P. Kaiser (Eds.), *Enhancing children's communication: Research foundations for intervention* (pp. 187–199). Baltimore: Brookes.

Walker, H. M., Ramsey, E., & Gresham, F. M. (2004). *Antisocial behavior in school: Evidence-based practices* (2nd ed.). Belmont, CA: Wadsworth.

Wallis, D., Musselman, C., & MacKay, S. (2004). Hearing mothers and their deaf children: The relationship between early, ongoing mode match and subsequent mental health functioning in adolescence. *Journal of Deaf Studies and Deaf Education, 9*(1), 2–14.

Walter, G., MacLeod-Gallinger, J., & Stuckless, R. (1987). *Outcomes for graduates of secondary education programs for deaf students: Early findings of a cooperative national longitudinal study.* Rochester, NY: Rochester Institute of Technology.

Walton, J. P., & Hendricks-Munoz, K. (1991). Profile and stability of sensorineural hearing loss in persistent pulmonary hypertension of the newborn. *Journal of Speech and Hearing Research, 34,* 1362–1370.

Wang, Y., Trezek, B., Luckner, J., & Paul, P. (2008). The role of phonology and phonologically related skills in reading instruction for students who are deaf or hard of hearing. *American Annals of the Deaf, 153*(4), 396–407.

Washington State School for the Deaf. (1972). An *introduction to manual English.* Vancouver, WA: Author.

Waters, G. S., & Doehring, D. G. (1990). Reading acquisition in congenitally deaf children who communicate orally: Insights from an analysis of component reading, language, and memory skils. In T. H. Carr & B. A. Levy (Eds.), *Reading and its development* (pp. 323–373). San Diego, CA: Academic Press.

Watson, L. (1998). Oralism: Current policy and practice. In S. Gregory et al. (Eds.), *Issues in deaf education* (pp. 69–76). London: David Fulton Publisher.

Waugh, N. C., & Norman, D. A. (1965). Primary memory. *Psychological Review, 72,* 89–104.

Waxman, R., & Spencer, P. (1997). What mothers do to support infant visual attention: Sensitivities to age and hearing status. *Journal of Deaf Studies and Deaf Education, 2,* 104–114.

Weaver, S. E., Coleman M., & Ganong, L. H. (2003). The sibling relationship in young adulthood: Sibling functions and relationship perceptions as influenced by sibling pair composition. *Journal of Family Issues, 24,* 245–263.

Wechsler, D. (1974). *Wechsler intelligence scale for children-revised.* New York: Psychological Corporation.

Weinrich, J. E. (1972). Direct economic costs of deafness in the United States. *American Annals of the Deaf, 117,* 446–454.

Weisel, A. (1988). Parental hearing status, reading comprehension skills and social-emotional adjustment. *American Annals of the Deaf, 133,* 356–359.

Weisel, A., Most., T., & Efron, C. (2005). Initiations of social interactions by young hearing impaired preschoolers. *Journal of Deaf Studies and Deaf Education, 10,* 161–170.

Welch, O. M. (2000). Building a multicultural curriculum: Issues and dilemmas. In K. Christensen (Ed.), *Deaf plus: A multicultural perspective* (pp. 1–28). San Diego, CA: Dawn Sign Press.

Wellman, H. M. (1993). Early understanding of mind: The normal case. In S. Baron-Cohen, H. Tager-Flusberg, & D. Cohen (Eds.), *Understanding other minds: Perspectives from autism* (pp. 10–39). Oxford, England: Oxford University Press.

Wellman, H. M. (2002). Understanding the psychological world: Developing a theory of mind. In U. Goswami (Ed.), *Handbook of childhood cognitive development* (pp. 167–187). Oxford: Blackwell.

Wellman, H., & Liu, D. (2004). Scaling of theory of mind tasks. *Child Development, 75,* 523–541.

Wells, G. (1986). *Language development in the pre-school years.* Cambridge, England: Cambridge University Press.

Welsh, W. (1993). Factors influencing career mobility of deaf adults. *The Volta Review, 95,* 329–339.

Welsh, W., & Walter, G. (1988). The effect of postsecondary education on occupational attainments of deaf adults. *Journal of the American Deafness and Rehabilitation Association, 22,* 14–22.

Werker, J., & Tees, R. (1984). Cross-language speech perception: Evidence for perceptual reorganization during the first year of life. *Infant Behavior and Development, 7,* 49–64.

Wheeler, A., Archbold, S., Gregory, S., & Skipp, A. (2007). Cochlear implants: The young people's perspective. *Journal of Deaf Studies and Deaf Education, 12*(3), 303–316.

Wheeler-Scruggs, K. (2002). Assessing the employment and independendence of people who are deaf and low functioning. *American Annals of the Deaf, 147*(4), 11–17.

Wheeler-Scruggs, K. (2003). Discerning characteristics and risk factors of people who are deaf and low functioning. *Journal of Rehabilitation, 69,* 39–46.

White, K. R. (1997, October). The scientific basis for newborn hearing screening: Issues and evidence. Invited keynote address to the Early Hearing Detection and Intervention (EHDI) Workshop sponsored by the Centers for Disease Control and Prevention, Atlanta, GA. Retrieved February 2, 2009, from www.infanthearing.org/resources/fact.pdf

White, K. R. (2003). The current status of EHDI programs in the United States. *Mental Retardation and Developmental Disabilities Research Reviews, 9,* 79–88.

White, K. R., Vohr, B. R., Meyer, S., Widen, J. E., Johnson, J. L., Gravel, J.S, et al. (2005). A multisite study to examine the efficacy of the otoacoustic emission/automated auditory brainstem response newborn hearing screening protocol: Research design and results of the study. *American Journal of Audiology, 14* S187 – S199.

Whitmore, K. (2000). Adolescence as a developmental phase: A tutorial. *Topics in Language Disorders, 20*(2), 1–14.

Wiig, E., & Secord, W. (1992). From word knowledge to world knowledge. *Clinical Connection, 6*(3), 12–14.

Wilbur, R. (1979). *American sign language and sign systems.* Boston: College-Hill Press.

Wilbur, R. (2000). The use of ASL to support the development of English and literacy. *Journal of Deaf Studies and Deaf Education, 5,* 81–104.

Wilbur, R. B. (1987). *American Sign Language: Linguistic and applied dimensions.* San Diego, CA: College-Hill Press.

Wilbur, R. B. (2008). Success with deaf children: How to prevent education failure. In K. A. Lindgren, D. DeLuca, & D. Napoli (Eds.), *Signs and voices: Deaf culture, identity, language, and arts* (pp. 117–138). Washington, DC: Gallaudet University Press.

Wilkens, C. P., & Hehir, T. P. (2008). Deaf education and bridging social capital: A theoretical approach. *American Annals of the Deaf 153*(3), 275–284.

Wilson, K. (1979). *Inference and language processing in hearing and deaf children.* Unpublished doctoral dissertation, Boston University.

Wilson, M., & Emmorey, K. (1997). A visuospatial "phonological loop" in working memory: Evidence from American Sign Language. *Memory and Cognition, 25,* 313–320.

Wilson, M., & Emmorey, K. (1998). A "word length effect" for sign language: Further evidence for the role of language in structuring working memory. *Memory & Cognition, 26*(3), 584–590.

Wilson, M., & Emmorey, K. (2003). The effect of irrelevant visual input on working memory for sign language. *Journal of Deaf Studies and Deaf Education, 8*(2), 97–103.

Wilson-Costello, D., Friedman, H., Minich, N., Fanaroff, A. A., & Hack, M. (2005). Improved survival rates with increased neurodevelopmental disability for extremely low birth weight infants in the 1990s. *Pediatrics, 115*(4), 997–1003.

Winston, E. (1994). An interpreted education: Inclusion or exclusion? In R. C. Johnson & O. P. Cohen (Eds.), *Implications and complications for deaf students of the full inclusion movement* (pp. 55–62). Washington, DC: Gallaudet Research Institute and Conference of Educational Administrators Serving the Deaf.

Winter, S., Autry, A., Boyle, C., & Yeargin-Allsopp, M. (2002). Trends in the prevalence of cerebral palsy in a population-based study. *Pediatrics, 110*(6), 1220–1225.

Witter-Merithew, A., & Johnson, L. J. (2005). *Toward competent practice: Conversations with stakeholders.* Alexandria, VA: RID, Inc.

Wolf, M., & Katzir-Cohen, T. (2001). Reading fluency and its intervention. *Scientific Studies of Reading, 5*(3), 211–238.

Wood, D. (1989). Social interaction as tutoring. In M. Bornstein & J. Bruner (Eds.), *Interaction in human development* (pp. 59–80). Hillsdale, NJ: Erlbaum.

Woolfe, T. (2001). The self esteem and cohesion to family members of deaf children in relation to the hearing status of their parents and siblings. *Deafness and Education International, 3*(2), 80–95.

Woolsey, M., Satterfield, S., & Roberson, L. (2006). Visual phonics: An English code buster? *American Annals of the Deaf, 151,* 434–440.

Woolsey, M. L., Harrison, T. J., & Gardner, R. (2004, August). A preliminary examination of instructional arrangements, teaching behaviors, levels of academic responding of deaf middle school students in three different educational settings. *Education and Treatment of Children, 27*(3), 263–279.

Wright, E. (1999). Full inclusion of children with disabilities in the regular classroom: Is it the only answer? *Social Work in Education, 21*(I), 11–22.

Wrightstone, J., Aronow, M., & Moskowitz, S. (1963). Developing reading test norms for deaf children. *American Annals of the Deaf, 108,* 311–316.

Yambert, G. B., & Van Craeynest, R. (1975). *Sign language and social networks: Grapevine communication in the deaf community.* Paper presented at the Annual Meeting of the Southwestern Anthropological Association, San Francisco, California.

Yarger, C. C., & Luckner, J. L. (1999). Itinerant teaching: The inside story. *American Annals of the Deaf, 144*(4), 309–314.

Yeargin-Allsopp, M., Rice, C., Karapurkar, T., Doernberg, N., Boyle, C., & Murphy, C. (2003). Prevalence of autism in a US metropolitan area. *Journal of the American Medical Association, 289*(91), 49–55.

Yell, M. L. (2006). The law and special education (2nd ed.). Upper Saddle River, NJ: Pearson.

Yell, M. L., & Drasgow, E. (2009). *No child left behind: A guide for professionals* (2nd ed.). Boston: Pearson.

Yetman, M. (2000). *Peer relations and self-esteem among deaf children in a mainstream school environment.* Doctoral dissertation, Gallaudet University, Washington, DC. *Dissertation Abstracts International, 63,* AAT3038028.

Yoshinaga-Itano, C. (2006). Early identification, communication modality, and the development of speech and spoken language skills: Patterns and considerations. In P. Spencer & M. Marschark (Eds.), *Advances in the spoken language development of deaf and hard-of-hearing children* (pp. 298–327). New York: Oxford University Press.

Yoshinaga-Itano, C., & Snyder, L. (1985). Form and meaning in the written language of hearing impaired children. *The Volta Review, 87,* 75–90.

Young, A. R., & Beitchman, J. H. (2007). Learning disabilities. In G. O. Gabbard (Ed.), *Gabbard's treatments of psychiatric disorders* (4th ed., pp. 119–127). Washington, DC: American Psychiatric Publishing.

Zazove, P., Meador, H., Derry, H., Gorenflo, D., Burdick, S., & Saunders, E. (2004). Deaf persons and computer use. *American Annals of the Deaf, 148*(5), 376–384.

Zwiebel, A., & Mertens, D. M. (1985). A comparison of intellectual structure in deaf and hearing children. *American Annals of the Deaf, 130,* 27–31.

Zwiebel, A. (1987). More on the effects of early manual communication on the cognitive development of deaf children. *American Annals of the Deaf, 132,* 16–20.

Zwolan, T. A. (2009). Cochlear implants. In J. Katz (Ed.), *Handbook of clinical audiology* (6th ed., pp. 912–933). Philadelphia: Lippincott Williams & Wilkins.

INDEX